Survival Analysis

Second Edition

Survival Analysis
A Practical Approach

Second Edition

DAVID MACHIN

Division of Clinical Trials and Epidemiological Sciences
National Cancer Centre, Singapore
UK Children's Cancer Study Group
University of Leicester, UK
Medical Statistics Group
School of Health and Related Sciences, University of Sheffield, UK

YIN BUN CHEUNG

MRC Tropical Epidemiology Group
London School of Hygiene and Tropical Medicine, UK
Division of Clinical Trials and Epidemiological Sciences
National Cancer Centre, Singapore

MAHESH KB PARMAR

Cancer Group
MRC Clinical Trials Unit, UK
National Cancer Research Network Coordinating Centre
University of Leeds, UK

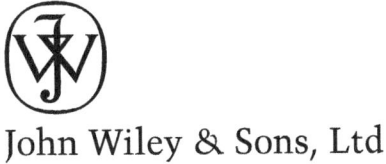

John Wiley & Sons, Ltd

Other Wiley Editorial Offices

John Wiley & Sons Inc., 111 River Street, Hoboken, NJ 07030, USA

Jossey-Bass, 989 Market Street, San Francisco, CA 94103-1741, USA

Wiley-VCH Verlag GmbH, Boschstr. 12, D-69469 Weinheim, Germany

John Wiley & Sons Australia Ltd, 42 McDougall Street, Milton, Queensland 4064, Australia

John Wiley & Sons (Asia) Pte Ltd, 2 Clementi Loop #02-01, Jin Xing Distripark, Singapore 129809

John Wiley & Sons Canada Ltd, 22 Worcester Road, Etobicoke, Ontario, Canada M9W 1L1

Wiley also publishes its books in a variety of electronic formats. Some content that appears in print may not be
available in electronic books.

Library of Congress Cataloging in Publication Data

Machin, David.
   Survival analysis : a practical approach / David Machin, Yin Bun Cheung, M.K.B. Parmar. — 2nd ed.
      p. ; cm.
   Rev. ed. of: Survival analysis : a practical approach / Mahesh K.B. Parmar and
   David Machin. c1995.
   Includes bibliographical references and index.
   ISBN 0-470-87040-0 (cloth : alk. paper)
   1. Survival analysis (Biometry) I. Cheung, Yin Bun. II. Parmar, Mahesh K.B.
   III. Parmar, Mahesh K.B. Survival analysis. IV. Title.
   [DNLM: 1. Survival Analysis. 2. Proportional Hazards Models. WA 950 M149s 2006]
   R853.S7P37 2006
   610.72—dc22   2005033616

British Library Cataloguing in Publication Data

A catalogue record for this book is available from the British Library

ISBN-10 0-470-87040-0
ISBN-13 978-0-470-87040-2

Typeset in 10/12pt Times by Integra Software Services Pvt. Ltd, Pondicherry, India

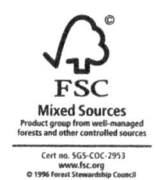

To
Annie Machin
Wong Oi Ming
Ambaben B. Parmar

Contents

Preface to the First Edition

Survival methods are used in many circumstances in medical and allied areas of research. Our objective here is to explain these methods in an accessible and nontechnical way. We have assumed some familiarity with basic statistical ideas, but we have tried not to overwhelm the reader with details of statistical theory. Instead, we have tried to give a practical guide to the use of survival analysis techniques in a variety of situations by using numerous examples. A number of these arise from our own particular field of interest—cancer clinical trials—but the issues that arise in the analysis of such data are common to trials in general and to epidemiological studies.

There are many people whom we would like to thank: these include past and present members of the Medical Research Council Cancer Therapy Committee and its associated working parties, colleagues of the Human Reproduction Programme of the World Health Organization, the European School of Oncology and the Nordic School of Public Health.

Particular thanks go to Vicki Budd, Maria Dasseville, Vivien Ellen and Vicki Greaves for typing the many drafts of each chapter, to Philippa Lloyd for detailed comments on the final draft and Lesley Stewart for providing a general assessment of the book's accessibility. We also thank John Machin, Caroline Mallam and Andrea Bailey for their statistical computing, and John Machin again for keeping us organised.

Mahesh K.B. Parmar and David Machin

Cambridge, 1995

Preface to the Second Edition

Since the first edition of this book there have been many developments in the statistical methods associated with survival techniques and, very importantly, parallel developments in computer software programs to implement the methodologies. The latter enable quite technical methods to be implemented by a wide range of users and not confined to statisticians alone. The object of this second edition is to refocus the presentation of the basic survival analysis techniques and to introduce some of the new developments while maintaining a 'practical' emphasis so that the book remains targeted at the practitioner rather than the research statistician.

Principal amongst the changes introduced, is a greatly expanded chapter on parametric modelling using the Weibull and other distributions of survival time and several extensions of the Cox model. Other new material introduced concerns more model diagnostic techniques, cure models, clustered and multiple failure time, and competing risks analysis. These have resulted in a major restructuring of the book and a substantial revision of the majority of the material of the first edition.

We would like to thank colleagues in Leicester, London, and Sheffield, UK, Singapore, and Skövde, Sweden for encouragement and advice.

David Machin
Yin Bun Cheung
Mahesh KB Parmar

Southover, Dorset and London

April 2005

1 Introduction and Review of Statistical Concepts

Summary

In this chapter we introduce some examples of the use of survival methods in a selection of different areas and describe the concepts necessary to define survival time. The chapter also includes a review of some basic statistical ideas including the Normal distribution, hypothesis testing and the use of confidence intervals, the χ^2 and likelihood ratio tests and some other methods useful in survival analysis, including the median survival time and the hazard ratio. The difference between clinical and statistical significance is highlighted. The chapter indicates some of the computing packages that can be used to analyse survival data and emphasises that the database within which the study data is managed and stored must interface easily with these.

1.1 INTRODUCTION

There are many examples in medicine where a survival time measurement is appropriate. For example, such measurements may include the time a kidney graft remains patent, the time a patient with colorectal cancer survives once the tumour has been removed by surgery, the time a patient with osteoarthritis is pain-free following acupuncture treatment, the time a woman remains without a pregnancy whilst using a particular hormonal contraceptive and the time a pressure sore takes to heal. All these times are triggered by an initial event: a kidney graft, a surgical intervention, commencement of acupuncture therapy, first use of a contraceptive or identification of the pressure sore. These initial events are followed by a subsequent event: graft failure, death, return of pain, pregnancy or healing of the sore. The time between such events is known as the 'survival time'. The term *survival* is used because an early use of the associated statistical techniques arose from the insurance industry, which was developing methods of costing insurance premiums. The industry needed to know the risk, or average survival time, associated with a particular type of client. This 'risk' was based on that of a large group of individuals with a particular age, gender and possibly other characteristics; the individual was then given the risk for his or her group for the calculation of their insurance premium.

There is one major difference between 'survival' data and other types of numeric continuous data: the time to the event occurring is not necessarily observed in all subjects. Thus in the above examples we may not observe for all subjects the events of

Survival Analysis Second Edition   David Machin, Yin Bun Cheung, Mahesh K.B. Parmar
© 2006 John Wiley & Sons, Ltd   ISBN: 0-470-87040-0

graft failure (the graft remains functional indefinitely), death (the patient survives for a very long time), return of pain (the patient remains pain-free thereafter), pregnancy (the woman never conceives) or healing of the sore (the sore does not heal), respectively. Such non-observed events are termed 'censored' but are quite different from 'missing' data items.

The date of 1 March 1973 can be thought of as the 'census day', that is, the day on which the currently available data on all patients recruited to the transplant programme were collected together and summarised. Typically, as in this example, by the census day some patients will have died whilst others remain alive. The survival times of those who are still alive are termed *censored survival times*. Censored survival times are described in Section 2.1

The probability of survival without transplant for patients identified as transplant candidates is shown in Figure 1.1. Details of how this probability is calculated using the Kaplan-Meier (product-limit) estimate, are given in Section 2.2. By reading across from 0.5 on the vertical scale in Figure 1.1 and then vertically downwards at the point of intersection with the curve, we can say that approximately half (see Section 2.3) of such patients will die within 80 days of being selected as suitable for transplant if no transplant becomes available for them.

Historically, much of survival analysis has been developed and applied in relation to cancer clinical trials in which the survival time is often measured from the date of randomisation or commencement of therapy until death. The seminal papers by Peto, Pike, Armitage *et al.* (1976, 1977) published in the *British Journal of Cancer* describing the design, conduct and analysis of cancer trials provide a landmark in the development and use of survival methods.

Example – *survival time* – *patients awaiting and received heart transplant*

One early example of the use of survival methods has been in the description of the subsequent survival experience and identification of risk factors associated with patients requiring heart transplants. Table 1.1, adapted from Turnbull, Brown and Hu (1974), reproduces some of the earliest heart transplant data published. The ultimate aim of a heart transplant programme is to restore the patient to the level of risk of his or her healthy contemporaries of the same age.

In this heart transplant programme, patients are assessed for transplant and then, if suitable, have to await a donor heart. One consequence of this wait is that patients may die before a suitable donor has been found (survival time X in Table 1.1). Thirty patients, of the 82 summarised in Table 1.1, did not receive a transplant. Of these, 27 died before a donor heart became available and four remained alive and were still waiting for a suitable transplant heart at 1 March 1973, after 1400, 118, 91 and 427 days respectively. For those who receive a transplant their survival time is measured from the date of assessment of suitability and consists of their waiting time to transplant, Y, plus their survival time from their transplant until death, Z. Thus, for the third patient who received a transplant, the waiting time to a transplant is $Y = 50$ days and the survival post transplant is $Z = 624$ days. This patient, therefore, lived for $Y + Z = 50 + 624 = 674$ days from admission to the transplant programme.

Table 1.1 Number of days to transplant and survival times for 82 patients selected for the Stanford Heart Transplantation Program (From Turnbull, Brown and Hu, 1974. Reprinted with permission from *Journal of the American Statistical Association*. Copyright 1974 by the American Statistical Association. All rights reserved.)

Patients not receiving a transplant		Patients receiving a transplant					
X	State*	Y	Z	State	Y	Z	State
49	D	0	15	D	82	663	A
5	D	35	3	D	31	253	D
17	D	50	624	D	40	147	D
2	D	11	46	D	9	51	D
39	D	25	127	D	66	479	A
84	D	16	61	D	20	322	D
7	D	36	1350	D	77	442	A
0	D	27	312	D	2	65	D
35	D	19	24	D	26	419	A
36	D	17	10	D	32	362	A
1400	A	7	1024	D	13	64	D
5	D	11	39	D	56	228	D
34	D	2	730	D	2	65	D
15	D	82	136	D	9	264	A
11	D	24	1379	A	4	25	D
2	D	70	1	D	30	193	A
1	D	15	836	D	3	196	A
39	D	16	60	D	26	63	D
8	D	50	1140	A	4	12	D
101	D	22	1153	A	45	103	A
2	D	45	54	D	25	60	A
148	D	18	47	D	5	43	A
1	D	4	0	D			
68	D	1	43	D			
31	D	40	971	A			
1	D	57	868	A			
20	D	0	44	D			
118	A	1	780	A			
91	A	20	51	D			
427	A	35	710	A			

*A = alive, D = dead;
 X = days to death or census date of 01 March 1973;
 Y = days to transplant;
 Z = days from transplant to death or census date

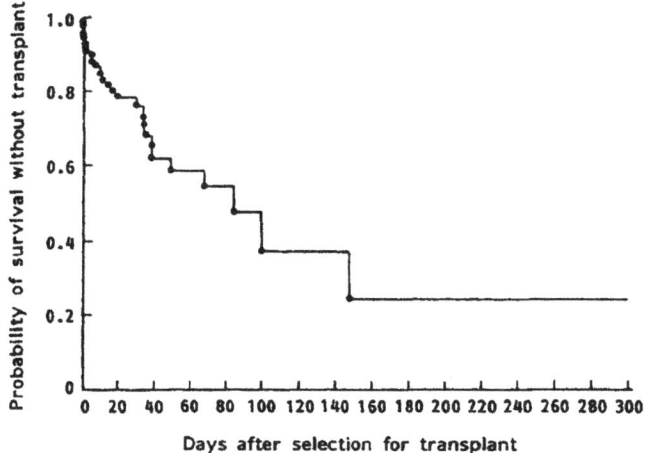

Figure 1.1 Probability of survival without transplant for transplant candidates. Estimated from all pre-transplant experience by the Kaplan-Meier method (From Turnbull, Brown and Hu, 1974. Reprinted with permission from *Journal of the American Statistical Association*. Copyright 1974 by the American Statistical Association. All rights reserved.)

Example – survival time – patients with chronic granulocytic leukaemia

Peto, Pike, Armitage *et al.* (1977) describe the survival experience of 102 patients with chronic granulocytic leukaemia (CGL) measured from the time of first treatment following diagnosis of their disease to the date of their death. The 'life-table' or 'actuarial' estimate of the percentage surviving is given in Figure 1.2 and shows that most patients have died by 300 weeks or approximately six years. The method of calculating such a survival curve is described in Section 2.2.

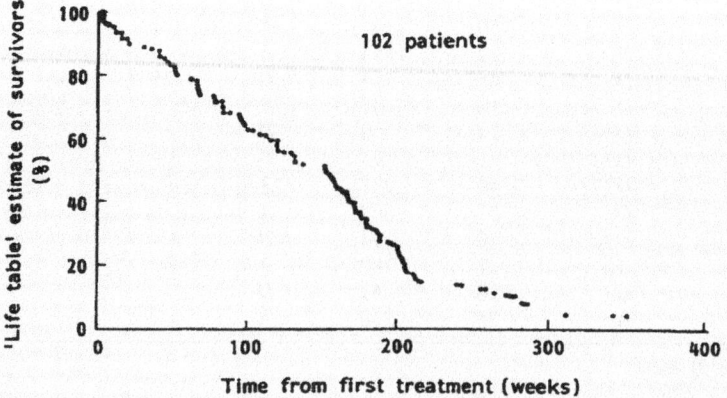

Figure 1.2 Life-table for all patients in the Medical Research Council's first CGL trial. The number of patients alive and under observation at entry and annually thereafter were: 102, 84, 65, 50, 18, 11 and 3 (reproduced from Peto, Pike, Armitage, *et al.*, 1977, by permission of The Macmillan Press Ltd)

These patients with CGL were randomly allocated to receive either chemotherapy, in the form of busulphan, or radiotherapy treatment for their disease. The life-table estimate of survival for each of the two treatment groups is shown in Figure 1.3 and suggests that the patients who received busulphan therapy lived, on average, longer than those who received radiotherapy.

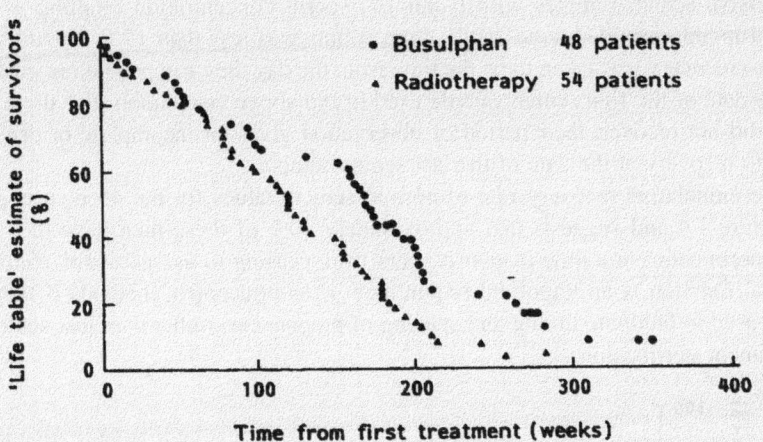

Figure 1.3   Life-tables for the two separate treatment groups in the Medical Research Council's first CGL trial. The numbers of patients alive and under observation at entry and annually thereafter were: Busulphan 48, 40, 33, 30, 13, 9 and 3; and Radiotherapy 54, 44, 32, 20, 3, 2 and 0 (reproduced from Peto, Pike, Armitage, *et al.*, 1977, by permission of The Macmillan Press Ltd)

The method of making a formal comparison of two survival curves with the Logrank test is described in Chapter 3.

One field of application of survival studies has been in the development of methods of fertility regulation. In such applications alternative contraceptive methods either for the male or female partner are compared in prospective randomised trials. These trials usually compare the efficacy of different methods by observing how many women conceive in each group. A pregnancy is deemed a failure in this context.

Survival time methods have been used extensively in many medical fields, including trials concerned with the prevention of new cardiovascular events in patients who have had a recent myocardial infarction (Wallentin, Wilcox, Weaver *et al.*, 2003), prevention of type 2 diabetes mellitus in those with impaired glucose tolerance (Chiasson, Josse, Gomis *et al.*, 2002), return of post-stroke function (Mayo, Korner-Bitensky and Becker, 1991), and AIDS (Bonacini, Louie, Bzowej, *et al.*, 2004).

Example – time to recovery of sperm function- men who are azoospermic

It has been shown that gossypol, a plant extract, can lower the sperm count to render men temporarily sterile (azoospermic) and hence may be useful as a male contraceptive method. In a study of 46 men who had taken gossypol, and as a consequence had become azoospermic, their time to recovery of sperm function was recorded by Meng, Zhu, Chen, *et al.* (1988). Recovery was defined as: "three successive semen samples with (summed) sperm concentration totalling at least $60 \times 106/\text{ml}$, provided none of the three counts was less than $15 \times 106/\text{ml}$". The time to recovery was taken to be the time from the day they stopped taking gossypol to the date of the first semen sample used in the above calculation. For those men who did not recover, their period of observation gives an incomplete or censored time to recovery at the date of the last semen sample.

The cumulative recovery rate to normal semen values for the 46 men is given in Figure 1.4 and suggests that approximately 70% of these men have recovered full sperm count in a little over two years from ceasing to use gossypol. Return to normal function is an important requirement of contraceptive methods if they are to be used to facilitate timing and spacing of pregnancies rather than just achieving permanent sterilisation.

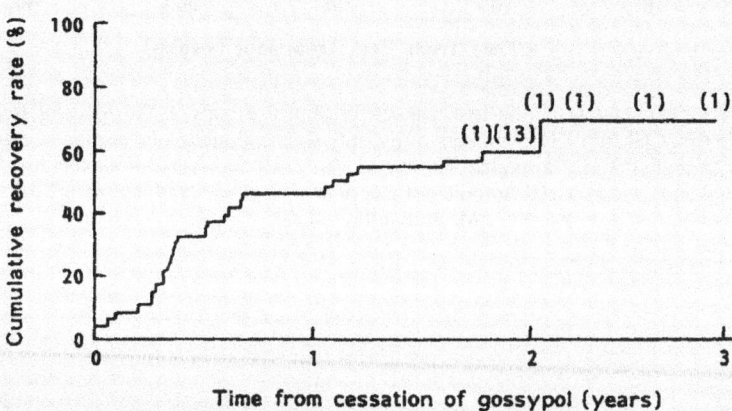

Figure 1.4 Cumulative recovery rate to threshold sperm function. Figures in parentheses indicate the follow-up time of the 18 men not yet recovered (reproduced from Meng, Zhu, Chen, *et al.*, 1988, by permission of Blackwell Science)

1.2   DEFINING TIME

In order to perform survival analysis one must know how to define the time-to-event interval. The endpoint of the interval is relatively easy to define. In the examples in Section 1.1, they were graft failure, return of pain, pregnancy, healing of the sore, recovery of sperm function, and death. However, defining the initial events that trigger the times is sometimes a more difficult task.

INITIAL EVENTS AND THE ORIGIN OF TIME

The origin of time refers to the starting point of a time interval, when $t = 0$. We have mentioned the time from the surgical removal of a colorectal cancer to the death of the patient. So the initial event was surgery and $t = 0$ corresponds to the date of surgery. However, a quite common research situation in cancer clinical trials is that after surgery, patients are randomised into receiving one of two treatments, say two types of adjuvant chemotherapy. Should the initial event be surgery, randomisation, or the start of chemotherapy? How does one choose when there are several (starting) events that can be considered? There are no definite rules, but some considerations are as follows.

It is intuitive to consider a point in time that marks the onset of exposure to the risk of the outcome event. For example, when studying ethnic differences in mortality, birth may be taken as the initial event as one is immediately at risk of death once born. In this case, survival time is equivalent to age at death. However, in studies of hospital readmission rates, a patient cannot be readmitted until he or she is first of all discharged. Therefore the latest discharge is the initial event and marks the origin of the time interval to readmission.

In randomised trials, the initial event should usually be randomisation to treatment. Prior to randomisation, patients may have already been at risk of the outcome event (perhaps dying from their colorectal cancer before surgery can take place), but that is not relevant to the research purpose. In randomised trials the purpose is to compare the occurrences of the outcome *given* the different assigned interventions. As such, the patient is not considered to be at risk until he or she is randomised to receive an intervention. In the colorectal cancer trial example, time of surgery is not a proper choice for the time origin. However, some interventions may not be immediately available at the time of randomisation, for example, treatments that involve waiting for a suitable organ donor or heavily booked facilities. In these cases a patient may die after randomisation but before the assigned treatment begins. In such circumstances would the date that the treatment actually begins form a better time origin? Most randomised clinical trials follow the 'intention-to-treat' (*ITT*) principle. That is, the interventions are not the treatments per se, but the clinical intention is to care for the patients by the particular treatment strategies being compared. If a treatment involves a long waiting time and patients die before the treatment begins, this is the weakness of the intervention and should be reflected in the comparisons made between the treatment groups at the time of analysis. In such situations it is correct to use randomisation to mark the time origin.

DELAYED ENTRY AND GAPS IN EXPOSURE TIME

Delayed entry, or late entry to the risk set, refers to the situation when a subject becomes at risk of the outcome event at a point in time after time zero. If, for example, ethnic differences in all cause mortality are being investigated, everyone becomes at risk of death at the time of birth ($t = 0$) so there is no delayed entry. An example of delayed entry is a study of first birth where no girl is at risk until menarche, the age of which varies from individual to individual. A common way of defining time in such circumstances is to 'reset the clock' to time zero at the age of menarche and time to first birth is counted from there. This is the approach used in Section 2.1 in the context of clinical trials. There is an alternative approach to defining time in the presence of delayed entry, which tends to be more useful in epidemiological studies and will be discussed in Section 7.4.

In certain circumstances a subject may be within the risk set for a period of time, leave the risk set, only to rejoin the risk set again. For example, a cohort may be recruited comprising all of the workforce at a particular factory at one point in time and these workers are then monitored for their exposure to a potential hazard within the work place. Some may leave the risk set later, perhaps for maternity leave, but will subsequently return once the baby is born. Such intermittent absences from the risk set leave gaps in the exposure time. If they are ignored, the event rate will be incorrectly estimated. The technique to handle these gaps in the 'at risk' time is similar to that for delayed entry and will also be discussed in Section 7.4.

FAILURE TIME MUST BE LARGER THAN ZERO

A logically valid survival time must be larger than zero. If survival time is measured in days and both the initial and outcome events take place on the same day, the survival time may be *recorded* as zero. For instance, in Table 1.1, a patient who did not receive a transplant had $X = 0$. Such values should usually be interpreted as a survival time smaller than one but larger than zero. Hence one may consider replacing the zero survival time value with a value of 0.5 days. In circumstances when time intervals are wide, say months, and the exact times of the initial and outcome events are not recorded, then one may assume that, on average, the initial event takes place at the middle of the time unit, and that the outcome event takes place at the middle between the time of the initial event and the end of that time unit. In this case, one might replace the zero survival time with 0.25. Other small values may also be considered depending on the context. The problem of survival time recorded as zero also highlights the importance of measuring survival time as precisely as practicable. Computer packages generally refuse to analyse observations with negative failure time (usually a data error) or those equal to zero.

1.3   BASIC STATISTICAL IDEAS

The aim of nearly all studies, including those involving 'survival' data, is to extrapolate from observations made on a sample of individuals to the population as a whole. For example, in a trial of a new treatment for arthritis it is usual to assess the merits of the therapy on a sample of patients (preferably in a randomised controlled trial) and try to deduce from this trial whether the therapy is appropriate for general use in patients with arthritis. In many instances, it may be that the target population is more exactly specified, for example by patients with arthritis of a certain type, of a particular severity, or patients of a certain gender and age group. Nevertheless, the aim remains the same: the inference from the results obtained from a sample to a (larger) population.

MEDIAN SURVIVAL

A commonly reported summary statistic in survival studies is the median survival time. The median survival time is defined as the value for which 50% of the individuals in the study have longer survival times and 50% have shorter survival times. A more formal definition is given in Section 2.3 The reason for reporting this value rather than the mean survival time (the mean is defined in equation (1.1) below) is that the distributions of survival time data often tend to be skew, sometimes with a small number of long-term

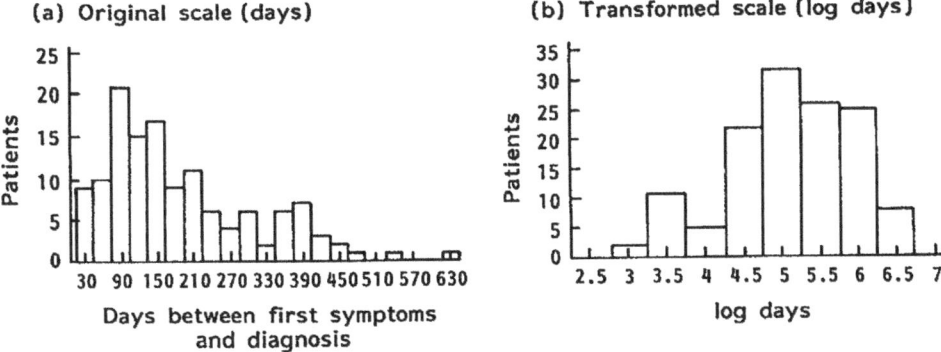

Figure 1.5 Distribution of the delay from first symptom to diagnosis of cervical cancer in 131 women: (a) Original scale (days), (b) Transformed scale (log days)

'survivors'. For example, the distribution shown in Figure 1.5(a) of the delay between first symptom and formal diagnosis of cervical cancer in 131 women, ranging from 1 to 610 days, is not symmetric. The median delay to diagnosis for the women with cervical cancer was 135 days. The distribution is skewed to the right, in that the right-hand tail of the distribution is much longer than the left-hand tail. In this situation the mean is not a good summary of the 'average' survival time because it is unduly influenced by the extreme observations.

In this example, we have the duration of the delay in diagnosis for all 131 women. However, the approach used here for calculating the median should not be used if there are censored values amongst our observations. This will usually be the case with survival-type data. In this instance the method described in Section 2.3 is appropriate.

THE NORMAL DISTRIBUTION

For many types of medical data the histogram of a continuous variable obtained from a single measurement on different subjects will have a characteristic 'bell-shaped' or Normal distribution. For some data which do not have such a distribution, a simple transformation of the variable may help. For example, if we calculate $x = \log t$ for each of the $n = 131$ women discussed above, where t is the delay from first symptom to diagnosis in days, then the distribution of x is given in Figure 1.5(b). This distribution is closer to the Normal distribution shape than that of Figure 1.5(a) and we can therefore calculate the arithmetic mean—more briefly the mean—of the x's by

$$\bar{x} = \sum x/n \qquad (1.1)$$

to indicate the average value of the data illustrated in Figure 1.5(b). For these data, this gives $\bar{x} = 4.88$ log days and which corresponds to 132 days.

Now that the distribution has an approximately Normal shape we can express the variability in values about the mean by the standard deviation (SD). This is given by

$$SD = \sqrt{[\Sigma(x - \bar{x})^2/(n - 1)]}. \qquad (1.2)$$

For the women with delay to diagnosis of their cervical cancer, equation (1.2) gives $SD = 0.81$ log days. From this we can then calculate the standard error (*SE*) of the mean as

$$SE(\bar{x}) = SD/\sqrt{n}. \tag{1.3}$$

This gives $SE(\bar{x}) = 0.81/\sqrt{131} = 0.07$ log days.

CONFIDENCE INTERVALS

For any statistic, such as a sample mean, $\bar{x}$, it is useful to have an idea of the uncertainty in using this as an estimate of the underlying true population mean, μ. This is done by constructing a (confidence) interval—a range of values around the estimate—which we can be confident includes the true underlying value. Such a confidence interval (*CI*) for μ extends evenly either side of $\bar{x}$ by a multiple of the standard error (*SE*) of the mean. Thus, for example, a 95% *CI* is the range of values from $\bar{x} - (1.9600 \times SE)$ to $\bar{x} + (1.9600 \times SE)$, while a 99% *CI* is the range of values from $\bar{x} - (2.5758 \times SE)$ to $\bar{x} + (2.5758 \times SE)$. In general a $100(1 - \alpha)$% CI, for μ is given by

$$\bar{x} - z_{1-\alpha/2} \times SE(\bar{x}) \quad \text{to} \quad \bar{x} + z_{1-\alpha/2} \times SE(\bar{x}). \tag{1.4}$$

Here $z_{1-\alpha/2}$ and $-z_{1-\alpha/2}$ are the upper and lower $1 - \alpha/2$ points of the standard Normal distribution of Figure 1.6, respectively.

Example – *confidence interval for a mean* – *time to diagnosis of cervical cancer*

For the data of Figure 1.5(b) suppose we require a 95% *CI* for log μ, the log of the true underlying mean. Then $\alpha = 0.05$ and $1 - \alpha/2 = 0.975$. From Table T1 locating the cell 0.0500 or in Table T2 using two-sided $\alpha = 0.0500$, we obtain $z_{0.975} = 1.9600$. Substituting $\bar{x} = 4.88$, $SE = 0.07$ and $z_{0.975} = 1.9600$ in equation (1.4) gives a 95% CI for log μ as 4.7428 to 5.017 log days. To obtain a 95% CI for μ, as opposed to log μ, we antilog the lower and upper values of our *CI* to obtain $\exp(4.7428) = 115$ and $\exp(5.017) = 151$ days, respectively.

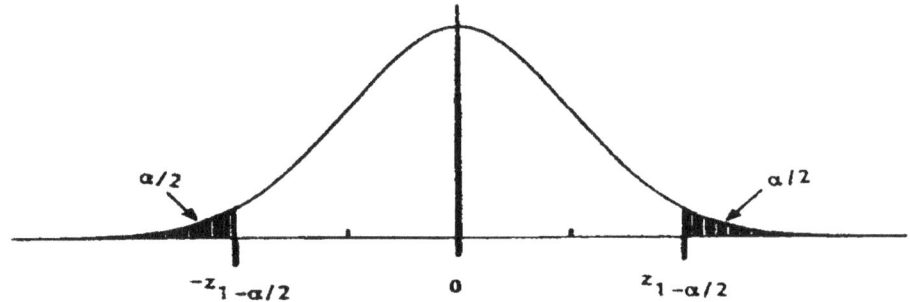

Figure 1.6 Upper and lower $\alpha/2$ points of the standard Normal distribution

Table 1.2 Some summary statistics and their standard errors (SE)

Statistic	Population value	Estimate	Standard error (SE)
Mean	μ	$\bar{x} = \sum x/n$	$SD/\sqrt{n}$
Difference between two means	$\delta = \mu_A - \mu_B$	$diff = \bar{x}_A - \bar{x}_B$	$\sqrt{\dfrac{SD_A^2}{n_A} + \dfrac{SD_B^2}{n_B}}$
Proportion	π	$p = r/n$	$\sqrt{\left[\dfrac{p(1-p)}{n}\right]}$
Difference between two proportions	$\delta = \pi_A - \pi_B$	$diff = p_A - p_B$	$\sqrt{\dfrac{p_A(1-p_A)}{n_A} + \dfrac{p_B(1-p_B)}{n_B}}$

We can increase the probability of including the true mean in the CI to, say, 99% by multiplying the SE in equation (1.4) by 2.5758 from Table T2 in place of 1.9600. Similarly we could reduce the probability to 90% by multiplying the SE by 1.6449 from Table T2, which, in turn, reduces the width of the interval. For no other reason than convention, it is common to report 95% CIs.

The expressions for the summary statistics and their SEs are different for different situations and some of these are listed in Table 1.2. Thus if a CI is required for the proportion of responses to a particular therapy, then we require to estimate this proportion by $p = r/n$, where r is the number of responses in n patients, and the $SE(p) = \sqrt{[p(1-p)/n]}$ as indicated in Table 1.2. These are then substituted in equation (1.4) in place of $\bar{x}$ and $SE(\bar{x})$, respectively, to obtain a CI. Further details of the calculation and use of CIs are given by Altman, Machin, Bryant and Gardner (2000).

A particularly important application of the use of estimation is to make a statement about relative treatment efficacy in a randomised clinical trial of, say, a new therapy compared to a standard or control treatment for a particular condition. The CI provides a range of values in which the true effect is likely to lie. That is, there is a small chance that this range will not contain the true effect. With a 95% CI there is a 5% chance that the true effect does not lie within it, while with a 99% CI there is only a 1% chance.

***Example** – comparison of two proportions – patients with severe burns*

The results of a clinical trial conducted by Ang, Lee, Gan, *et al.* (2001) comparing two forms of dressing for patients with severe burns are summarised in Table 1.3. Of 112 patients recruited 54 received MEBO (open) dressing (M) and 58 Conventional (covered) dressing (C) and the proportions healed to 75% of their initial wound are, respectively, 43% and 67%.

In an obvious notation $n_C = 58$, $p_C = a/(c+a) = 0.4310$, $n_M = 54$ and $p_M = b/(d+b) = 0.6667$. The observed difference between treatments is $diff = p_M - p_C = 0.6667 - 0.4310 = 0.2357$. The corresponding SE of $diff$ is given in Table 1.2 as

$$SE(diff) = \sqrt{\frac{p_C(1-p_C)}{n_C} + \frac{p_M(1-p_M)}{n_M}} = 0.09134.$$

From equation (1.4) the 95% CI around the difference in proportions healed at three weeks is 0.0567 to 0.4147 or 6% to 41%.

Table 1.3 Percentage of burns healed to 75% of the initial wound at three weeks by treatment group (based on Ang, Lee, Gan, *et al.*, 2001)

| Dressing | Healed | | | |
	Yes	No	Total	Healed (%)
Conventional (C)	25 (a)	33 (c)	58 ($m=c+a$)	43.10
MEBO (M)	36 (b)	18 (d)	54 ($n=d+b$)	66.67
Total	61 (r)	51 (s)	112 (N)	

1.4   THE HAZARD RATIO (HR)

The hazard ratio (HR) has been specifically developed for survival data, and is used as a measure of the relative survival experience of two groups. It is described in detail in Chapter 3. In brief, if the observed number of deaths in group A is O_A and the corresponding expected number of deaths (under the hypothesis of no survival difference between the groups under study) is E_A then the ratio O_A/E_A is the relative death rate in group A. Similarly O_B/E_B is the relative death rate in group B. The HR is the ratio of the relative death rates in the two groups, that is

$$HR = \frac{O_A/E_A}{O_B/E_B}. \tag{1.5}$$

It is important to note that for the HR the 'expected' deaths in each group are calculated using the Logrank method described in Chapter 3. This method allows for the censoring which occurs in nearly all survival data. The HR gives an estimate of the overall difference between the survival curves as discussed in Section 3.3. If there is no difference between two groups the value of $HR = 1$, and this can be tested by means of the Logrank test of Section 3.2.

However, summarising the difference between two survival curves into one statistic can also have its problems. One particularly important consideration for its use is that the ratio of the relative event rates in the two groups should not vary greatly over time. Sections 4.1 and 5.5 describe a graphical approach to assessing this.

RELATIVE RISK (RR)

The term relative risk (RR) has been defined for use in prospective epidemiological or cohort studies, in which groups of subjects with different exposures to a potential hazard

Table 1.4 General representation of the results of a prospective epidemiological study in the form of a 2 × 2 table

	Mesothelioma diagnosed		
Asbestos exposure	Yes	No	Total
Type I	*a*	*c*	$m = (c + a)$
Type II	*b*	*d*	$n = (d + b)$
Total	*r*	*s*	*N*

are followed to see whether or not an event of interest occurs. Thus Table 1.4 represents the notation for a prospective study in which two groups of industrial workers are likely to be exposed to different types of asbestos. They are then followed in time to see if they do or do not develop mesothelioma (the event under study). We assume here that all these workers are examined for evidence of the disease at, say, 15 years following their first exposure, and only presence or absence of the disease noted at that time.

A total of N subjects have been followed, $(c + a)$ who were exposed to Type I asbestos and $(d + b)$ exposed to Type II asbestos. The proportions of subjects in which mesothelioma subsequently develops, as recorded 15 years later, are $a/(c + a)$ and $b/(d + b)$ for Types I and II asbestos respectively. The *RR* is the ratio of these two proportions and is a measure of increased (or decreased) risk in one group when compared with the other. Thus

$$RR = \frac{a/(c + a)}{b/(d + b)} = \frac{a(d + b)}{b(c + a)}.\tag{1.6}$$

If there is no difference between the two exposure groups, i.e. the type of asbestos exposure does not influence the proportion of individuals subsequently developing mesothelioma, the expected value of the $RR = 1$.

Example – *relative risk – patients with severe burns*

To illustrate the calculation of a *RR* we use the data of Table 1.3, although this summarises a clinical trial rather than an epidemiological investigation. These data give, from equation (1.6), $RR = (25 \times 54)/(36 \times 58) = 0.6466$ or approximately 0.6. This suggests that those patients receiving Conventional dressing are approximately half as likely as those who receive MEBO to have their burns healed by three weeks.

ODDS RATIO (*OR*)

Using the same layout as in Table 1.4 we can define the odds of developing to not developing mesothelioma with Type I asbestos as $a{:}c$ or a/c and similarly as $b{:}d$ or b/d for Type II asbestos. The odds ratio (OR) is defined as their ratio which is:

$$OR = \frac{a/c}{b/d} = \frac{ad}{bc}. \tag{1.7}$$

If there is no difference in the odds of developing mesothelioma in the two asbestos groups then the expected value of $OR = 1$.

***Example** – odds ratio – patients with severe burns*

In the example of Table 1.3 we have $a = 25, b = 36, c = 33$ and $d = 18$. Hence a/c is 25/33 and b/d is 36/18, giving an $OR = (25 \times 18)/(36 \times 33) = 0.3787$ or approximately 0.4.

In this example, an $OR < 1$ indicates fewer healed burns with Conventional dressing as we had concluded when we calculated the $RR \approx 0.6$. In this example, the values of the RR and OR are not too different.

RELATIONSHIP BETWEEN THE HR, RR AND OR

If we go back to Table 1.4 but consider situations when the event is rare, i.e. assume relatively few individuals will develop mesothelioma from a large number of workers exposed to asbestos, then the number a will be small compared with the number c. In this case $a/(c + a)$ will be approximately equal to a/c. Similarly $b/(d + b)$ will be approximately equal to b/d. As a consequence, in this situation, equation (1.6) for the RR is approximately

$$RR \approx \frac{a/c}{b/d} = \frac{ad}{bc} = OR. \tag{1.8}$$

Both the OR and RR can be calculated in the situation of Table 1.3 and, if this were a rare event case in that the proportion healed was small in both groups, then they would be numerically close.

However, in a retrospective case-control study, only the OR can be estimated. This is because, if the numerical procedure of equation (1.6) is used to calculate the RR directly in a case-control study, the result obtained depends on the proportion of cases to controls selected by the design. For example, if one doubles the number of controls (equivalent to replacing a by $2a$ and b by $2b$ in Table 1.4) the OR remains the same since we double both the numerator and denominator in equation (1.7), but the value obtained for the RR will be different. Nevertheless, in situations in which the event is rare, the OR may provide an estimate of the corresponding RR.

We have seen that the OR and RR can be numerically similar, and that the OR can provide an estimate of the RR when the event rates are small. There is also a link between the HR and RR and in special situations the HR can be the same as the RR.

> **Example** – *healing time* – *patients with severe burns*
>
> In fact Ang, Lee, Gan, *et al.* (2001) recorded the actual time to burn healing from the date at which treatment started (which is also the date of randomisation as this is a clinical trial of emergency care) in their patients, but our illustration so far has ignored this fact. In this case, those patients with healed ulcers within three weeks would be included as healed in Table 1.3 but those that heal after this time will not be counted.

If we were to analyse these data using standard methods for a 2×2 table then under the (null) hypothesis of no difference in outcome in the two groups, the expected proportion of unhealed burns in the two groups will be estimated, using the same notation as before, by $(a + b)/N = r/N$. Of these, we would expect $E_C = (c + a) \times (r/N) = r(c + a)/N$ to occur in those patients treated with Conventional dressing and $E_M = (d + b) \times (r/N) = r(d + b)/N$ to occur in those treated with MEBO dressing. Now the actual numbers of *healed burns* in groups C and M are $O_C = a$ and $O_M = b$, respectively. Hence if we were then to use equation (1.5), as if for a HR, we would have

$$
\frac{O_C/E_C}{O_M/E_M} = \frac{a/[r(c + a)/N]}{b/[r(d + b)/N]}
$$
$$
= \frac{a/(c + a)}{b/(d + b)} = \frac{a(d + b)}{b(c + a)} = RR.
$$

Reference to equation (1.6) shows that this is just the expression for the RR. Thus, when there is no censoring (see Section 2.1) and when the actual time an event occurs is not considered important, and is not therefore used, the HR and RR are equivalent.

There is some confusion in the appropriate use of the RR and OR and this extends to the use of the HR. The HR is specifically defined for survival studies in which the time between two critical events is recorded. In these circumstances, the HR is the estimate that should always be used and reported.

Despite this many researchers still refer to the 'HR' as the 'RR'. This is poor practice and we prefer to use the terminology of HR for survival studies and reserve the term RR for situations in which both censoring, and the time at which the critical event occurs, are not relevant.

1.5 SIGNIFICANCE TESTS

THE z-TEST

A central feature of statistical analysis is the test of the null hypothesis of 'no difference'. For example, in a clinical trial of a new treatment versus a standard treatment the null hypothesis that is to be tested is that there is no difference between the new and standard treatments in their efficacy.

To test the null hypothesis, often denoted by H_0 and often expressed as the true difference $\delta = 0$, we compare the group of patients receiving the new treatment with the group receiving the standard, with the goal of rejecting the null hypothesis in favour of an alternative hypothesis, should a difference in efficacy be observed. Such an alternative hypothesis, often denoted H_A, implies that $\delta \neq 0$ and therefore there is a real difference between the new and the standard therapies in their efficacy.

The z-test, which is used as the significance test of the null hypothesis, takes the form

$$z = \frac{\text{(Observed difference)} - \text{(Difference anticipated by the null hypothesis)}}{SE\text{(Observed difference)}}. \qquad (1.9)$$

In many circumstances, the estimate of the effect anticipated by the null hypothesis is zero, so that equation (1.9) becomes in such cases,

$$z = \frac{\text{(Observed difference)}}{SE\text{(Observed difference)}} = \frac{diff}{SE(diff)}. \qquad (1.10)$$

Once the test statistic z is calculated, this value is then referred to Table T1 of the Normal distribution to obtain the p-value.

The resulting p-value is defined as the answer to the question: what is the probability that we would have observed the difference, *or a more extreme difference*, if the null hypothesis were true?

Example *– significance test – patients with severe burns*

In the context of the trial of two treatments for burns by Ang, Lee, Gan *et al.* (2001) the null hypothesis is that both Conventional and MEBO dressings are equally effective in healing burns. The observed difference between the treatments is expressed in terms of $diff = 0.2357$. The corresponding null hypothesis of no treatment difference is stated as δ, the true difference, equals zero.

Thus, use of equation (1.10) with the Observed difference $diff = 0.2357$ and the SE(Observed difference) $= SE(diff) = 0.09134$, gives $z = 0.2357/0.09134 = 2.5805$. Reference to Table T1, with $z = 2.581$, gives a total area in the tails of the distribution, by combining that to the left of $z = -2.58$ with that to the right of $z = +2.58$, of approximately 0.0099. This area is termed the p-value.

If the p-value is small, say < 0.001, then we may conclude that the null hypothesis is unlikely to be true. On the other hand, if the p-value is large, say > 0.5, we would be reluctant to conclude that it is not true.

However, somewhere between these two clear possibilities there is likely to be a grey area in which it is hard to decide. For this reason, it has become something of a convention to report a 'statistically significant' result if the p-value < 0.05, and a 'highly statistically significant' result if the p-value < 0.01. However, the exact value of the p-value obtained in these circumstances should always be quoted. It is a somewhat unfortunate convention to use 'not statistically significant' if the p-value > 0.05. It is particularly important in this latter situation to quote the exact p-value, the value of the estimate of the difference (or *OR*, *RR* or *HR* as appropriate) and the corresponding *CI*.

***Example** – p-value – patients with severe burns*

In the case of the p-value $= 0.0099$, obtained from the significance test from the data on burns patients, then this is clearly < 0.05. From this we may conclude that there is a statistically significant difference between the healing rates of the two dressings.

For consistency we have to specify at the planning stage a value, α, so that once the study is completed and analysed, a p-value below this would lead to the null hypothesis being rejected. Thus if the p-value obtained from a comparative study is $\leq \alpha$, then one rejects the null hypothesis and concludes that there is a statistically significant difference between groups. On the other hand, if the p-value is $> \alpha$ then one does not reject the null hypothesis. Although the value of α is arbitrary, it is often taken as 0.05 or 5%.

SIGNIFICANCE TESTS AND CONFIDENCE INTERVALS

In the context of a randomised trial, the observed difference between the treatments obtained with the trial data is termed the estimated effect size and is the best estimate of the true or population difference between them. Further, the *CI* provides a range of values, in particular plausible minimum and maximum values within which the effect is likely to lie. In contrast, a hypothesis test does not tell us about the actual size of the effect, only whether it is likely to be different from zero.

Although the two approaches of *CI*s and significance tests do apparently address different questions, there is a close relationship between them. For example, whenever the 95% *CI* for the estimate excludes the value zero, i.e. the *CI* lies either entirely above or entirely below zero, then the corresponding hypothesis test will yield a p-value < 0.05. Similarly if the 99% *CI* for the estimate excludes zero then the p-value < 0.01.

As for the significance level of a statistical test, α, it is important to specify at the design stage of a study whether 95% or 99% *CI*s will be used at the analysis. If the context is very clear, one can replace 'p-value $= 0.0099$' by the shortened form '$p = 0.0099$'.

CLINICAL AND STATISTICAL SIGNIFICANCE

It is important to distinguish between a 'clinically significant' result and a 'statistically significant' result. The former is an effect, which if established, is likely to make a real (clinical) impact. For example, if the difference in efficacy between two treatments, as established by a randomised clinical trial, is substantial then the better of the two treatments, if given to all future patients, will have clinical impact and is therefore 'clinically significant'. In certain circumstances, even small differences that are firmly established may have clinical impact. For example, the impact of aspirin in reducing the risk of second attacks in patients who have suffered a myocardial infarction is not dramatic, but the modest benefit gained through its use has been shown to save many lives annually since the disease is common. Hence, although the effect for an individual is small, that is proportionally few will be saved from a second attack, the result is of considerable 'clinical significance' to the population as a whole.

In contrast, a 'statistically significant' result does not automatically imply a clinically important consequence of that result. For example, suppose we demonstrate that a new therapy provides a small but statistically significant improvement in survival over the standard therapy: however, the new therapy is so toxic, difficult and costly that the small improvement in survival is not sufficient to make it clinically worthwhile to use the new therapy in patients. Consequently, the trial has produced a statistically significant result of little clinical significance.

It is also necessary to appreciate that one should not dismiss a result that is 'not statistically significant' as therefore 'not clinically important'. For example, a study may be too small to reliably detect and measure important differences between two groups. In this situation the study may provide an estimate of the difference which, had it been reliably shown and measured, would have been of clinical or scientific importance. In such circumstances it may be that the study should be repeated, perhaps in a larger group of patients. We discuss the choice of sample sizes for survival studies in Chapter 9.

We now introduce two additional methods for performing significance tests which form the basis of many of the tests used in the remainder of the book.

1.6   OTHER SIGNIFICANCE TESTS

THE χ^2 TEST

We have seen earlier, that the analysis of data from a randomised trial comparing two groups can be expressed in terms of observed (O) and expected (E) values. In the notation of Table 1.3, often termed a (2×2) contingency table with $R = 2$ rows and $C = 2$ columns, we have observed for the four cells of the table, $O_1, = a, O_2 = b, O_3 = c$ and $O_4 = d$. The corresponding expected values, calculated on the assumption of the null hypothesis of no difference, are $E_1 = r(c + a)/N$, $E_2 = r(d + b)/N$, $E_3 = s(c + a)/N$ and $E_4 = s(d + b)/N$. To obtain the χ^2 test these values are then substituted into

$$\chi^2 = \Sigma(O - E)^2/E \tag{1.11}$$

where the summation is over the four cells of Table 1.3. We use a similar equation to (1.11) when describing the Logrank test in Chapter 3.

Example – χ^2 *test – patients with severe burns*

Using the data of Ang, Lee, Gan *et al.* (2001), $O_1 = 25, O_2 = 36, O_3 = 33$ and $O_4 = 18$. The corresponding expected values are $E_1 = 31.5893, E_2 = 29.4107, E_3 = 26.4107$ and $E_4 = 24.5893$. This gives

$$\chi^2 = \frac{(25 - 31.5893)^2}{31.5893} + \frac{(36 - 29.4107)^2}{29.4107} + \frac{(33 - 26.4107)^2}{26.4107}$$
$$+ \frac{(18 - 24.5893)^2}{24.5893} = 6.2605.$$

The value $\chi^2 = 6.26$ is then referred to Table T3 of the χ^2 distribution with degrees freedom (df) equal to one. This gives the p-value ≈ 0.01. An exact value can be obtained in this case, since $df = 1$, by referring $z = \sqrt{\chi^2} = 2.502$ to Table T1. Hence the p-value ≈ 0.0123. We note that 2.502 is close to $z = 2.581$ obtained from the use of equation (1.10). In fact, the two approaches are algebraically similar but not identical.

The basic concept of a χ^2 test, in the form of equation (1.11), can be extended to a general $R \times C$ contingency table. The number of degrees of freedom is now $df = (R-1)(C-1)$. The χ^2 test statistic obtained from the calculation corresponding to the $R \times C$ table is referred to Table T3 with the appropriate df.

LIKELIHOOD RATIO (LR) TEST

In some situations, an alternative approach to testing hypotheses is required. One such method is termed the likelihood ratio (LR) test. Such a test compares the probability or likelihood of the data under one hypothesis with the likelihood under an alternative hypothesis. To illustrate this procedure it is first necessary to define the likelihood of the data.

Suppose we are estimating the probability of response to treatment in a group of n patients with a particular disease and the true or population value for this probability is π. Then an individual patient will respond with probability π and fail to respond with probability $(1 - \pi)$. Here π must take a value between 0, the value when no patients ever respond, and 1, in which all cases respond.

If, in our study, r of these patients respond and $(n - r)$ do not respond, then the probability of this outcome is

$$\ell = \pi^r (1 - \pi)^{(n-r)}. \tag{1.12}$$

Here ℓ is termed the likelihood. If we then calculate $L = \log \ell$ then this is termed the log likelihood and we have

$$L = \log \ell = r \log \pi + (n - r) \log(1 - \pi). \tag{1.13}$$

It turns out that if we estimate π by $p = r/n$ then this corresponds to the value for π which maximises the value of ℓ in equation (1.12) or, equivalently, the maximum possible value of L in equation (1.13). We therefore state that $p = r/n$ is the maximum likelihood estimate of π.

To obtain this estimate in a formal way, it is necessary to differentiate equation (1.13) with respect to π and equate the result to zero. The solution of this equation gives the estimate as $\pi = r/n$ which is hence the maximum likelihood estimate.

The LR test calculates the likelihood under two different hypotheses and compares these. For convenience, we term these the likelihood under the null hypothesis, ℓ_0, and the likelihood under the alternative hypothesis, ℓ_a. The likelihood ratio test is then

$$LR = -2\log(\ell_0/\ell_a) = -2(L_0 - L_a). \tag{1.14}$$

A large value of LR would indicate that the assumption of equal treatment efficacy is unlikely to be consistent with the data. If the null hypothesis were true we would expect a small value of the LR. In fact, it can be shown that the LR in equation (1.14) is approximately distributed as a χ^2 variable with the appropriate df.

The df corresponds to the difference between the number of parameters (see below) estimated under the alternative hypothesis, m_A, minus the number of parameters estimated under the null hypothesis, m_0, that is $df = m_A - m_0$. The value of the LR statistic is then referred to the χ^2 distribution, using the appropriate row in Table T3 for the df, to give the p-value. As we noted earlier, in the case of $df = 1$ and only in this case, $z = \sqrt{\chi^2}$ and so Table T1 can be used.

Example – *likelihood ratio (LR) – patients with severe burns*

For the trial of Ang, Lee, Gan, *et al.* (2001) the null hypothesis is that $\pi_C = \pi_M = \pi_0$. In this case we have one parameter π_0 which is estimated, using the notation of Table 1.3, by $r/N = 61/112$. Therefore, under the null hypothesis, equation (1.13) becomes

$$L_0 = r \log \pi_0 + (N - r) \log(1 - \pi_0)$$
$$= 61 \times \log(61/112) + 51 \times \log(51/112) = -77.1855.$$

In contrast, under the alternative hypothesis that the two treatments differ, the parameters π_C and π_M are estimated separately by 25/58 and 36/54, respectively. In this case L_A, the log likelihood corresponding to equation (1.13), becomes the sum of L_C and L_M. That is,

$$L_A = L_C + L_M = 25 \log(25/58) + 33 \log(33/58) + 36 \log(36/54) + 18 \log(18/54)$$

$$= -74.0208.$$

Substituting these values for L_0 and L_A into equation (1.14) gives $LR = -2(-77.1855 + 74.0208) = 6.3294$. Reference to Table T3 with $df = 1$ gives a p-value between 0.01 and 0.02 for this observed LR. To obtain a more precise figure for the p-value, in the case of $df = 1$ only, we calculate $z = \sqrt{LR} = 2.516$ and refer this to Table T1 to obtain a p-value ≈ 0.0119.

Finally we note that $z = 2.516$ is close to the $z = 2.581$ we obtained earlier using equation (1.10). These will often be close, although the two approaches are not algebraically equivalent. In our example, the z, χ^2 and LR tests yield much the same conclusion.

The advantage of the LR test of equation (1.14), over the z test of equation (1.9), is that the method extends to comparisons of more than two groups. For example, if we were comparing three treatments, then we would estimate three parameters, π_1, π_2 and π_3, under the alternative hypothesis and one parameter, π_0, under the null hypothesis. In this case $df = m_A - m_0 = 3 - 1 = 2$ and to obtain a p-value $= 0.05$, for example, in Table T3 we require a value of $\chi^2 = 5.99$ as opposed to $\chi^2 = 3.84$ when $df = 1$.

The maximum likelihood estimates of the parameters of some distributions of survival are given in Chapter 4 and further discussion of the LR statistic is given in Section 5.6.

1.7 STATISTICAL COMPUTING

Many statistical packages now include procedures that enable the techniques described in this book to be implemented. Unfortunately much of what we describe cannot be implemented without this support. A comprehensive review of the use the statistical package SAS for survival analysis is given by Collett (2003) and the whole textbook by Allison (1995) is devoted to this topic. Other packages that have survival analysis facilities include EGRET, EPI-INFO, SYSTAT and Stata. Cleves, Gould and Gutierrez (2002) extensively describe the use of Stata. For more advanced users the book by Venables and Ripley (1999) provides a useful guide to the use of S-Plus in this and other contexts.

It is important that the data you collect can interface with these statistical packages. In many situations, particularly in clinical trials and longitudinal follow-up studies in epidemiology, the data do not come neatly packaged in a rectangular array, free of missing values and with complete information on the relevant endpoints for all subjects. Typically such studies have ragged data files of variable length for each subject. For example, those patients that die early following diagnosis of their disease will have a correspondingly short data file, while those that survive will have a long period of observation and a data file which continues to expand with time. Such ragged data files usually have to be converted to a flat file for transport to a statistical package.

In studies in which times between successive events are important, database facilities must be readily available to calculate survival times by subtraction of two dates. Thus, in a patient recruited to a clinical trial with a fatal disease, the date of entry (DOE) to a trial therapy (first event) may be recorded, the patient is then followed up (FU) at successive clinical visits, each of which will have a date, DFU(1), DFU(2), ..., until their eventual death (DOD), which is the second (critical) event. The database package must then have the facility to calculate the survival time in days by $t = \mathrm{DOD} - \mathrm{DOE}$. For those patients who have not died at the time of analysis (these create censored observations, see Section 2.1) it is necessary to identify the last follow-up visit for each patient and determine that date. This is then used to calculate the (censored) survival time by $T^+ = \mathrm{DFU}\,(\mathrm{Last}) - \mathrm{DOE}$. Statistical packages often have functions to define dates in terms of the number of days from an anchorage date, usually 01 January 1960. Hence 02 January 1960 is 1, 31 December 1959 is -1, 31 December 2004 is 16 436 etc. By defining dates as such, subtraction can be done easily.

1.8 BIBLIOGRAPHY

As already indicated, important papers describing survival time applications in clinical trials are those by Peto, Pike, Armitage *et al.* (1976, 1977). These papers describe not only appropriate statistical methodology, including the Logrank test, but also many practical aspects relevant to the conduct of clinical trials. There are several explanatory papers presenting statistical methods for survival studies, including a description of the Cox regression model, and these include the series of papers published in the *British Journal of Cancer* by Bradburn, Clark, Love and Altman (2003a, b), Clark, Bradburn, Love and Altman (2003a, b) and Pocock, Clayton and Altman (2002) who describe good practice in terms of the graphical presentation of survival data.

Kaplan and Meier (1958) first described the product-limit estimator of the survival curve (Chapter 2). The paper by Cox (1972) introducing the proportional hazards model (Chapter 5) has led to a revolution in the analysis of survival data. There are several texts which describe survival analysis techniques but more from a technical perspective and they include, in approximate order of mathematical complexity, Marubini and Valsecchi (1995), Collett (2003), Cox and Oakes (1984) and Kabfleisch and Prentice (2002). These papers and books are written, however, for a more mathematical audience and may be heavy going for the general reader.

Basic statistical texts include Campbell, Machin and Walters (2006), Bland (2000) and Altman (1991) and these are ordered here in terms of their relative complexity and detail. The first is for beginners, the last for medical researchers. The book by Machin and Campbell (2005) focuses on design issues for a wide range of medical studies.

A full description of the use and calculation of *CI*s, including a computer package for implementation, is given by Altman, Machin, Bryant and Gardner (2000).

Programs for the calculation of the appropriate size of a study (Chapter 9) for survival-time endpoints are given by Machin, Campbell, Fayers and Pinol (1997) and Elashoff (2000).

2 Survival Curves

Summary

In this chapter we describe the basic methods that can be used to describe and analyse survival data involving censored observations. In particular, we present the method of calculating the Kaplan-Meier survival curve and associated confidence intervals. We also describe the calculation of the median survival time and introduce the use of the hazard rate.

2.1 SURVIVAL TIME DATA

In a clinical trial or medical investigation, patients are often entered into the study over a period of time and then followed beyond the treatment or intervention period and assessed for the endpoint of interest some time later. However, as noted in Chapter 1, this endpoint may not always be observed for all patients. For example, in a randomised trial of tamoxifen in the treatment of inoperable hepatocellular carcinoma (HCC) conducted by the Asia-Pacific Hepatocellular Carcinoma Trials Group as reported by Chow, Tai, Tan *et al.* (2002), 329 eligible patients were entered between 04 April 1997 and 08 June 2000. Thus recruitment to the trial lasted for over two years. The focus in this trial was to establish the impact of treatment on the length of patient survival from commencement of treatment until death. This event, that is, the 'death', was considered the 'principal outcome measure' of the trial. An analysis of this trial was performed in late 2001, at which time patients had differing times in the trial depending on their actual date of recruitment and hence the start of therapy. A total of 20 of the 296 patients were still alive at this analysis date. Although this is generally a fatal disease, for the analysis and reporting of the trial results it was unrealistic to wait until these 20 patients had died as some patients can live for a long time following diagnosis.

However, each of the 20 patients alive at the time of analysis had individual survival times from commencement of treatment. These ranked from relatively short periods for those who entered rather late in the recruitment period, to 36 months (three years) for one patient entered in the early stages of the trial. Thus for the patient who has survived 36 months, and is still alive, all we know is his total survival time from start of treatment to death will exceed 36 months. We denote this as 36+ months. If the analysis had been delayed until all the patients had died, the investigators may have had to wait for some considerable time, particularly if any patient entered late into the trial also lived to beyond 36 months. Clearly, to wait for such an event would not have been advisable as it is important to report the conclusions from a study as soon as it is practically possible.

Survival Analysis Second Edition   David Machin, Yin Bun Cheung, Mahesh K.B. Parmar
© 2006 John Wiley & Sons, Ltd   ISBN: 0-470-87040-0

Further, some patients who have 'not yet died' may have actually 'left' the trial, perhaps moving to a different locality or country. In such cases the investigators may never observe an 'event' for them. These patients are often termed 'lost to follow-up'.

Survival time is measured from one event, here start of treatment, to a subsequent event, here patient death. Patients for whom we have not observed the event of interest are said to provide 'censored' data. All we know about these patients is that they have survived a certain length of time. The reasons for this censoring are either that the patient has not yet died or that the patient has been lost to follow-up.

For the heart transplant patients of Chapter 1, the 'survival' times may be the time from the date of diagnosis to the date a donor heart becomes available or, for those who received a transplant, the time from surgery until rejection of the donor heart.

The flow of patients recruited to a typical prospective clinical trial involving patient accrual and observation over time is illustrated in Figure 2.1. The study has a recruitment and observation phase, an observation only phase, and an analysis time.

In this trial, recruitment has been over a period of one year, further observations made for the next two years and the definitive analysis undertaken three years from the start of the trial. The maximum possible (observable) survival time for the two patients entered in early January 2001 is three years, whilst for the one recruited in late December 2001 it is only two years.

Figure 2.1 shows that five patients died and two were still alive at the end of the study. A further five patients were lost from observation before the time of analysis. We often do not need to distinguish between these patients lost to follow-up, and for whom we could obtain no further information, and the two known to be alive at the date of analysis but who could be observed beyond the analysis date if necessary. In doing this we are assuming that the reason for the five patients being lost to follow-up has nothing to do with their outcome after treatment. We thus have five firm survival times and seven censored times. The patient

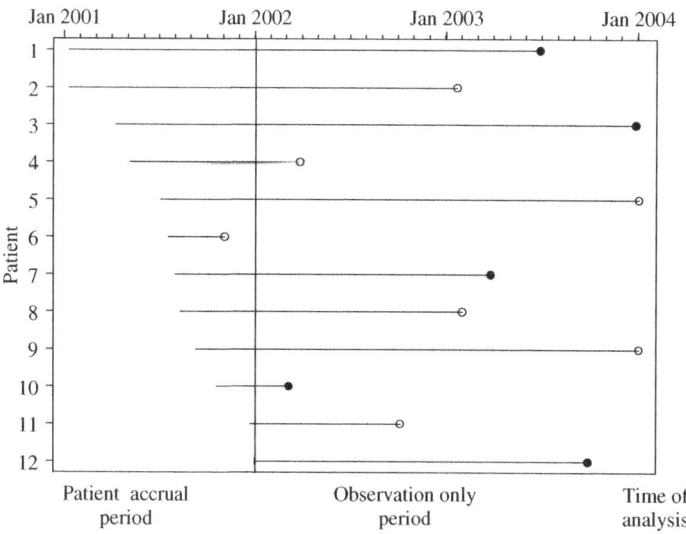

Figure 2.1 Patients entering a prospective clinical study at different times with the known (●) and censored (○) survival times indicated

Table 2.1 Survival times for patients shown in Figure 2.1

Patient	Date of entry (dd.mm.yyyy)	Time at entry (days)	Time at death or censoring since 01.01.2001 (days)	Death (D) or censored (C)	Survival time t or T+ (days)
1	01.01.2001	0	910	D	910
2	01.01.2001	0	752	C	752+
3	26.03.2001	84	1090	D	1006
4	26.04.2001	115	451	C	336+
5	23.06.2001	173	1096	C	923+
6	09.07.2001	189	307	C	118+
7	22.07.2001	202	816	D	614
8	02.08.2001	213	762	C	549+
9	01.09.2001	243	1097	C	854+
10	07.10.2001	279	431	D	152
11	14.12.2001	347	644	C	297+
12	26.12.2001	359	1000	D	641

recruitment dates, time at entry and time at death measured in days from 01 January 2001, and total survival time, are as shown in Table 2.1. The plus sign (+) denotes a censored survival time.

In many circumstances the different starting times of the patients are not relevant to the analysis of survival data, and neither is it necessary for the details in the third and fourth columns of the table to be formally recorded. However, for purposes of hand calculation, (computer packages do this without one being aware of this fact), it is necessary to order (or rank) the patient observations by the duration of the individual 'survival' times and Figure 2.2 shows the data of Figure 2.1 rearranged in rank order.

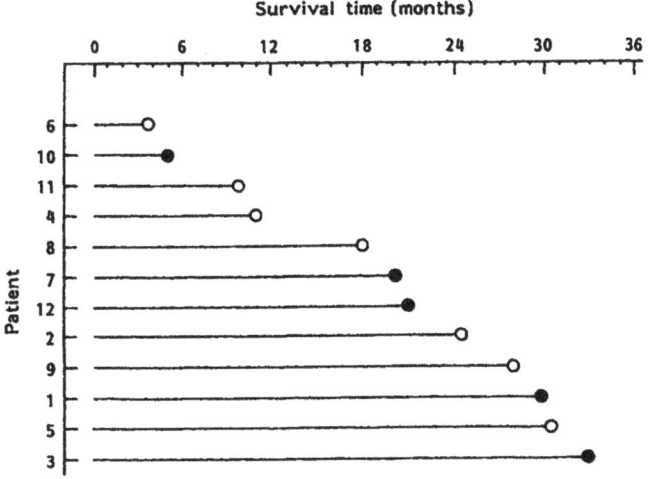

Figure 2.2 The data of Figure 2.1 ordered by length of observed survival time with (•) representing a known survival time and (o) a censored survival time

Example – *survival times* – *patients with colorectal cancer*

McIllmurray and Turkie (1987) report the ordered survival times of 24 patients with Dukes' C colorectal cancer as 3+, 6, 6, 6, 6, 8, 8, 12, 12, 12+, 15+, 16+, 18+, 18+, 20, 22+, 24, 28+, 28+, 28+, 30, 30+, 33+ and 42 months. These data, in the ordered format of Figure 2.2, are illustrated in Figure 2.3.

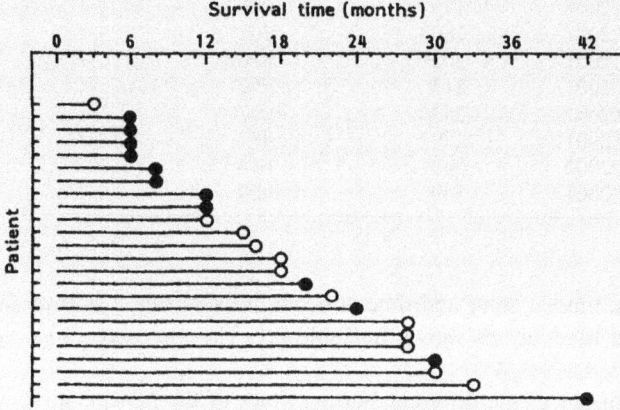

Figure 2.3   Ordered survival time of 24 patients with Dukes' C colorectal cancer (From McIllmurray and Turkie, 1987. Reproduced by permission of *British Medical Journal* **294**: 1260 and **295**: 475. Published by BMJ Publishing Group)

These same data are detailed again in Table 2.2. We will show in Chapter 9 that, for assessing studies, which involve patient follow-up, it is the number of critical events observed which is the determinant of statistical power (see Section 9.2) considerations, rather than the number of patients actually recruited. Thus, all other things being equal, the study by McIllmurray and Turkie (1987) lacks statistical power, as only 12 patients (50%) had died at the time of analysis and reporting, while the remaining 12 (50%) were still alive. However, even if the authors had awaited the deaths of these patients the study would still have involved relatively few events (deaths). This contrasts with the Asia-Pacific Hepatocellular Carcinoma Trials Group trial in which there were 329 patients amongst whom 296 (91%) deaths had occurred at the time of analysis.

The survival times of the patients with Dukes' C colorectal cancer in the McIllmurray and Turkie study are given to the nearest month resulting in, for example, four patients having the same recorded survival time of six months. Such observations are termed tied. It is usually better to avoid tied observations, if possible, and here if survival times had been reported in days then these four patients would be more likely to have different survival times, each of approximately six months. This would have allowed these four survival times to be placed in rank order, leading to the possibility of a more sensitive analysis.

Table 2.2 Survival data by month for the 24 patients with Dukes' C colorectal cancer randomly assigned to receive control treatment (from McIllmurray and Turkie, 1987. Reproduced by permission of *British Medical Journal* **294**: 1260 and **295**: 475. Published by BMJ Publishing Group)

Rank	Survival time t (months)	Number at risk n_t	Observed deaths d_t	$p_t = 1 - \dfrac{d_t}{n_t}$	Survival proportion $S(t)$
–	0	24	0	1.0000	1
1	3+	24	0		
2	6				
3	6	23	4	0.8261	0.8261
4	6				
5	6				
6	8	19	2	0.8947	0.7391
7	8				
8	12	17	2	0.8824	0.6522
9	12				
10	12+	15	0		
11	15+	14	0		
12	16+	13	0		
13	18+	12			
14	18+				
15	20	10	1	0.9000	0.5780
16	22+	9	0		
17	24	8	1	0.8750	0.5136
18	28+				
19	28+	7	0		
20	28+				
21	30	4	1	0.7500	0.3852
22	30+	3	0		
23	33+	2	0		
24	42	1	1	0.0000	0

Another feature of these data is the three patients with survival times of 12 months. Two of these patients have died at this time and the third is still alive. In ranking survival times it is a convention to give the censored observations in such a situation the higher rank. The assumption here is that the censored individual at, say, 12 months is likely to live longer than the patient who has died at 12 months even though the observation periods (as far as the study is concerned) are the same for these two individuals. The three survival times would thus be recorded as 12, 12 and 12+, having ranks 8, 9 and 10, respectively.

NOTATION

It is convenient to denote the observed survival time by (lower case) t for those observations in which the critical (second) event has occurred. However, as already indicated, there are often censored survival times in such studies which correspond to individuals in which the second event has not occurred. We denote their censored survival times by (capital) $T+$. We might have used $t+$ for this but, for expository purposes only, we use $T+$ to give added emphasis to the fact that they are censored observations. Individual survival times are distinguished by using a subscript to either t or $T+$ as appropriate.

To illustrate the use of this notation consider the data of Table 2.1, which gives $t_1 = 910$, $T_2^+ = 752+$, $t_3 = 1006$, and so on until $t_{12} = 641$ days. Once these survival times are ordered (ranked) in increasing magnitude, they are relabelled by $T_{(1)}^+ = 118+$, since the shortest survival time observed is censored, $t_{(2)} = 152$, $T_{(3)}^+ = 297+$ and so on until $t_{(12)} = 1006$ days. The parentheses, (.), around the subscript indicate that the data are now in rank order.

If there are tied observations (either all censored or all events) then they are each given the mean rank; for example, if $t_{(4)} = t_{(5)} = t_{(6)}$, then each is relabelled $t_{(5)}$, $t_{(5)}$ and $t_{(5)}$, respectively.

2.2   ESTIMATING SURVIVAL

SURVIVAL AT A FIXED TIME-POINT

Before introducing the method of estimating the survival curve as a whole, we review methods that have been suggested but which are not recommended. At their worst these methods can give a very misleading impression of the true situation.

One method is to report the proportion of patients alive at a fixed time-point. Thus, for the McIllmurray and Turkie (1987) data of Figure 2.3 eight of 24 patients are known to have died by 12 months, giving a one year survival rate of 16/24 or 66.7%. However, this calculation presumes that the patient who is censored at 3+ months will be alive at one year. If, on the other hand, the patient dies before one year the estimate decreases to 15/24 or 62.5%. Of course, when calculating this estimate we do not know which of these will turn out to be the case.

Another possibility is only to use information on those patients that have reached a fixed point in the observation time or that have died before this time. This 'reduced sample' estimate at one year, for example, would exclude the patient who has a censored survival time $T_{(1)}^+ = 3+$, and would give the survival rate estimate at one year as 15/23 or 65.2%. One can well imagine that excluding patients, perhaps who are alive at 364 days (just short of one year) by this process, will give a distorted pattern of the survival experience of all those recruited to the study.

KAPLAN-MEIER (K-M)

In a clinical study a question of central interest is: what is the probability that patients will survive a certain length of time? For example, in the Stanford heart transplant data from Turnbull, Brown and Hu (1974) presented in Table 1.1, we may be interested in estimating the probability of a patient surviving for one year following heart transplant. This probability can be calculated in the following way. The probability of surviving 365 days (one year) is the probability of surviving the 365th day having already survived the previous 364 days. Clearly one must have survived this day before one can have the possibility to survive the next day. Survival into day 365 is therefore conditional on surviving the whole of day 364. Similarly, the conditional probability of surviving for 364 days is the probability of surviving the 364th day having already survived for 363 days. This argument clearly continues for each preceding day of the one year.

In more formal terms we define

p_1 = probability of surviving for at least one day after transplant;

p_2 = conditional probability of surviving the second day after having survived the first day;

p_3 = conditional probability of surviving the third day after having survived the second day;

.

.

.

p_{365} = conditional probability of surviving the 365th day after having survived day 364.

The overall probability of surviving 365 days after a heart transplant, $S(365)$, is then given by the product of these probabilities. Thus

$$S(365) = p_1 \times p_2 \times p_3 \times \cdots \times p_{364} \times p_{365},$$

and, in general, the probability of survival to time t is

$$S(t) = p_1 \times p_2 \times \cdots \times p_t. \tag{2.1}$$

To calculate $S(t)$ we need to estimate each of p_1, p_2, p_3, ... and p_t. We can obtain an estimate of any particular one, say p_{365}, by

$$p_{365} = \frac{\left[\begin{array}{c} \text{Number} \cdot \text{of} \cdot \text{patients} \cdot \text{followed} \cdot \text{for} \cdot \text{at} \cdot \text{least} \cdot 364 \cdot \text{days} \\ \text{and} \cdot \text{who} \cdot \text{survive} \cdot \text{day} \cdot 365 \end{array}\right]}{[\text{Number} \cdot \text{of} \cdot \text{patients} \cdot \text{alive} \cdot \text{at} \cdot \text{end} \cdot \text{of} \cdot \text{day} \cdot 364]}$$

In a similar way, we can calculate for any time t

$$p_t = \frac{\left[\begin{array}{c} \text{Number} \cdot \text{of} \cdot \text{patients} \cdot \text{followed} \cdot \text{for} \cdot \text{at} \cdot \text{least} \cdot (t-1) \cdot \text{days} \\ \text{and} \cdot \text{who} \cdot \text{survive} \cdot \text{day} \cdot t \end{array}\right]}{[\text{Number} \cdot \text{of} \cdot \text{patients} \cdot \text{alive} \cdot \text{at} \cdot \text{end} \cdot \text{of} \cdot \text{day} \cdot (t-1)]} \tag{2.2}$$

Example *– conditional probability of surviving – patients with colorectal cancer*

To illustrate the process we calculate p_{12} for the Dukes' C colorectal cancer data summarised in the second column of Table 2.2. It can be seen that seven patients have either died or been lost to follow-up before the 12th month; of these six have died and one is censored at 3+ months. This leaves the number of patients at risk of death at the beginning of the 12th month as $24 - 7 = 17$. In the 12th month, however, two die but the remainder, including the censored patient with a survival of 12+ months, survive the month, leaving 15 patients alive, who will die at a later stage. Using equation (2.2), but now expressed in units of a month, we have

$$p_{12} = \frac{\begin{bmatrix} \text{Number} \cdot \text{of} \cdot \text{patients} \cdot \text{who} \cdot \text{are} \cdot \text{followed} \cdot \text{for} \cdot 11 \cdot \text{months} \\ \text{and} \cdot \text{who} \cdot \text{survive} \cdot \text{month} \cdot 12 \end{bmatrix}}{[\text{Number} \cdot \text{of} \cdot \text{patients} \cdot \text{alive} \cdot \text{at} \cdot \text{the} \cdot \text{end} \cdot \text{of} \cdot \text{month} \cdot 11]}$$

$$= \frac{15}{17} = 0.8824.$$

Thus 88% of the patients, who survive month 11, are alive at the end of month 12.

For convenience of presentation, in what follows we will assume time is measured in days but it could be seconds, minutes, hours, months or years, depending on the context.

It is convenient to think of the time, t, as denoting the start of a short time interval ending at time $(t+1)$. We then use n_t as the number of patients alive at the start of the interval and therefore at risk of death during that short interval afterwards. We denote the number of patients dying in the short time interval just after t as d_t. The number of patients surviving the interval is therefore $(n_t - d_t)$. This number in turn becomes the number starting interval $(t+1)$, which we denote by n_{t+1}. This notation enables us to write equation (2.2) as

$$p_t = \frac{(n_t - d_t)}{n_t} \tag{2.3}$$

or,

$$p_t = 1 - \frac{d_t}{n_t}. \tag{2.4}$$

It follows from equation (2.4) that $p_t = 1$ at times (days) when nobody dies, as $d_t = 0$, since the number at risk of death at the beginning of that day is the same as the number at risk at the end of that day.

Thus the value of $S(t)$, the overall probability of survival to time t, changes only at times (days) on which at least one person dies. As a consequence, we can skip over the times (days) when there are no deaths when calculating equation (2.1).

We can rewrite equation (2.1) by using equation (2.4) as

$$S(t) = \left(1 - \frac{d_1}{n_1}\right)\left(1 - \frac{d_2}{n_2}\right) \cdots \left(1 - \frac{d_t}{n_t}\right)$$

or more briefly as

$$S(t) = \prod_t \left(1 - \frac{d_t}{n_t}\right), \tag{2.5}$$

where $\prod_t$ denotes the product of all the terms following this symbol, up to and including that of time t.

The successive overall probabilities of survival, $S(1)$, $S(2), \ldots, S(t)$, are known as the Kaplan-Meier (K-M) or product-limit estimates of survival.

It is useful to note from equation (2.1) that $S(t) = S(t-1) \times p_t$, or

$$S(t) = S(t-1) \left(1 - \frac{d_t}{n_t} \right). \tag{2.6}$$

This result enables each successive survival probability to be obtained by successive multiplication by equation (2.4). It is necessary to specify that when $t = 0$, $S(0) = 1$, that is, all patients are assumed alive at time zero.

Example *– calculating the Kaplan-Meier (K-M) survival curve – patients with colorectal cancer*

The calculations necessary to obtain the K-M estimate of the survival curve with the data from the Dukes' C colorectal cancer patients of McIllmurray and Turkie (1987) are summarised in Table 2.2. We note that in this example survival time is being measured in months.

The patient survival times are first ranked, as we have indicated earlier, in terms of increasing survival. These are listed in the first column of the table. The number of patients at risk at the start, $t = 0$, is $n_0 = 24$. As time progresses, no deaths or patient losses occur until month three, when a censored value is observed, that is $T_{(1)}^+ = 3+$. As a consequence, in the next month we are not able to observe the progress of this particular patient. This leaves $n_4 = n_0 - 1 = 23$ patients potentially at risk in the following (fourth) month.

Prior to this time the number 'at risk' does not change and $n_1 = n_2 = n_3$ all equal n_0, the number of patients at risk at commencement, since the number of deaths and losses is zero. As a consequence $p_1 = p_2 = p_3 = 1$ for these months. In the months that follow $n_4 = n_5 = n_6 = 23$ remain the same, but in the sixth month the first death occurs and there are four deaths in total that month, so that $d_6 = 4$. Thus although $p_4 = p_5 = 1$, we have

$$p_6 = 1 - \frac{d_6}{n_6} = 1 - \frac{4}{23} = 0.8261,$$

and by use of equation (2.5) we have therefore

$$S(6) = p_1 p_2 p_3 p_4 p_5 p_6 = 1 \times 1 \times 1 \times 1 \times 1 \times 0.8261 = 0.8261.$$

Following these deaths at six months, $n_7 = n_6 - d_6 = 23 - 4 = 19$ and $n_8 = 19$ also. There are then two deaths in month eight, giving $d_8 = 2$. Hence, while $p_7 = 1$, since there are no deaths in month seven, $p_8 = 1 - (2/19) = 0.8947$. From these we obtain

$$S(8) = p_1 p_2 p_3 p_4 p_5 p_6 p_7 p_8$$

$$= S(6) \times p_7 p_8$$

$$= 0.8261 \times 1 \times 0.8947$$

$$= 0.7391$$

In a similar way

$$S(12) = S(8) \times p_9 p_{10} p_{11} p_{12}$$
$$= 0.7391 \times 1 \times 1 \times 1 \times 0.8824$$
$$= 0.6522$$

and so on.

The completed calculations for $S(t)$ are summarised in the last column of Table 2.2. It is worth noting that the estimate of survival beyond 42 months is zero from these data as no patient has lived (so far) beyond that time.

In contrast to the calculations of survival at a fixed time-point and by the reduced sample estimate, all available information, including that from those individuals with censored survival times, is included in the K-M estimate. For this reason the K-M estimate of survival is the one that should always be used.

2.3   THE SURVIVAL CURVE

GRAPHICAL DISPLAY

The graph of $S(t)$ against the number of days, t, gives the K-M estimate of the survival curve and provides a useful summary of the data. $S(t)$ will start from 1 (100% of patients alive) since $S(0) = 1$, and progressively decline towards 0 (all patients have died) with time. It is plotted as a step function, since the estimated survival curve remains at a plateau between successive patient death times. It drops instantaneously at each time of death to a new level. The graph will only reach 0 if the patient with the longest observed survival time has in fact died. Were such a patient still alive then the K-M curve would have a plateau commencing at the time of the last death and continuing until the censored survival time of this longest surviving patient.

Example – K-M survival curve – patients with colorectal cancer

The resulting survival curve from the calculations of Table 2.2 is shown in Figure 2.4. This curve starts at one and continues horizontally until the first (four) deaths at six months; at this time it then drops to 0.8261 and then again continues horizontally once more. Subsequently two deaths occur at month eight and so the curve drops to 0.7391 then continues horizontally until the next death. The longest (known) survival time is for a patient who in fact died at 42 months, which is longer than any censored survival time. The K-M estimate is therefore zero at, and beyond, that time.

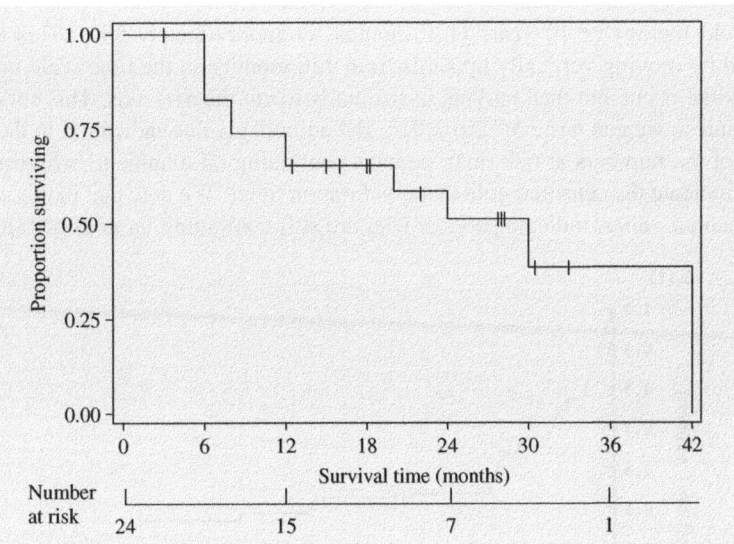

Figure 2.4 Kaplan-Meier estimate of the survival curve of 24 patients with Dukes' C colorectal cancer (From McIllmurray and Turkie, 1987. Reproduced by permission of *British Medical Journal*, **294**, 1260 and **295**, 475. Published by BMJ Publishing Group)

We have indicated the number of patients remaining at risk as time passes under the curve at convenient (annual) time points. This information is crucial for a sensible interpretation of any survival curve. Also marked are the censored survival times, with bold vertical lines cutting the curve. Marking censored survival times on the curve in this way can be informative, but it is sometimes omitted because this makes the graphics more complex, cluttered and difficult to read, especially when there are a large number of censored observations.

It is clear from the vertical lines that if, after a further period of observation of these patients, a death is observed amongst the (so far) censored observations, then the shape of the *K-M* curve (to the right of that point) could be substantially affected. Thus any new follow-up information on the patients with censored survival times could influence the interpretation of this study, perhaps in a substantial way. This is because there is a large proportion censored, and many with less than 24 months of follow-up which is an important time-point in this disease.

Example – K-M duration of therapy curve – patients with rheumatoid arthritis

Samanta, Roy and Woods (1991) reported on the duration of intramuscular gold therapy in 78 patients with rheumatoid arthritis. They calculated the Kaplan-Meier 'survival' curve which is shown in Figure 2.5.

For these patients the initial event is the start of gold therapy for their rheumatoid arthritis and the outcome event (endpoint) is cessation of this therapy for whatever reason. From the survival curve the authors estimate that the proportion continuing with gold therapy at 10 years (120 months) is approximately 50%. This can be verified by moving vertically upwards from 120 months on the time scale until the *K-M* curve is cut and then moving horizontally to cut the *S*(*t*) axis. This cut occurs at 0.5 and so we can write *S*(120) = 0.5. The authors give no indication in their text figure of the numbers at risk (here patients continuing on treatment) with time and do not indicate the censored gold therapy duration times. We note that in this context the censored values indicate patients who are still continuing on gold therapy.

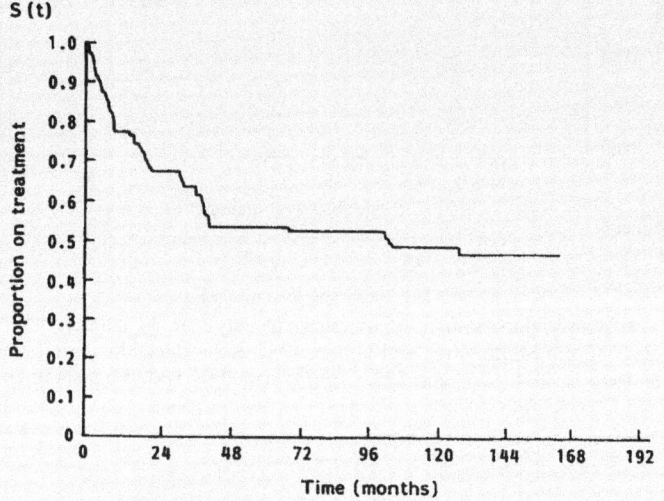

Figure 2.5 Time on intramuscular gold therapy for 78 patients with rheumatoid arthritis (Reprinted from *The Lancet*, **338**, Samanta, Roy and Woods, Gold therapy in rheumatoid arthritis, 642, © 1991, with permission from Elsevier)

In certain circumstances a graph of [1 − *S*(*t*)], rather than *S*(*t*), is plotted against *t* to give the cumulative death curve. Such a plot can be seen from the *S*(*t*) plot by first turning the page over and holding the upside-down page to the light. This method of plotting is sometimes chosen if the outcome event is relatively rare or is of benefit to the patient. Thus the healing of an ulcer, achieving a pregnancy if you are being treated for infertility, and discharge (fit) from hospital are all examples of successful outcomes. This plot has the advantage of starting from 0 on the vertical axis and so is easier to scale for presentation purposes if the maximum value attained for [1 − *S*(*t*)] is much smaller than one.

Example – cumulative healing rates – patients with venous ulceration

Moffatt, Franks, Oldroyd, *et al.* (1992) calculated the Kaplan-Meier cumulative rates, 1 − *S*(*t*), of healing of limbs with venous ulceration for different groups of patients. The solid line in Figure 2.6 shows the cumulative healing rate for those

349 patients whose ulcers have areas of less than 10 cm^2 at presentation. Approximately 50% of these ulcers have healed by 7 weeks. The authors quote the numbers of patients observed up to and including 12 and 24 weeks in parentheses, and so the remaining numbers at risk of 72 and 37 can be calculated for this group. Those patients with large ulcers (>10 cm^2), denoted by the hatched line, appear to heal more slowly, as one might expect.

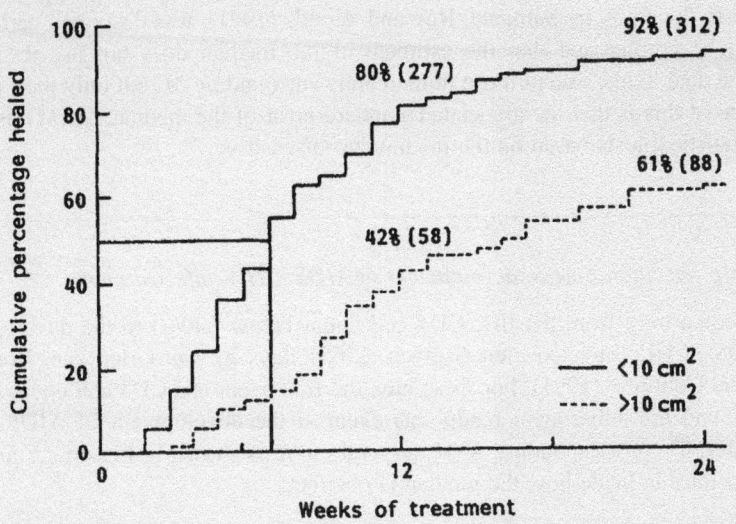

Figure 2.6   Cumulative rate of healing of limbs with venous ulceration of area less than or greater than 10 cm^2 (after Moffatt, Franks, Oldroyd, et al., 1992)

Although it is desirable to indicate the censored observations, in situations such as Figure 2.6, presenting these in an uncluttered way when there are many censored observations is not easy.

MEDIAN SURVIVAL TIME

If there are no censored observations, for example all the patients have died on a clinical trial, then the median survival time, M, is estimated by the middle observation of the ranked survival times, $t_{(1)}, t_{(2)}, \ldots, t_{(n)}$ if the number of observations, n, is odd, and by the average of $t_{(n/2)}$ and $t_{(n/2+1)}$ if n is even, that is

$$M = t_{([n+1]/2)} \text{ if } n \text{ is odd}$$

$$= 1/2[t_{(n/2)} + t_{(n/2+1)}] \text{ if } n \text{ is even} \qquad (2.7)$$

In the presence of censored survival times the median survival is estimated by first calculating the Kaplan-Meier survival curve, then finding the value of M that satisfies the equation

$$S(M) = 0.5. \tag{2.8}$$

This can be done by extending a horizontal line from $S(t) = 0.5$ (or 50%) on the vertical axis of the $K\text{-}M$ survival curve, until the actual curve is met, then moving vertically down from that point to cut the horizontal time axis at M, the median survival time.

A parallel calculation, to estimate the proportion continuing on gold therapy at 120 months or 10 years in the study by Samanta, Roy and Woods (1991), was described earlier.

It should be emphasised that the estimate of the median does not use the individual values of the data items, except those immediately surrounding M, but only their ranks. One consequence of this is that the associated standard error of the median, $SE(M)$, is large and therefore statistical tests based on the median are insensitive.

Example – *median time to development of AIDS – HIV infected men*

The median time from the first CD4 cell count below 200/μl to the development of AIDS in HIV-infected men is given as 651 days by van Griensven, Boucher, Ross and Coutinho (1991). For these men the first event is a CD4 cell count below 200/μl and the subsequent (endpoint) event is the development of AIDS some time later. The corresponding $K\text{-}M$ survival curve is shown in Figure 2.7 and the hatched lines indicate how the median is obtained.

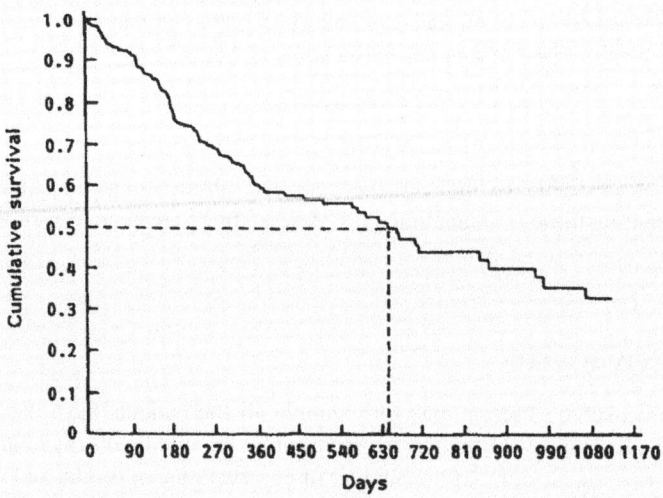

Figure 2.7 Probability of freedom from AIDS (expressed as survival) among 161 homosexual men with CD4 count below 200/μl (Reprinted from *The Lancet*, **338**, van Griensven *et al.*, Expansion of AIDS case definition, 1012–1013, © 1991, with permission from Elsevier)

Example – median infusion time – patients from a general surgical unit

Khawaja, Campbell and Weaver (1988) estimate the median survival-time of the
infusion as 127 hours in 170 patients from a general surgical unit randomised to
receive transdermal glyceryl trinitrate. The object of the therapy was to increase the
length of time of the infusion. In contrast, the median survival-time of the infusion
in the 170 patients randomised to a placebo infusion was only 74 hours.

In a similar way the median survival time of the patients with Dukes' C colorectal cancer
is estimated from Figure 2.4 as 30 months. The seven week median healing time of the
limb ulcers, reported by Moffatt, Franks, Oldroyd, *et al.* (1992), of less than 10 cm^2 at
presentation was indicated earlier. This latter example uses the cumulative estimate of the
death curve, $1 - S(t)$, but the median is unchanged, since $[1 - S(t)] = 0.5$ at the same time
point as $S(t) = 0.5$. The median healing of those ulcers >10 cm^2 is approximately 20 weeks.

INTERPRETATION OF THE SURVIVAL CURVE

The Kaplan-Meier estimate of the survival curve is the best description of times to death of
a group of patients using all the data currently available. If all the patients have died before
the data are analysed the estimate is exactly the same as the proportion of survivors plotted
against time. In this case the proportions are plotted at each death time and the size of the
downward part of the step will be $1/n_0$ at every death time, where n_0 is the initial number
of patients under observation, unless there are tied observations when two or more patients
die with the same survival time. In this circumstance the step down will be that multiple of
$1/n_0$. Each step starts at each successive death time and the process continues until the final
death, which will have the longest survival time.

The overall survival curve is much more reliable than the individually observed conditional
survival probabilities, p_t, of which it is composed. Nevertheless spurious (large) jumps or
(long) flat sections may sometimes appear. These are most likely to occur if the proportion
of censored observations is large and in areas in the extreme right of the curve when the
number of patients still alive and being followed up may be relatively small.

*Example – features of K-M survival curve – time to development of AIDS in HIV
infected men*

In the data of van Griensven, Boucher, Roos and Coutinho (1991), describing the
probability of remaining free of AIDS after the first CD4 count below 200/μl, there
is a section beyond 720 days in Figure 2.7 when the steps are deeper than in other
sections of the curve. There is also a suggestion of some levelling off (plateauing)
beyond this time, with relatively long gaps between successive events.

Both of these features may be spurious as there is very little information in
this part of the curve. Thus the suggestion of the beginnings of a plateau may be

explained by the relatively few subjects still on follow-up and so far without AIDS at and beyond two years and the rather larger steps here may result from a single patient developing AIDS at this stage, amongst the few that have been followed to that time.

Other spurious features can also occur, thus the apparent rapid drop close to 180 days (six months) may not be that the rate of development of AIDS is faster around this period of time but is more likely to be a feature of prearranged clinic visits. Thus if individuals are being tested for AIDS at a prearranged six month visit, and are then found to have AIDS on examination, it is the clinic visit date that is recorded as the date of (proven) onset of AIDS. However, the true onset of the, as yet, undetected AIDS is likely to have occurred at an earlier date.

As indicated earlier, a guide to the reliability of different portions of the survival curve can be obtained by recording the number of patients at risk at various stages beneath the time axis of the survival curve, as we illustrated in Figure 2.4. The 'number at risk' is defined as the number of patients who are known to be alive at that time-point and therefore have not yet died nor been censored before the time-point. At time zero, which is the time of entry of patients into the study, all patients are at risk and hence the number 'at risk' recorded beneath $t = 0$ is n_0, the number of patients entered into the study. The patient numbers obviously diminish as time elapses, both because of deaths and censoring, and thereby their number also indicates the diminishing reliability of the K-M estimate of $S(t)$ with increasing t.

It is difficult to judge precisely when the right-hand tail of the survival curve becomes unreliable. However, as a rule of thumb, the curve can be particularly unreliable when the number of patients remaining at risk is less than 15. The width of the CIs (see Section 2.4), calculated at these and other time-points, will help to decide this in a particular circumstance. Nevertheless, it is not uncommon to see the value of $S(t)$, corresponding to the final plateau, being quoted for example for patients with cancer as the 'cure' rate—especially if the plateau is long. This can be seriously misleading as the rate will almost certainly be reduced with further patient follow-up. We discuss the topic of 'cure models' in Chapter 10.

FOLLOW-UP MATURITY

In any study with a survival-type endpoint there will usually be a mixture of subjects in which the critical event has been observed and those in which it has not. As a consequence it is often useful to have a measure which will help to give a brief summary of the maturity of the data being analysed. Mature data are those in which most of the events that can be anticipated have been observed. The numbers at risk at various stages along the K-M survival curve and an indication of the censored data on these curves do fulfil this purpose to some extent (see for example Figure 2.4), and the addition of the SEs at specific time-points may give further clarity. However, these do not give a concise means of assessing follow-up maturity. Simple summaries, which have been suggested for this purpose, include the median follow-up time of those individuals still alive, together with the minimum and maximum follow-up times of these individuals.

Example – follow-up maturity – patients with colorectal cancer

In Table 2.2 there are 12 surviving from the 24 patients with Dukes' C colorectal cancer of McIllmurray and Turkie (1987), with corresponding ordered censored survival times of 3+, 12+, 15+, 16+, 18+, 18+, 22+, 28+, 28+, 28+, 30+ and 33+ months. Thus 50% of the potential events have not yet been observed and follow-up in seven patients is less than 24 months, which suggests that these data were not really mature enough for reliable reporting of outcome. The minimum follow-up of those still alive is three months, the median follow-up is $(18 + 22)/2 = 20$ months and the maximum follow-up is 33 months. The median rather than mean follow-up time is chosen since, as already indicated, the distributions of survival time data are usually skewed.

A more complete graphical method has been suggested in which follow-up information on all patients, both dead and alive, is used. The first step is to construct a Kaplan-Meier 'follow-up' curve. To do this, we label those patients who have 'died' as actually being 'censored' on their date of death, and those patients who are still alive as having an 'event' on the date they were censored. That is, we reverse the censoring. The reason for this is that since our principal attention is now on a different 'endpoint', that of follow-up, those patients who have died could theoretically have provided more follow-up, while those who have actually been censored have reached the end of their follow-up (as far as the current data set is concerned). The estimated median follow-up can be read off the curves in the same way as the median survival.

Example – K-M estimate of follow-up maturity – patients with colorectal cancer

The Kaplan-Meier follow-up curve for the 24 patients with colorectal cancer is shown in Figure 2.8. From this we obtain the median follow-up as 28 months, which contrasts with the 20 months given earlier using the alive patients only.

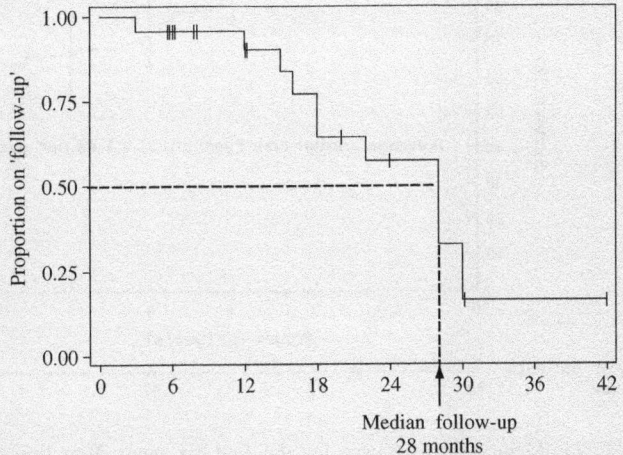

Figure 2.8   The Kaplan-Meier 'follow-up curve' for patients with Dukes' C colorectal cancer

We should point out, however, that such an approach, and indeed the whole concept of measuring median follow-up by whatever method, has been criticised by Shuster (1991), who states: "median follow-up is not a valid or useful scientific term". He gives examples of how it can be misleading, particularly since it can be low with excellent follow-up or high with poor follow-up when recruitment to a study is still ongoing. Nevertheless, although it may have its drawbacks when describing only one group, the graphical method just described may have greater use when comparing two or more groups when recruitment to a study is complete and patients are in the follow-up phase of the study.

2.4   CONFIDENCE INTERVALS

CONFIDENCE INTERVALS FOR $S(t)$

We have indicated earlier that *CI*s calculated at key points along the *K-M* survival curve will give an indication of the reliability of the estimates at those points. These can be calculated for the time-point of interest using the usual format for *CI*s of equation (1.4) by assuming a Normal distribution for the *K-M* estimates, $S(t)$. Thus, the 95% *CI* at time t is

$$S(t) - 1.96 \ SE[S(t)] \text{ to } S(t) + 1.96 SE[S(t)]. \tag{2.9}$$

Example – CI at a fixed time-point – patients with retinal infarction

Hankey, Slattery and Warlow (1991) calculate the *K-M* survival curve of 99 patients following retinal infarction without prior stroke. Their survival curve is shown in Figure 2.9 and illustrates the 95% *CI* calculated at each year. The width of these intervals widens with successive years, reflecting the reduced number of patients at risk as time passes.

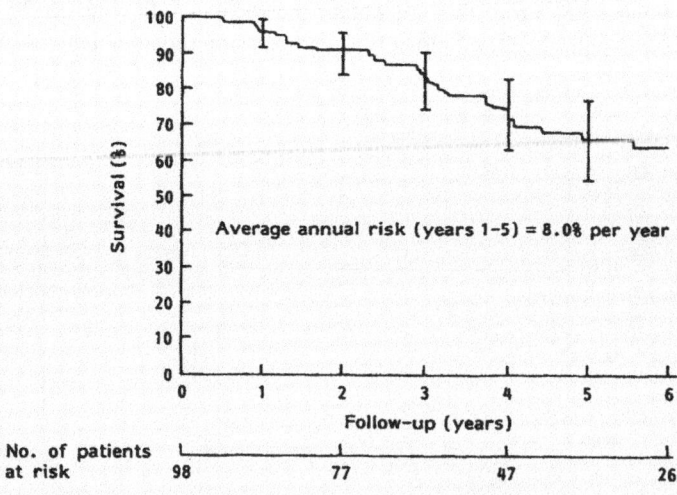

Figure 2.9   Kaplan-Meier survival curve for the first six years after retinal infarction. Bars at each year are 95% confidence intervals (From Hankey, Slattery and Warlow, 1991. Reproduced by permission of *British Medical Journal*, **302**, 499–504.)

Greenwood's method

There are several ways in which an estimate of $SE[S(t)]$ can be obtained and one is that given by M Greenwood (1880–1949), which is

$$SE_{Gr}[S(t)] = S(t) \left(\sum_{j=0}^{t-1} \frac{d_j}{n_j(n_j - d_j)} \right)^{1/2}. \tag{2.10}$$

Here d_j is the number of deaths on day j and n_j is the number of patients alive and on follow-up at the beginning of day j. Just as we noted, prior to equation (2.5) when describing the K-M calculations, equation (2.10) too is only affected on days that at least one death occurs.

***Example** – Greenwood CI at a fixed time-point – patients with colorectal cancer*

To illustrate the calculation of $SE_{Gr}[S(t)]$ and the corresponding 95% *CI* we use the data from the patients with Dukes' C colorectal cancer summarised in Table 2.2. For example, at $t = 12$ months the K-M estimate of the proportion alive is $S(12) = 0.6522$ or 65%, and since there are four deaths at six months and two deaths at eight months prior to this time, we have from equation (2.10) that

$$SE_{Gr}[S(12)] = 0.6522 \left[\frac{4}{23(23-4)} + \frac{2}{19(19-2)} \right]^{1/2}$$

$$= 0.6522 \, (0.009153 + 0.006192)^{1/2}$$

$$= 0.6522 \times 0.12387$$

$$= 0.0808$$

We note here that, although $n_0 = 24$ patients were recruited to this study, one of these is censored at $T^+ = 3+$ months before any death occurs. Consequently the number at risk, before any death, is reduced to $n_0 - 1 = 23$, which is the figure used in the above calculation.

The 95% *CI* for $S(12)$, using the *SE* estimated by $SE_{Gr}[S(12)]$, is therefore from $0.6522 - 1.96 \times 0.0808 = 0.4938$ to $0.6522 + 1.96 \times 0.0808 = 0.8106$. The wide *CI*, of 49% to 81% survival, gives some indication of how little information is available on the survival rate of these patients at this time.

Peto's Method

Greenwood's formula is only accurate for large numbers of subjects alive at the time-point under consideration and so strictly was not very appropriate in our example. In particular, the Greenwood method tends to underestimate the *SE*, especially in the tail of the survival curve, so that its use only provides a guide to the minimum width of the corresponding *CI*.

A more reliable estimate of the SE, and one which is easier to calculate, is given by Peto (1984). This is

$$SE_{Peto}[S(t)] = \left\{ \frac{S(t)[1-S(t)]}{R_t} \right\}^{1/2},$$ (2.11)

where R_t is the number of patients recruited to the trial minus the number censored by the time under consideration. Thus $R_t = n_0 - c_t$, where c_t is the number of patients censored before time t. R_t is sometimes termed the 'effective' sample size.

If there are no censored observations before this time-point then this SE is the same as that for the SE given in Table 1.2. In our context we replace p by $S(t)$, thus $SE = \sqrt{\{S(t)[1-S(t)]/n_0\}}$.

Example – Peto CI at a fixed time-point – patients with colorectal cancer

If we use equation (2.11) in place of equation (2.10) with the data from the colorectal cancer patients we have $R_{12} = 24 - 1 = 23$ and therefore $SE_{Peto}[S(12)] = [0.6522 \times (1-0.6522)/23]^{1/2} = 0.0993$. Here SE_{Peto} is a little larger than that given by the Greenwood (SE_{Gr}). The corresponding 95% CI for $S(12)$ of 0.4575 to 0.8468 or 46% to 85% is therefore a little wider than that of the previous calculation.

It should be emphasised that the CIs just calculated are approximate and have equal width above and below the estimate $S(t)$. The technically 'correct' CIs should only be symmetric about $S(t)$ when $S(t)$ is close to 0.5. However, these approximations will usually be satisfactory provided $S(t)$ is neither close to one or close to 0, that is, near the beginning or end of the K-M curve. In such situations the CI is restricted by, for example, the horizontal time axis as negative values of the lower confidence limit are not possible. Similarly, values within the CI beyond unity (100% survival) are not possible.

Transformation Method

An alternative method, and one we recommend, of calculating a CI is to first transform $S(t)$ onto a scale which more closely follows a Normal distribution. It can be shown that the complementary logarithmic transformation of $S(t)$ or $\log\{-\log[S(t)]\}$ has an approximately Normal distribution, with SE given by

$$SE_{Tr}[S(t)] = \frac{\left[\sum_{j=0}^{t-1} \frac{d_j}{n_j(n_j - d_j)} \right]^{1/2}}{\left[-\sum_{j=0}^{t-1} \log\left(\frac{n_j - d_j}{n_j} \right) \right]}.$$ (2.12)

Use of equation (2.9) then gives, on this transformed scale, a 95% CI of

$$\log\{-\log[S(t)]\} - 1.96 SE_{Tr} \text{ to } \log\{-\log[S(t)]\} + 1.96 SE_{Tr}$$ (2.13)

To return to the untransformed scale we have to antilog the lower and upper values of this *CI* given by equation (2.13), take the negative of these and then antilog again. The result of this quite involved process is summarised by

$$S(t)^{\exp(+1.96SE_{Tr})} \text{ to } S(t)^{\exp(-1.96SE_{Tr})}. \tag{2.14}$$

Note that the signs attached to 1.96 in equation (2.14) are correct.

Since $S(t)$ is confined to values between 0 and 1, and since further $\exp(+1.96SE_{Tr})$ and $\exp(-1.96SE_{Tr})$ are both larger than 0, the *CI* of equation (2.14) will then always be in the range of 0 and 1 also. This is an important advantage of the transformation method.

Example – *transformation method CI at a fixed time-point – patients with colorectal cancer*

Repeating the earlier example for $S(12) = 0.6522$, we have from equation (2.12), that

$$SE = \sqrt{\left[\frac{4}{23(23-4)} + \frac{2}{19(19-2)}\right] / \left[-\log\left(\frac{23-4}{23}\right) - \log\left(\frac{19-2}{19}\right)\right]}$$

$$= \sqrt{[(0.014345)/(+0.191055 + 0.111226)]}$$

$$= 0.4098.$$

From this $\exp(+1.96SE_{Tr}) = 2.2327$, $\exp(-1.96SE_{Tr}) = 0.4479$ and finally the 95% *CI* is $S(t)^{2.2327} = 0.3851$ to $S(t)^{0.4479} = 0.8258$ or 39% to 83%

This *CI* is not symmetric around $S(12) = 0.6522$ (65%) and is wider than that for all the methods presented earlier.

However, all but the Peto method are computationally complex and really require appropriate statistical software for their implementation.

CONFIDENCE INTERVAL FOR A MEDIAN

The calculations required for the *CI* of a median are quite complicated and an explanation of how these are derived is complex. Collett (2003) gives a clear description of the technical aspects. He gives an expression for the *SE* of the median as:

$$SE_{Median} = SE_{Gr}[S(M)]\{(t_{Small} - t_{Large}) / [S(t_{Large}) - S(t_{Small})]\} \tag{2.15}$$

where t_{Small} is the smallest observed survival time from the *K-M* curve for which $S(t)$ is less than or equal to 0.45, while t_{Large} is the largest observed survival time from the *K-M* curve for which $S(t)$ is greater than 0.55.

The expression for the 95% *CI* is

$$M - 1.96SE_{Median} \quad to \quad M + 1.96SE_{Median} \tag{2.16}$$

Example – *CI for the median survival time – Dukes' C colorectal cancers*

If we use the *K-M* estimate of the survival time of patients with Dukes' colorectal cancer then, from Figure 2.4, the median $M = 30$ months approximately. Reading from Table 2.2 at $S(t)$ less than 0.45 gives $t_{Small} = 30$ months also and for $S(t)$ greater than 0.55 we have $t_{Large} = 20$ months.

We then need an estimate of the *SE* of $S(t)$ which is

$$SE_{Gr}[S(30)] = 0.5 \left[\frac{4}{23(23-4)} + \frac{2}{19(19-2)} + \frac{2}{17(17-2)} + \frac{1}{10(10-1)} \right.$$
$$\left. + \frac{1}{8(8-1)} \right]^{1/2}$$
$$= 0.5(0.009153 + 0.006192 + 0.007843 + 0.011111 + 0.017857)^{1/2}$$
$$= 0.5 \times 0.228377 = 0.114188.$$

Therefore

$$SE_{Median} = 0.114188 \times [(30-20)/(0.5780-0.3852)]$$
$$= 0.114188 \times 51.8672 = 5.92.$$

The corresponding 95% *CI* is $30 - (1.96 \times 5.92) = 18.40$ to $30 + (1.96 \times 5.92) = 41.60$ months or approximately 18 to 42 months.

However, we must caution against the uncritical use of this method for such small data sets, since as we have indicated before the value of SE_{Gr} is unreliable in such circumstances, and also the values of t_{Small} and t_{Large} will be poorly determined.

Example – *CI for median survival time – development of AIDS*

As indicated in Figure 2.7 the median time in the development of AIDS given by van Griensven, Boucher, Roos and Coutinho (1991) in their study was 651 days (21 months) with a 95% *CI* of 429 to 865 days or 14 to 32 months. So even in a study involving 161 individuals, this leaves considerable uncertainty with respect to the median's true value.

2.5   THE HAZARD RATE

In many situations it is important to know how the risk of a particular outcome changes with time. For example, it is well known that infant mortality is highest in the few days following birth and thereafter declines very rapidly. Similarly, there is usually additional (short-term) risk following some medical procedures.

Example – risk changing with time – pelvic inflammatory disease

Farley, Rosenberg, Rowe *et al.* (1992) show how the risk of pelvic inflammatory disease (PID) associated with the use of an intrauterine device (IUD) for contraceptive purposes is at its greatest in the immediate post-insertion period. This risk reduced from 9.4 to 1.4 per 1000 woman years after the first 20 days and remained at 1.4 per 1000 for up to eight years. Their PID incidence rates are shown in Figure 2.10.

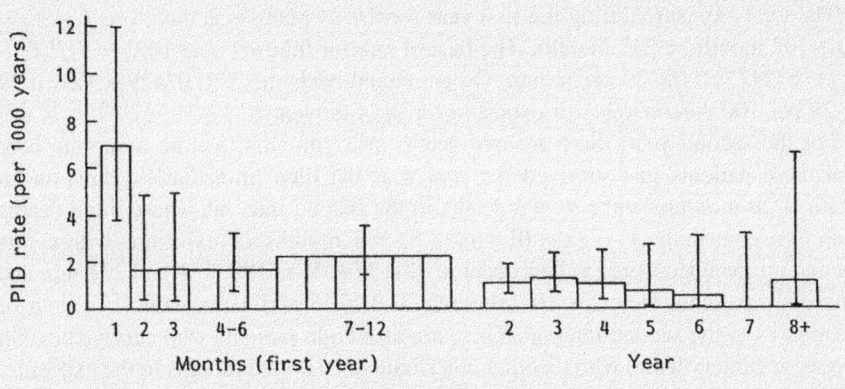

Figure 2.10   PID incidence and 95% confidence intervals by time since insertion of an IUD (Reprinted from *The Lancet*, **339**, Farley, Rosenberg, Rowe, *et al.*, Intrauterine devices and pelvic inflammatory disease: an international perspective, 785–788, © 1992, with permission from Elsevier)

The risk or hazard rate, λ, can be estimated, within specific time intervals, by dividing the total period of survival into time segments, counting the number of events arising in the segment and dividing by the number of patients at risk during that segment. When the unit of time is a day, it is the probability of the event occurring within the (next) day, given that you have survived to the beginning of that day. In a survival time context the hazard rate can be interpreted as the risk of dying on that particular day. In this framework, if the time segment is short, it is sometimes referred to as the instantaneous death rate.

Example – risk changing with time – patients with colorectal cancer

We illustrate the idea of the (annual) hazard rate using the data of Table 2.2. We first calculate the total months of exposure for all patients during the first year.

Six patients (d_1) died during the first year: four at six months and two at eight months. We define their total exposure during the first year as f_1, where

$$f_1 = (4 \text{ patients} \times 6 \text{ months}) + (2 \text{ patients} \times 8 \text{ months})$$

$$= 40 \text{ months of exposure.}$$

Of the patients alive, one was censored at three months while 17 survive the 12 months. The exposure time contributed by these 18 patients is F_1, where

$$F_1 = (1 \times 3) + (17 \times 12)$$

$$= 207 \text{ months of exposure.}$$

The total exposure during the first year for the 24 patients is therefore $f_1 + F_1 = 40 + 207$ months $= 247$ months. The hazard rate for the first year is $\lambda_1 = d_1/(f_1 + F_1) = 6/247 = 0.02429$ per month. On an annual basis this is $0.02429 \times 12 = 0.29$ or 29 per 100 person years of exposure for the first year.

For the second year, there are two deaths at 12 months (we are assuming here that these patients just survived the first year but died immediately after) and a death at 20 months, hence $d_2 = 3$ deaths in the second interval. These three deaths therefore contribute $f_2 = (2 \times 0) + (1 \times 8) = 8$ months of exposure within this second interval. Censored values occur at 12+, 15+, 16+, 18+, 18+ and 22+ months. These six patients therefore contribute 0, 3, 4, 6, 6 and 10 months or a total of 29 months to the second interval. There are also eight patients who survive beyond the second interval and who together contribute $8 \times 12 = 96$ months to the exposure. Collectively these 14 patients contribute $F_2 = 29 + 96 = 125$ months of exposure within the second interval. The total exposure is therefore, $f_2 + F_2 = 8 + 125 = 133$ months, and the hazard is $\lambda_2 = d_2/(f_2 + F_2) = 3/133 = 0.02256$ per month. On an annual basis this is 0.23 or 23 per 100 person years for the second year.

Similar calculations give $\lambda_3 = 2/33 = 0.06061$ and $\lambda_4 = 1/6 = 0.16667$ per month or 73 and 200 per 100 person years, for the third and fourth years, respectively.

In this example, the values we obtain for λ_1 and λ_2 depend rather critically on how we deal with the deaths at the boundaries of the intervals. Such problems only arise if there are several tied events at the boundaries. In the above example, two deaths at 12 months occur at the break of the interval. If we ascribe these deaths to the first interval then $\lambda_1 = d_1/(f_1 + F_1) = 8/247 = 0.03239$ per month. On an annual basis this is 0.39 or 39 per 100 person years for the first year. These two deaths will not of course now occur in the second interval but the death at 24 months is now counted in the interval. Consequently, $d_2 = 2$ and $\lambda_2 = d_2/(f_2 + F_2) = 2/133 = 0.01504$ per month. On an annual basis this is 0.18 or 18 per 100 person years.

With such a small data set we should not be too surprised at the above changes. They do emphasise, however, that survival time is best recorded in small time units so that events can then be assigned to the appropriate interval without ambiguity.

The above hazards of 29, 23, 73 and 200 per 100 person years are sometimes expressed as 29%, 24%, 73% and 200% respectively, although they are strictly not percentages.

Example – daily hazard – patients with small cell lung cancer

Stephens, Girling and Machin (1994) calculated the daily hazard obtained from data on more than 2000 patients with small cell lung cancer. These data are shown in Figure 2.11 and show that except for a period between eight and 14 days from start of treatment the daily hazard appears to be approximately constant. Outside of this time period there appear to be random fluctuations, which are to be expected because the one-day unit of time is small. The authors suggest that the increased hazard rates during the eight to 14 day period may be due to a treatment-induced mortality.

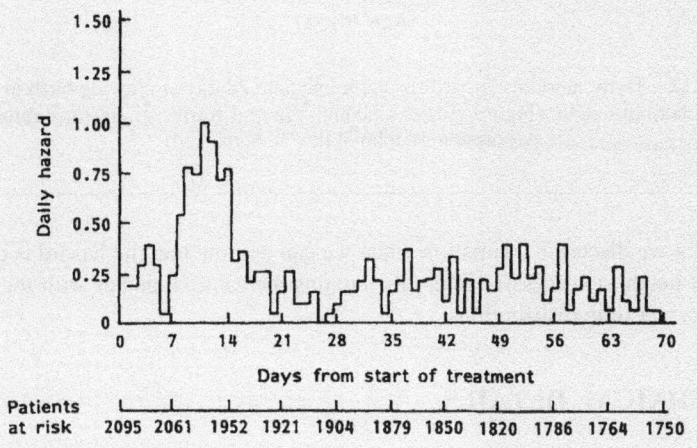

Figure 2.11   Estimated daily hazard from start of treatment in patients with small cell lung cancer (after Stephens, Girling and Machin, 1994)

Example – daily risk of death – first 28 days after birth

In a study that involved about 1.3 million live births and 2000 neonatal deaths, Cheung, Yip and Karlberg (2001a) investigated the risk of death in the first 28 days of life in relation to size at birth and gestational duration. For instance, among full term babies with a normal body length, the daily hazard was about 0.00024 in the first day, which sharply declined to a stable level of about 0.000002 from day seven to day 28. These values provide the step function plotted in Figure 2.12. The smoothed hazard curve shown is based on a parametric model (see Chapter 4) for the daily hazards.

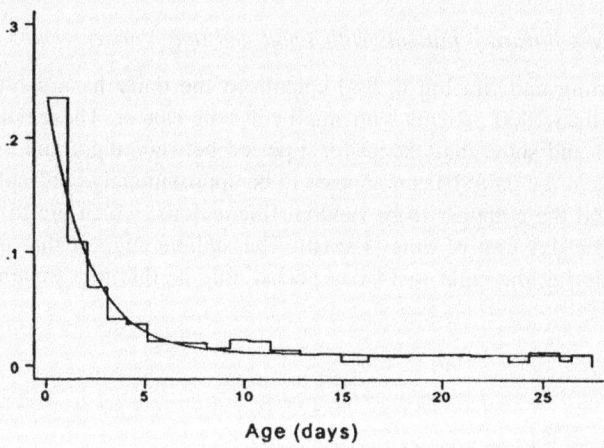

Figure 2.12 Daily mortality hazard for the immediate 28 days following birth in full term babies of normal length. (Figure 1(d) of Cheung, Yip and Karlberg, 2001a. Reproduced by permission of John Wiley & Sons, Ltd)

In Chapter 4 we discuss the situation when we can assume that the hazard is constant, that is, the rate of death in successive intervals remains the same, together with the Exponential and other survival time distributions.

2.6 TECHNICAL DETAILS

It is convenient to think of the survival times in a particular context of having a distribution. In Figure 2.13 we sketch the form that this might take. We can then interpret $S(t)$, for any given time t, as the proportion of the total area under the curve, to the right of t. The total area under the curve is unity. The height of the distribution at a particular time, denoted $\phi(t)$, is known as the probability density function. We introduced in Section 2.5 the hazard rate, λ, which in some circumstances may vary with time. In these cases we denote it by $\lambda(t)$. There are mathematical relationships between $S(t)$, $\phi(t)$ and $\lambda(t)$.

The distributional form of survival times may be presented by either the survivor function (previously called the survival curve) $S(t)$, the hazard function $\lambda(t)$, or the probability density function $\phi(t)$.

The probability density function is the probability of a death occurring at time t which is contained in a very small time interval between τ and $\tau + \Delta\tau$. That is

$$\phi(t) = \lim_{\Delta\tau \to 0} \left\{ \frac{\text{Prob}[\text{death} \cdot \text{in} \cdot \text{interval}(\tau, \tau + \Delta\tau)]}{\Delta\tau} \right\} \qquad (2.17)$$

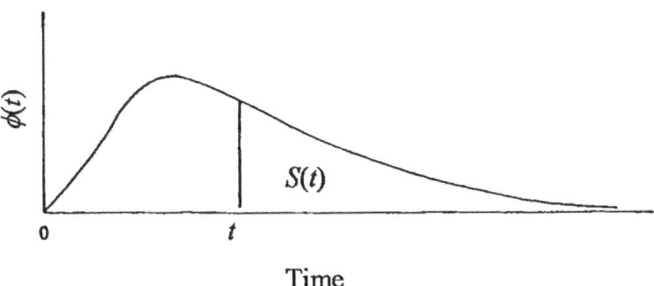

Figure 2.13 A typical distribution of survival times

The survival function, $S(t)$ = Prob(individual survives longer than time t). This is the probability of surviving at least as long as t, which is one minus the integral of $\phi(t)$ up to time t, that is

$$S(t) = 1 - \int_0^t \phi(u)\mathrm{d}u = 1 - \Phi(t). \tag{2.18}$$

Finally, the hazard function is the instantaneous failure rate at t, which is the probability of dying in the next small interval, having already survived to the beginning of the interval. This is defined as

$$\lambda(t) = \lim_{\Delta\tau \to 0} \left\{ \frac{\mathrm{Prob}[\tau < t < \tau + \Delta\tau | \tau \le t]}{\Delta\tau} \right\}. \tag{2.19}$$

The hazard and survival functions can be expressed in terms of each other, since

$$\phi(t) = \frac{d}{dt}[1 - S(t)]$$

and

$$\lambda(t) = \frac{\phi(t)}{S(t)} = -\frac{d}{dt}[\log S(t)]. \tag{2.20}$$

The hazard, survival and probability density functions are therefore alternative forms of describing the distribution of survival times. The survival function is most useful for comparing the survival progress of two or more patient groups. The hazard function, since it is an instantaneous measure, gives a more useful graphical description of the risk of failure at any time-point t. It is not necessarily always increasing or decreasing.

3 Comparison of Survival Curves

Summary

This chapter describes the Logrank test to compare Kaplan-Meier (K-M) survival curves. The hazard ratio (HR) is introduced as a useful single measure for summarising the differences between two survival curves. Methods of calculation of confidence intervals for the HR are described. The Logrank test is extended to a stratified analysis in which, for example, the influence of a prognostic variable is taken into account, and to the comparison of three or more groups. For situations where there is a natural ordering of the groups a test for trend is described. The particular situation of a factorial design structure for the groups is included. The Mantel-Haenszel alternative to the Logrank test for a three-group comparison is also described.

3.1 INTRODUCTION

In Chapter 2, we described how the Kaplan-Meier (K-M) estimate of a single survival curve is obtained. However, in many applications, there will often be several survival curves to compare. Thus we may wish to compare the survival experiences of patients who receive different treatments for their disease, or compare the discontinuation rates in women using one of two types of intrauterine device for fertility control. In such circumstances, for two groups we require a procedure analogous to that of the Student's t-test for normally distributed data. Before we describe the methods available to compare two survival curves, we note that it is inappropriate and usually very misleading to compare survival curves at a particular point of the curve, for example, making comparisons of one year survival rates. The reason for this is that each individual point on the curve is not in itself a good estimate of the true underlying survival. Thus comparing two such point estimates (one from each of the two curves) gives an unreliable comparison of the survival experience of the two groups. Further, it makes very poor use of all the data available by concentrating on particular points of each curve and ignoring the remainder of the survival experience.

3.2 THE LOGRANK TEST

We have given in Chapter 2 several examples of the K-M survival curves. There are many situations, particularly in the context of randomised trials and epidemiological studies, in which we may wish to compare two or more such curves. The Logrank test, also referred to as the Mantel-Cox test, is the most widely used method of comparing two survival curves and can easily be extended to comparisons of three or more curves.

Survival Analysis Second Edition   David Machin, Yin Bun Cheung, Mahesh K.B. Parmar
© 2006 John Wiley & Sons, Ltd   ISBN: 0-470-87040-0

Example – *K-M survival curves by treatment group and the Logrank test* – *patients with chronic heart failure*

The *K-M* estimates of the survival curves for patients with chronic heart failure receiving treatment with either placebo or milrinone reported by Packer, Carver, Rodeheffer *et al.* (1991) are illustrated in Figure 3.1. The numbers of patients at risk, at three monthly intervals, are shown at the bottom of the figure.

The authors report the result of a Logrank test of significance for the comparison of these two groups and from this they conclude that there is a greater death rate amongst patients receiving milrinone. They state: "Mortality was 28% higher in the milrinone group than in the placebo group ($p = 0.038$)".

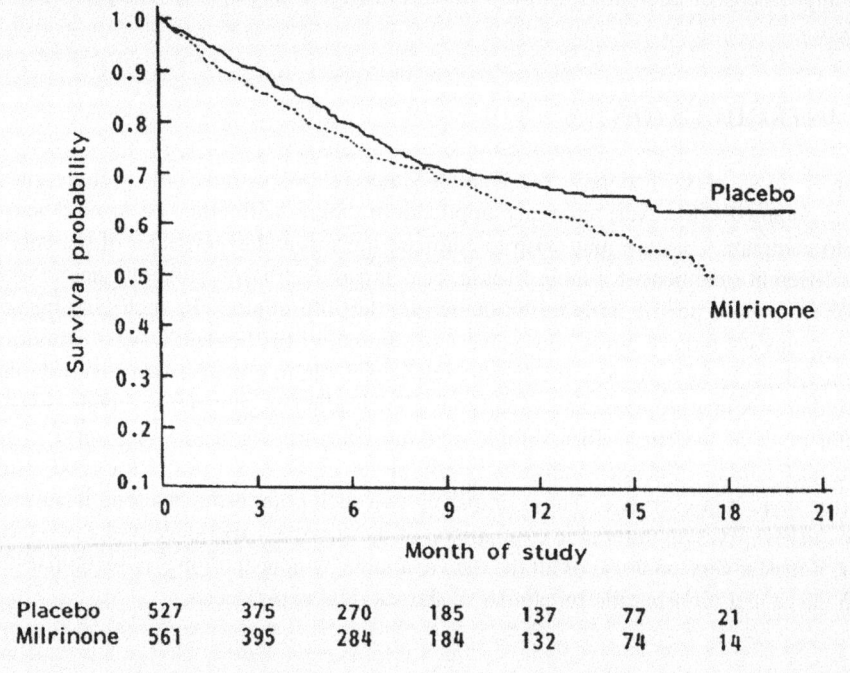

Placebo	527	375	270	185	137	77	21
Milrinone	561	395	284	184	132	74	14

Figure 3.1 Kaplan-Meier analysis showing survival in patients with chronic heart failure treated with milrinone or placebo (From Packer, Carver, Rodeheffer, *et al.*, 1991. Reprinted by permission of *New England Journal of Medicine*, **325**, 1468–75. © 1991 Massachusetts Medical Society. All rights reserved.)

To illustrate the Logrank test, Table 3.1 shows the survival times of 30 patients recruited to a randomised trial of the addition of a radiosensitiser to radiotherapy (New therapy, *B*) versus radiotherapy alone (Control, *A*) in patients with cervical cancer. Of these 30

Table 3.1 Survival by treatment group of 30 patients recruited to a trial in patients with cervical cancer. (Based on data from the Medical Research Council Working Party on Advanced Carcinoma of the Cervix, 1993. Reproduced by permission of *Radiotherapy Oncology*, **26**, 93–103.)

Control *A*			New therapy *B*		
Patient number	Survival time	Survival status	Patient number	Survival time	Survival status
2	1037	DEAD	1	1476+	ALIVE
4	1429	DEAD	3	827	DEAD
5	680	DEAD	7	519+	ALIVE
6	291	DEAD	8	1100+	ALIVE
9	1577+	ALIVE	10	1307	DEAD
11	90	DEAD	12	1360+	ALIVE
14	1090+	ALIVE	13	919+	ALIVE
15	142	DEAD	16	373	DEAD
17	1297	DEAD	18	563+	ALIVE
19	1113+	ALIVE	21	978+	ALIVE
20	1153	DEAD	22	650+	ALIVE
23	150	DEAD	25	362	DEAD
24	837	DEAD	27	383+	ALIVE
26	890+	ALIVE	28	272	DEAD
29	269	DEAD			
30	468+	ALIVE			

patients, 16 received *A* and 14 received *B*. These data are a subset of those obtained from 183 patients entered into a randomised Phase III trial conducted by the Medical Research Council Working Party on Advanced Carcinoma of the Cervix (1993). We refer to the treatments as *A* and *B* for ease and because we do not intend to draw conclusions on the relative effect of the two treatments in such a small subset of the patients.

Now if the two treatments are of equal efficacy, that is, the addition of the radiosensitiser to radiotherapy has no effect, then the corresponding survival curves should only differ because of chance variation. Thus, under the assumption of no difference between the two treatments, we anticipate that the two patient groups will have a similar survival experience. This should be the case, at least approximately, if allocation to treatment is random and the groups are of sufficient size.

We can check for balance between the treatment groups for known factors which are likely to influence prognosis (prognostic factors). For example, the age of the patient may be an important determinant of prognosis and we can check that the two groups have similar age distributions. However, we cannot check balance for unknown prognostic factors. Thus, any observed differences between the two survival curves, and which we would like to ascribe to differences between treatments, may be explained by chance differences due to a maldistribution of unknown prognostic factors.

For the trial in patients with cervical cancer, treatment was allocated at random but as the patient groups selected for the purposes of illustration are very small, with a total of only 30 patients, imbalances of known and unknown prognostic variables in the two groups are quite possible.

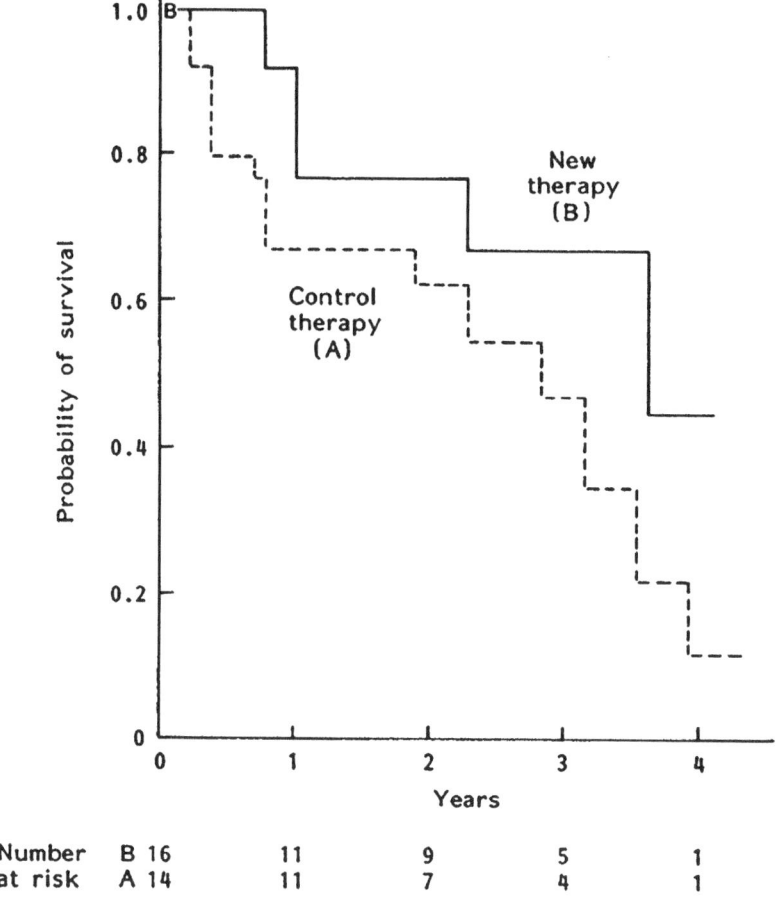

Figure 3.2 Kaplan-Meier survival curves calculated from the data of Table 3.1

The *K-M* survival curves for the groups *A* and *B* of Table 3.1 are shown in Figure 3.2 and appear to be quite different. However, how different do they have to appear to be before we can reliably attribute this difference to a treatment effect? How can we be sure that the difference is not due to an imbalance in known and unknown prognostic factors? How different must they be in order to reject the (null) hypothesis of 'no treatment difference'?

To make a formal comparison of these two survival curves we first rank the survival times of all 30 patients, using the convention already stated in Chapter 2, that if a 'death' and a 'censored' observation have the same numerical value we will allocate the censored time a higher rank. This ranking has been done in two stages: first the survival times are ranked within each treatment group as in Table 3.2 and then, for all data combined, irrespective of treatment, in the first two columns of Table 3.3. The two columns are separated, one for each treatment, only for the sake of clarity. Note that there is a tendency for those on treatment *B* to have a higher ranking and thus experiencing later deaths than those receiving *A*, as would be expected from Figure 3.2.

Table 3.2 Ranked within-treatment survival times of 30 patients recruited to a trial in patients with cervical cancer

	Control A			New therapy B	
Patient number	Survival time (days)	Survival status	Patient number	Survival time (days)	Survival status
11	90	DEAD	28	272	DEAD
15	142	DEAD	25	362	DEAD
23	150	DEAD	16	373	DEAD
29	269	DEAD	27	383+	ALIVE
6	291	DEAD	7	519+	ALIVE
30	468+	ALIVE	18	563+	ALIVE
5	680	DEAD	22	650+	ALIVE
24	837	DEAD	3	827	DEAD
26	890+	ALIVE	13	919+	ALIVE
2	1037	DEAD	21	978+	ALIVE
14	1090+	ALIVE	8	1100+	ALIVE
19	1113+	ALIVE	10	1307	DEAD
20	1153	DEAD	12	1360+	ALIVE
17	1297	DEAD	1	1476+	ALIVE
4	1429	DEAD			
9	1577+	ALIVE			

Before going into full details of how the Logrank test is calculated we illustrate the approach by examining the 2×2 table corresponding to the first death of Table 3.3 which occurred on day 90 to a patient receiving treatment A. This table is reproduced in Table 3.4 together with the notation we shall use to describe the Logrank test procedure.

From Table 3.2 (and Table 3.3) we see for this patient receiving treatment A who died on day 90 following randomisation that just before her death there were 30 patients alive: 16 on treatment A and 14 on treatment B. If we were told of the occurrence of one death at this stage (without knowledge of the particular treatment group in which the death occurred) then, under the null hypothesis of no difference in the treatments, we can calculate the odds of this death for A against B. This will take account of the number of patients known to be receiving A (m_{90}) and B (n_{90}). Thus for the one death at $t = 90$ days, we calculate the odds as m_{90} to n_{90} or 16: 14 and so the expected number of deaths on treatment A is $E_{A,90} = 16/(16 + 14) = 0.533333$ and the expected number of deaths on treatment B is $E_{B,90} = 14/(16 + 14) = 0.466667$. These are given in the top panel of Table 3.4. We discuss the definition and use of V_t in Section 3.3.

This calculation is equivalent to calculating the expected values in a standard 2×2 contingency table at $t = 90$, with $r_{90} = 1$, $m_{90} = 16$ and $N_{90} = 30$, as is indicated in the lower panel of Table 3.4. We then compare the observed number of deaths, $a_t = 1$ and $b_t = 0$, with these expected values. It is a common convention to call $a_t = O_{At}$ and $b_t = O_{Bt}$, respectively. Thus, there are more deaths under A (here $O_{At,90} = 1$ death) than expected (0.533333) but fewer under B (here $O_{Bt,90} = 0$ deaths) than expected (0.466667). If there is only one death at the time, then the expected number of deaths can also be interpreted as the probability of the death occurring in each treatment group.

Table 3.3 Ranked survival times of 30 patients with cervical cancer by treatment group

Patient number	Rank	Survival (days) A	B		Dead	Alive	Total	E_{At}	E_{Bt}	V_t
11	1	90		A	1	15	16			
				B	0	14	14			
					1	29	30	0.533333	0.466667	0.248889
15	2	142		A	1	14	15			
				B	0	14	14			
					1	28	29	0.517241	0.482759	0.249703
23	3	150		A	1	13	14			
				B	0	14	14			
					1	27	28	0.500000	0.500000	0.250000
29	4	269		A	1	12	13			
				B	0	14	14			
					1	26	27	0.481481	0.518519	0.249657
28	5		272	A	0	12	12			
				B	1	13	14			
					1	25	26	0.461538	0.538462	0.248521
22	6	291		A	1	11	12			
				B	0	13	13			
					1	24	25	0.480000	0.520000	0.249600
6	7		362	A	0	11	11			
				B	1	12	13			
					1	23	24	0.458333	0.541667	0.248264
25	8		373	A	0	11	11			
				B	1	11	12			
					1	22	23	0.478261	0.521739	0.249527
27	9		383+							
30	10	468+								
7	11		519+							
18	12		563+							
22	13		650+							
5	14	680		A	1	9	10			
				B	0	7	7			
					1	16	17	0.588235	0.411765	0.242215

3	15		827	A	0	9	9			
				B	1	6	7			
					1	15	16	0.562500	0.437500	0.246094
24	16	837		A	1	8	9			
				B	0	6	6			
					1	14	15	0.600000	0.400000	0.240000
26	17	890+								
13	18		919+							
21	19		978+							
2	20	1037		A	1	6	7			
				B	0	4	4			
					1	10	11	0.636364	0.363363	0.231405
14	21	1090+								
8	22		1100+							
19	23		1113+							
20	24	1153		A	1	3	4			
				B	0	3	3			
					1	6	7	0.571429	0.428571	0.244898
17	25	1297		A	1	2	3			
				B	0	3	3			
					1	5	6	0.500000	0.500000	0.250000
10	26		1307	A	0	2	2			
				B	1	2	3			
					1	4	5	0.400000	0.600000	0.240000
12	27		1360+							
4	28	1429		A	1	1	2			
				B	0	1	1			
					1	2	3	0.666667	0.333333	0.222222
1	29		1476+							
9	30	1577+								
Total				$O_A = 11$ $O_B = 5$ $E_A = 8.435382$ $E_B = 7.564618$ $V = 3.910995$						

This basic calculation is then repeated at each death time. For the second death at $t = 142$, we have $O_{A,142} = 1$ and $O_{B,142} = 0$. However, as with the $K\text{-}M$ estimate, we do not carry forward the patient receiving treatment A who died at $t = 90$, so the odds of death at $t = 142$ are divided in the ratio 15: 14 rather than the 16:14 at $t = 90$. This gives $E_{A,142} = 15/(15 + 14) = 0.517241$ and $E_{B,142} = 14/(15 + 14) = 0.482759$.

Table 3.4 Comparison of observed and expected deaths following the first death of a patient with cervical cancer at 90 days and the general notation used at time t

Treatment	Dead	Alive	Total	$O_{A,90}$	$O_{B,90}$	$E_{A,90}$	$E_{B,90}$	V_{90}
Time $t=90$								
A	1	15	16			—	—	—
B	0	14	14			—	—	—
Total	1	29	30	1	0	0.533333	0.466667	0.248889
Time t						$E_{A,t}$	$E_{B,t}$	V_t
A	a_t	c_t	m_t			—	—	—
B	b_t	d_t	n_t			—	—	—
Total	r_t	s_t	N_t	a_t	b_t	$\dfrac{r_t m_t}{N_t}$	$\dfrac{r_t n_t}{N_t}$	$\dfrac{m_t n_t r_t s_t}{N_t^2(N_t-1)}$

In general the expected number of deaths for A and B at death time t are calculated by

$$E_{At} = r_t m_t / N_t, \ E_{Bt} = r_t n_t / N_t \tag{3.1}$$

as indicated in Table 3.4. This takes into account the situation of tied observations when two or more deaths occur at a particular time t.

The process of calculating the expected values continues for every successive 2×2 table. There is one formed for each distinct time of death, with the margins of the table for either A or B or both decreasing death by death. In addition, if censored observations occur between death times then the respective marginal totals for A (m_t) and/or B (n_t) are reduced and the 2×2 table is formed at the next death with these reduced margins. This process is illustrated by considering the death on treatment B at 373 days: just before this death there are 23 patients still at risk. This death is followed by five censored observations: 168+ for treatment A, and 383+, 519+, 563+ and 650+ for treatment B (see Table 3.3). As a consequence, the next 2×2 table is formed at $t = 680$ and is made up from the 17 patients still at risk: 10 on treatment A and seven on treatment B.

Once these calculations are completed, that is, all deaths have been included, the observed and expected deaths are summed, to give

$$O_A = \Sigma O_{At}, O_B = \Sigma O_{Bt}, E_A = \Sigma E_{At}, \text{ and } E_B = \Sigma E_{Bt}. \tag{3.2}$$

Finally the Logrank statistic is calculated as

$$\chi^2_{Logrank} = \frac{(O_A - E_A)^2}{E_A} + \frac{(O_B - E_B)^2}{E_B}. \tag{3.3}$$

This format is similar to that for the standard χ^2 test of equation (1.11).

From Table 3.1 we obtain $O_A = 11$, $E_A = 8.435382$, $O_B = 5$ and $E_B = 7.564618$. These give $(O_A - E_A) = 2.564618$ indicating more deaths than expected on treatment A, and $(O_B - E_B) = -2.564618$ or fewer deaths than expected on treatment B. Finally

$$\chi^2_{Logrank} = (2.564618)^2 / 8.435382 + (-2.564618)^2 / 7.564618 = 1.649$$

In general for g treatment groups the $\chi^2_{Logrank}$ is compared with the χ^2 distribution with g - 1 degrees of freedom. Thus for two treatment groups $\chi^2_{Logrank}$ is compared with the χ^2 distribution with degrees of freedom $df = 2 - 1 = 1$. Using the first row of Table T3 we obtain an approximate p-value ≈ 0.2. In this situation, as indicated in Section 1.6, an exact p-value is obtained by referring $z = \sqrt{\chi^2_{Logrank}} = \sqrt{1.649} = 1.28$ to Table T1, which gives a p-value $= 0.2005$. Thus this result, although not conventionally statistically significant at the 5% level, suggests that treatment B may be better than treatment A. However, this is certainly not conclusive evidence. A larger study is required to reliably confirm or refute this result. We discuss in Section 3.4 how important it is to quote appropriate CIs to reflect the uncertainty in such situations.

It is useful to note, since E_A and E_B are the sums of a large number of small quantities, that it is practice to calculate the individual components, E_{At} and E_{Bt} to sufficient (many) decimal places just as for the calculations of the K-M estimate of the survival curves. Since $E_A + E_B$ must also equal the total number of deaths $O_A + O_B$, it is not strictly necessary to calculate the individual components of E_B since

$$E_B = (O_A + O_B) - E_A.$$

It is, however, a useful check on the arithmetic if E_B is calculated from the sum of the individual E_{Bt} rather than merely from this difference.

It is also important to note that in a study in which all the patients have died and, therefore, there is 100% mortality in both (all) groups, provided we have their survival times recorded, then the corresponding E can exceed O, the total number of patients (here also deaths), in a single group. This is because the expectations, E, are calculated using the assumption that the death rates are equal in the two (or more) groups and therefore the group with the largest summed survival time should 'expect' more deaths, in which case E_1 will be greater than O_1 for this group. On the other hand, the group in which the patients die more quickly will have the smallest summed survival time and should 'expect' fewer deaths under the null hypothesis, hence E_2 is less than the corresponding O_2 for this group. Nevertheless $E_1 + E_2 = O_1 + O_1$ in all circumstances.

***Example** – time to progression – patients with AIDS with low and high antibodies*

Cheingsong-Popov, Panagiotidi, Bowcock *et al.* (1991) compared the time to progression to Stage IV disease in patients with AIDS whose gag (p24) antibody levels are 1600 or more than those with fewer antibodies.

Their results are summarised in Figure 3.3, which suggests that the disease of patients with the fewer gag (p24) antibodies may progress more quickly. They quote a significance test with p-value $= 0.0008$, which would correspond to a $\chi^2_{Logrank} \approx 7.1$ with $df = 1$.

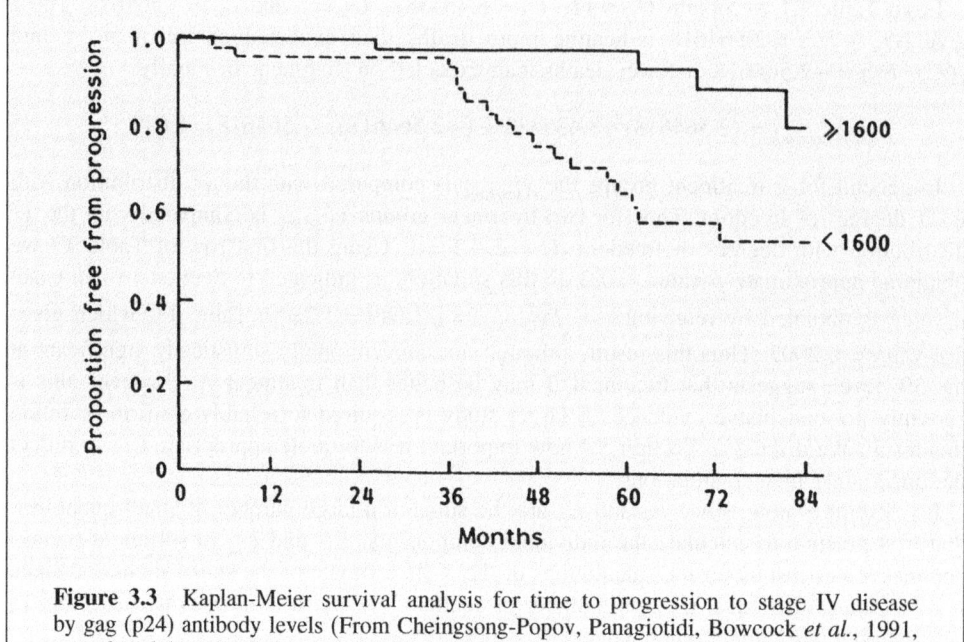

Figure 3.3   Kaplan-Meier survival analysis for time to progression to stage IV disease by gag (p24) antibody levels (From Cheingsong-Popov, Panagiotidi, Bowcock *et al.*, 1991, reproduced by permission of *British Medical Journal*, **302**, 23–26. Published by BMJ Publishing Group)

This example illustrates the use of the survival techniques for a between-group comparison where the group is defined by a characteristic of the individuals under study and not by the investigator as, for example, would be the case of the treatment given to a patient in a clinical trial.

Example – comparative cumulative discontinuation rates – women using two injectable contraceptives

The World Health Organization Task Force on Long-acting Systemic Agents for Fertility Regulation (1988) conducted an international multicentre randomised trial of two, once-monthly injectable contraceptives, HRP102 and HRP112, in 2328 women. Figure 3.4 shows the cumulative method discontinuation rates for all reasons by type of injectable contraceptive. In this situation losses to follow-up are not censored but are regarded as events (failure to continue with the method) since it is presumed that women who do not return to the clinic for the next injection are not satisfied with the method. They are not therefore 'true' losses to follow-up in this context. The trial only continues for one year, so that all subjects have this as the maximum observation time. The time of one year will provide a censored observation for all those women who continue method use up to this time. From these data there is little evidence of a difference between the discontinuation rates with either contraceptive method.

These tend to be summarised by the discontinuation rates at one year when the trial period closes for each woman. Of particular interest in this trial was the comparison of bleeding-related, including amenorrhoea, discontinuation rates. These were 6.3% and 7.5% at one year for HRP112 and HRP102, respectively although the Logrank test of this difference in discontinuation rates uses the times of the individual discontinuations to give $\chi^2_{\text{Logrank}} = 0.77$, $df = 1$, p-value $= 0.38$. For this analysis, the time to discontinuation for the competing other reasons is treated as censored.

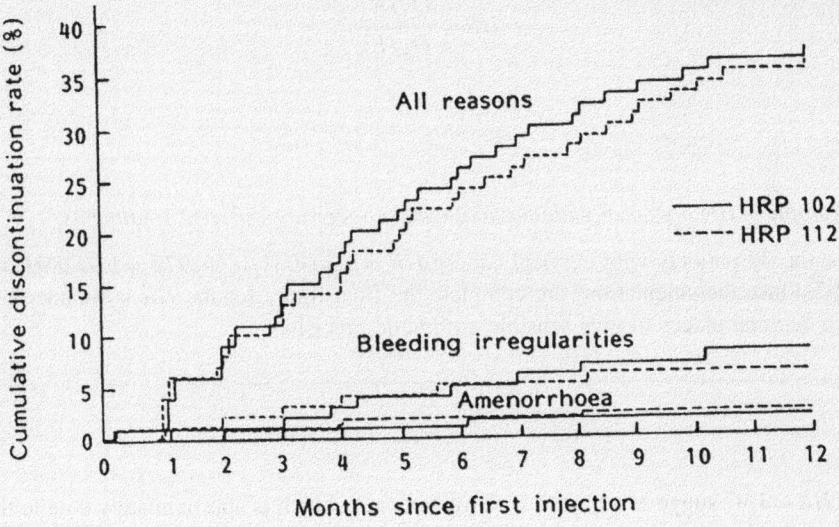

Figure 3.4 The cumulative discontinuation rates in women using two, once-monthly, injectable contraceptives for amenorrhoea, bleeding irregularities and all reasons including women lost to follow-up (From World Health Organization Task Force on Long-acting Systemic Agents for Fertility Regulation, 1988, with permission)

We note that equation (3.3) can be written as

$$\chi^2_{Logrank} = (O_A - E_A)^2 \left(\frac{1}{E_A} + \frac{1}{E_B} \right). \tag{3.4}$$

since $(O_A - E_A)^2 = (O_B - E_B)^2$. This format provides a direct comparison with equation (3.12) below and is one that we shall use later.

3.3   THE HAZARD RATIO (*HR*)

From the calculations summarised in Table 3.3 we can obtain the ratio $O_A/E_A = 11/8.435382 = 1.304031$, which is an estimate of the relative death rate in group A. The value being greater than unity suggests that there are more deaths in the treatment A group than would be expected under the null hypothesis of equal treatment efficacy. In contrast, patients receiving treatment B experience fewer deaths than expected. The relative death rate for them is $O_B/E_B = 5/7.564618 = 0.660972$. We can combine these rates into a single statistic which gives a useful summary of the results of a particular study. In particular, as shown in equation (1.5), we can calculate the hazard ratio (*HR*), defined as the ratio of these two relative death rates; that is,

$$HR = \frac{O_A/E_A}{O_B/E_B}.$$ (3.5)

Example – *HR* – *women with cervical cancer receiving different treatments*

For the 30 patients with cervical cancer $HR = 1.304031/0.660972 = 1.972899$ or 1.97. Once the calculations are complete the final figure for the *HR* is rounded to two decimal places to give sensible arithmetic precision.

The $HR = 1.97$ suggests a hazard with treatment A, which is approximately double that of treatment B. Alternatively the *HR* could have been defined as the ratio $(O_B/E_B)/(O_A/E_A) = 0.660972/1.304031 = 0.51$. In that case the result would be described as B having approximately half the hazard rate of treatment A. The choice of which to calculate is determined by the context in which the *HR* is to be used.

Table 3.5   Presentation of results following the Logrank test of the worked example of the survival time of 30 patients with cervical cancer

Treatment	Number of patients (*n*)	Number of deaths		*O/E*	*HR*	$\chi^2_{Logrank}$	*p*-value
		Observed (*O*)	Expected (*E*)				
A	16	11	8.44	1.30			
					1.97	1.65	0.20
B	14	5	7.56	0.66			
Total	30	16	16.00				

As already indicated, the *HR* of greater than unity emphasises the fact that the patients receiving *A* are dying at a faster rate than those who receive *B*. However, the Logrank test suggested that this excess was not statistically significant, since the *p*-value $= 0.2$, implying that these data are not inconsistent with the null hypothesis value of *HR* $= 1$.

Example – HR – patients with pressure sores receiving different types of ultrasound treatment

McDiarmid, Burns, Lewith and Machin (1985) recorded the time to complete healing of bedsores in 40 hospitalised patients randomised, in a double blind trial, to ultrasound (US) or mock-ultrasound (mock-US) therapy. They give *HR* $= 1.12$, which expresses the ratio of the healing rates in the two groups, with $\chi^2_{Logrank} = 0.1$, $df = 1$, *p*-value $= 0.8$, in favour of US.

However, the number of sores healed was only 18 since many patients were either discharged or died before complete healing could be observed, and so this trial does not provide reliable evidence that US is better than mock-US.

It is useful to summarise the results, following the calculation of the *HR* and the Logrank test, in a tabular form similar to that of Table 3.5, which uses the data from the worked example for the 30 patients with cervical cancer.

Example – HR – patients with severe pain receiving transcutaneous electrical nerve stimulus treatments

Nash, Williams and Machin (1990) compared the value of high- as opposed to low-frequency transcutaneous electrical nerve stimulation (TENS) for the relief of pain in a randomised trial. They measured the time taken, from the date of randomisation for the patients to achieve a 50% reduction in pain levels as compared to those levels recorded at admission to the trial. Pain was measured using a visual analogue scale (VAS). The cumulative pain relief rates are summarised in Figure 3.5 and Table 3.6.

Of the 200 patients recruited—100 randomised to low-frequency and 100 to high-frequency TENS—only 55 achieved the reduction in pain defined as the critical event of interest. The *HR* $= 1.41$ suggests a considerable advantage of the high-frequency therapy. However, this does not reach conventional statistical significance $(\chi^2_{Logrank} = 1.64$, $df = 1$, *p*-value $= 0.20)$. Here a *HR* > 1 is used to indicate the better of the two treatments.

Clearly, the number of events observed is relatively small, and because of this, although the estimate of the treatment effect suggests high-frequency therapy may be of considerable benefit to patients, this trial has not been able to provide reliable evidence to support this.

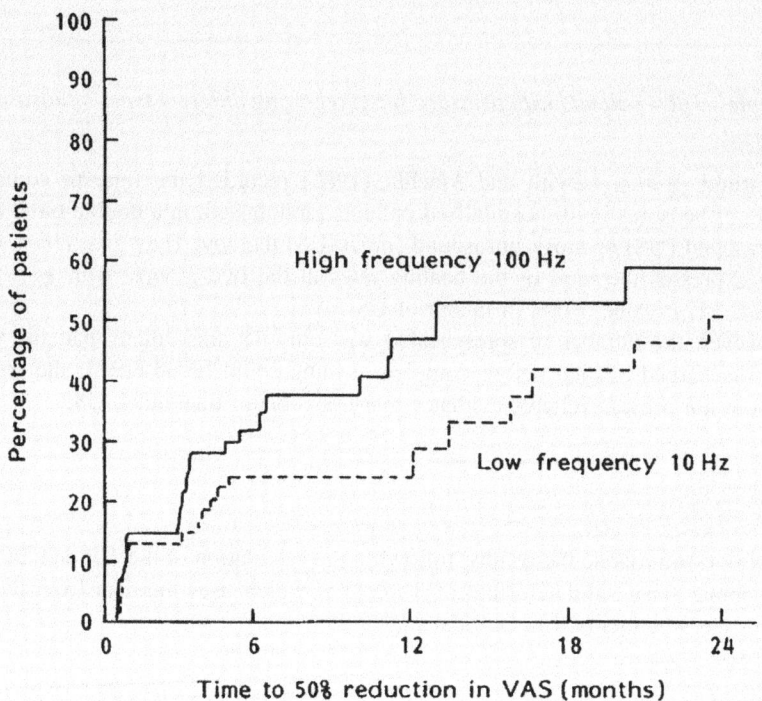

Figure 3.5 Percentage of patients achieving a 50% reduction in VAS pain levels with high- and low-frequency simulation (From Nash, Machin and Williams, 1990. Reproduced by permission of VSP International Science Publishers, an imprint of Brill Academic Publishers)

Table 3.6 Results of the trial comparing low- and high-frequency TENS (From Nash, Willliams and Machin, 1990. Reproduced by permission of VSP International Science Publishers, an imprint of Brill Academic Publishers)

| Frequency | Number of patients (n) | Number achieving relief | | O/E | HR | χ^2_{Logrank} | p-value |
		Observed (O)	Expected (E)				
Low	100	24	28.7	0.84			
					1.41	1.64	0.20
High	100	31	26.3	1.18			
Total	200	55	55.0				

Example – HR – patients with myeloblastic syndromes in two bone marrow blast level groups

A useful format for the summary of the calculations of the Logrank test and *HR*, together with the corresponding survival curves, is presented by Mufti, Stevens,

Osier *et al.* (1985) and is shown in Figure 3.6. Although they do not explicitly show the *HR*, this can be calculated as $HR = 3.69/0.71 = 5.20$. This shows a very adverse prognosis for patients with myelodysplastic syndromes with bone marrow blasts $\geq 5\%$. This is statistically significant with a *p*-value $= 0.00001$. In their paper they also give the median survival times for the two patient groups as 0.9 and 3.9 months for those with $< 5\%$ and $\geq 5\%$ bone marrow blasts, respectively.

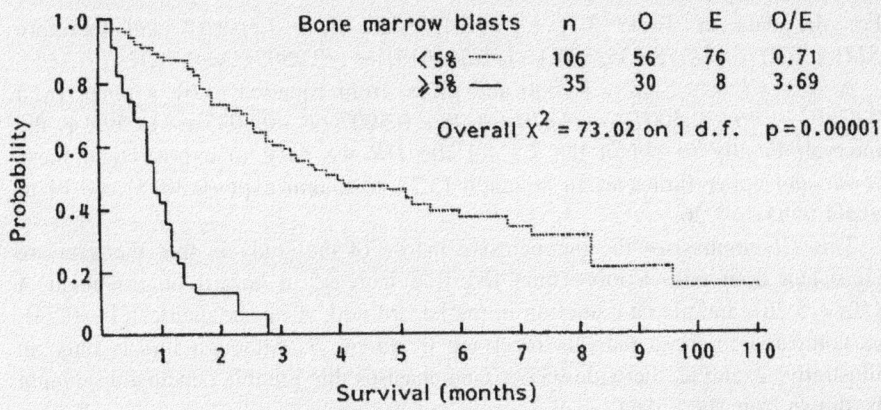

Figure 3.6 Survival in patients with myelodysplastic syndromes according to bone marrow blasts at presentation (From Mufti, Stevens, Oscier *et al.*, 1985. Reproduced by permission of *British Journal of Haematology* 59: 425–33.)

CONFIDENCE INTERVALS

Whenever an estimate of a difference between groups is given, it is useful to calculate a confidence interval (*CI*) for the estimate. Thus, for the *HR* obtained from any study, we would like to know a range of values which are not inconsistent with the observation.

In calculating *CI*s, it is convenient if the statistic under consideration can be assumed to follow an approximately Normal distribution. However, the estimate of the *HR* is not normally distributed. In particular it has a possible range of values from 0 to ∞, with the null hypothesis value of unity not located at the centre of this interval. To make the scale symmetric and to enable us to calculate *CI*s, we transform the estimate to make it approximately normally distributed. We do this by using log *HR*, rather than *HR* itself, as the basis for our calculation.

It is possible to show that a general $100(1 - \alpha)\%$ *CI* for the log *HR* is

$$\log HR - [z_{1-\alpha/2} \times SE(\log HR)] \quad \text{to} \quad \log HR + [z_{1-\alpha/2} \times SE(\log HR)], \qquad (3.6)$$

where $z_{1-\alpha/2}$ is the upper $(1 - \alpha/2)$ point of the standard Normal distribution (see Figure 1.6). The $100(1 - \alpha)\%$ CI for the HR itself is then

$$\exp[\log HR - [z_{1-\alpha/2} \times SE(\log HR)] \quad \text{to} \quad \exp[\log HR + [z_{1-\alpha/2} \times SE(\log HR)]. \quad (3.7)$$

In both these expressions

$$SE(\log HR) = \sqrt{\left(\frac{1}{E_A} + \frac{1}{E_B}\right)}. \quad (3.8)$$

Example – *confidence interval for the HR* – *patients with cervical cancer*

For the data of Table 3.3, $E_A = 8.435382$, $E_B = 7.564618$ and therefore $SE(\log HR) = \sqrt{[(1/8.435382) + (1/7.564618)]} = \sqrt{0.250743} = 0.5007$.

A 95% CI sets $z_{0.975} = 1.9600$ and gives, from equation (3.6), a range from $0.6780 - 1.96 \times 0.5007$ to $0.6870 + 1.96 \times 0.5007$ or -0.3035 to 1.6595 as the interval. Finally to obtain the CI for the HR we have to exponentiate these lower and upper limits, as in equation (3.7), to obtain $\exp(-0.3035) = 0.74$ to $\exp(1.6595) = 5.26$.

This CI emphasises the inconclusive nature of the study in that the data are consistent both with a more than five-fold increase in hazard on treatment A ($HR = 5.26$), and also a reduction in the hazard with A of one quarter $(1 - 0.74)$, as compared to those patients receiving treatment B. Although this is only an illustrative example, the wide 95% CI emphasises that reliable conclusions cannot be drawn from these data.

Example – *CI for the HR* – *patients with cervical cancer*

The full results of the trial in women with cervical cancer have been published by the Medical Research Council Working Party on Advanced Carcinoma of the Cervix (1993). They give for 183 patients randomised either to receive radiotherapy alone or radiotherapy plus a sensitizer (Ro-8799), the Logrank test, HR and associated CI using survival as the endpoint. Their results are summarised in Table 3.7. Despite a $HR = 1.58$ which suggests the death rate may be higher in the radiotherapy plus radiosensitiser group, the 95% CI for the HR of 1.01 to 2.48 (just) excludes the null hypothesis value of one.

Table 3.7 shows that only 77 (42%) of patients had died at the time of this analysis, which suggests that a more statistically powerful comparison of these treatments may have been obtained if analysis had been delayed. In fact the Medical Research Council Working Party on Advanced Carcinoma of the Cervix (1993) indicated this as an interim analysis of these data.

Table 3.7 Results from the Logrank test for treatment differences on survival in patients with cervical cancer (From the Medical Research Council Working Party on Advanced Carcinoma of the Cervix, 1993 *Radiotherapy Oncology*, **26**, 93–103. Reproduced with permission from Elsevier)

Treatment*	Number of patients (n)	Observed (O)	Expected (E)	O/E	HR	$\chi^2_{Logrank}$	p
RTX + R0-8799	91	45	36.20	1.24			
					1.58	4.05	0.044
RTX alone	92	32	40.80	0.78			
	183	77	77.00				

*The treatments are presented in reverse order to the illustration in Table 3.5.

***Example** – CI for the HR – patients with severe pain*

Nash, Williams and Machin (1990), in the example described earlier in Table 3.6 and Figure 3.5, give an $HR = 1.41$ and a 95% *CI* as 0.8 to 2.6. This interval includes $HR = 1$, the value we would expect if there was no difference between the two frequencies in their effect on pain relief. However, the interval is also consistent with, for example, $HR = 2$ or a large benefit of the high-frequency therapy.

HAZARD RATIO (*HR*) FROM MEDIAN SURVIVAL

If M_1 and M_2 are the respective median survival times of two groups calculated as indicated in section 2.3, then an estimate of the *HR* can be obtained from

$$HR_{Median} = M_2/M_1. \tag{3.9}$$

In this case, it is the inverse of the ratio of the two medians that estimates the *HR* for Group 1 as compared to Group 2.

A *CI* for this *HR* is given by

$$\exp\{\log(M_2/M_1) - \{z_{1-\alpha/2} \times SE[\log(M_2/M_1)]\}\}$$

to

$$\exp\{\log(M_2/M_1) + \{z_{1-\alpha/2} \times SE[\log(M_2/M_1)]\}\}. \tag{3.10}$$

Here the *SE* is given by

$$SE(\log M_2/M_1) = \sqrt{[(1/O_1) + (1/O_2)]}$$

where O_1 and O_2 are the observed numbers of deaths in the two groups. This method of estimating the HR and the associated CI assumes an Exponential distribution for the survival times, which we discuss in Chapter 4.

Example – CI for the median based estimate of HR – patients with cervical cancer

Reading the median survival times of patients with cervical cancer from Figure 3.2 for the two treatment groups with corresponding deaths $O_A = 11$ and $O_B = 5$ gives $M_A = 1037$ and $M_B = 1307$ days.

Hence from equation (3.9) the $HR_{Median} = M_B/M_A = 1307/1037 = 1.2604$. This gives log $HR_{Median} = \log(1.2604) = 0.2314$ and the $SE(\log HR_{Median}) = \sqrt{[(1/11) + (1/5)]} = 0.5394$. The 95% CI for this estimated HR is therefore exp[0.2314 − (1.96 × 0.5394)1 to exp[0.2314 + (1.96 × 0.5394)], that is, exp(−0.825824) = 0.4379 to exp(1.288624) = 3.6278 or 0.4 to 3.6. The width of the CI reflects the considerable uncertainty about the value of the HR.

THE MANTEL-HAENSZEL TEST

The estimate of the $SE(\log HR)$ given in equation (3.8) is not always reliable in situations when the total number of events in the study is small. A preferred estimate of the SE, albeit involving more extensive computation, requires the calculation of the variance, called the hypergeometric variance, at each death time. Summing these variances across all times leads to the Mantel-Haenszel version of the Logrank test.

Referring back to Table 3.4 the hypergeometric variance at time t is given by

$$V_t = \frac{m_t n_t r_t s_t}{N_t^2(N_t - 1)} \tag{3.11}$$

If all deaths occur at different times, that is, there are no tied observations, then $r_t = 1$, $s_t = N_t - 1$ and equation (3.11) simplifies to $V_t = m_t n_t / N_t^2$. The calculation of V_t at each time point, t, is shown in Table 3.3, for 30 of the patients recruited to the cervical cancer trial. The general calculation of V_t, from equation (3.11) is repeated in the lower panel of Table 3.4.

As for both E_{At} and E_{Bt}, we finally sum the individual V_t calculated at each distinct event time to obtain $V = \Sigma V_t$. The Mantel-Haenszel test statistic is then defined as

$$\chi^2_{MH} = \frac{(O_A - E_A)^2}{V}. \tag{3.12}$$

This has an approximate χ^2 distribution with $df = 1$ in the same way as the Logrank test of equation (3.3). It should be noted that χ^2_{MH} of equation (3.12) only differs from $\chi^2_{Logrank}$ of equation (3.4) by the expression for V.

It should also be noted that the numerator of equation (3.12) can be replaced by the corresponding expression for treatment B, since for the two-group comparison considered here, as $(O_B - E_B) = -(O_A - E_A)$. The difference in sign is removed once the square is taken.

In fact, it can be shown that the individual components of the numerator of equation (3.12) are $(O_{At} - E_{At})^2 = (n_t O_{At} - m_t O_{Bt})^2$. This format illustrates the symmetry of the equation with respect to treatments A and B more clearly.

Example – Logrank and Mantel-Haenszel tests – patients with cervical cancer

Using the calculations from Table 3.3 we have $O_A = 11$, $E_A = 8.435382$, $V = 3.910995$ and therefore, from equation (3.12), we have $\chi^2_{MH} = (2.564618)^2 / 3.910995 = 1.682$.

This is very similar to $\chi^2_{Logrank} = 1.649$ obtained earlier using equation (3.3) and, in this example, the extra calculation required for the Mantel-Haenszel statistic has little impact. However, in certain circumstances, especially if there are many ties in the data, the difference between the two can be much greater.

The use of the Mantel-Haenszel statistic to test for the difference between two groups also gives an alternative estimate of the *HR* to that of equation (3.5). This estimate is

$$HR_{MH} = \exp\left(\frac{O_A - E_A}{V}\right). \tag{3.13}$$

As already indicated, if there are ties in the data the estimates will diverge but, except in rather unusual circumstances, they will usually be close to each other. In fact if there are no ties in the data, as is the case in our example, the two methods lead to the same value except for rounding errors introduced by the different methods of calculation.

The corresponding *SE* of the Mantel-Haenszel log HR_{MH} is

$$SE(\log HR_{MH}) = 1/V^{1/2}. \tag{3.14}$$

This $SE(\log HR_{MH})$ can be used to give *CIs* derived from the Mantel-Haenszel estimate of the *HR* as

$$\exp[\log HR_{MH} - (z_{1-\alpha/2}/V^{1/2})] \quad \text{to} \quad \exp[\log HR_{MH} + (z_{1-\alpha/2}/V^{1/2})]. \tag{3.15}$$

Example – Logrank and Mantel-Haenszel estimates of the HR – patients with cervical cancer

Using the *HR* estimator of equation (3.13) gives, for the data of Table 3.3, $O_A - E_A = 2.564618$, $V = 3.910995$ and $HR_{MH} = \exp(2.564618/3.910995) = \exp(0.655746) = 1.93$. This is very close to the HR = 1.97 that we obtained using equation (3.5). Thus the two seemingly quite different estimates of the *HR* give almost identical results.

Further, equation (3.12) gives $SE(\log HR_{MH}) = 1/\sqrt{(3.910995)} = 0.5057$. This is very close to the previous value given by equation (3.8), which was 0.5007.

3.4   THE STRATIFIED LOGRANK TEST

As we have indicated earlier, in any clinical study the outcome for patients may be as much, if not more, influenced by characteristics of the patients themselves as by the treatments they receive. In contraceptive development trials, for example, cultural considerations may influence the continuation of use of new contraceptives as much as the 'efficacy' of the method itself. In cancer, it is well known that patients with a more advanced stage of the disease have a shorter expectation of life than patients with less advanced disease. Thus, patients with Stage III cervical cancer will (on average) do worse than those with Stage IIb.

When making comparisons between two groups receiving, for example, different treatments, we need to ensure as much as possible that any differences observed between groups is due to the treatments and not due to the fact that the groups have inherently differing prognoses. We thus may wish to adjust for potential imbalances of these prognostic variables when making comparisons between groups. In a trial of two treatments (A and B) in women with cervical cancer we can do this by first making a comparison of treatment A against treatment B within each cervical cancer stage separately. This ensures that 'like' is compared with 'like'. These individual comparisons are then combined to achieve an overall comparison of treatments. This is done by means of the stratified Logrank test.

To illustrate the method, stage of disease for each patient with cervical cancer is added, in Table 3.8, to the data previously outlined in Table 3.2. For example, the patient who died after 90 days had Stage III disease. The calculation of the stratified Logrank test proceeds exactly as that described earlier in Table 3.3, but first confining the comparison to within one of the strata. The first strata analysis is summarised in the Stage IIb section of Table 3.9 and gives $O_A = 3$, $E_A = 2.105129$, $O_B = 1$ and $E_B = 1.894871$. A similar analysis is then made within the second strata, here Stage III, to give $O_A = 8$, $E_A = 7.813810$, $O_B = 4$ and $E_B = 4.186190$. The next step is to combine the stratum-specific observed and expected values across the two strata, to obtain

$$\sum_s O_A = 3 + 8 = 11, \sum_s E_A = 2.105129 + 7.813810 = 9.918939$$

$$\sum_s O_B = 1 + 4 = 5, \sum_s E_B = 1894871 + 4.186190 = 6.081061$$

Here s beneath the Σ denotes the sum over the strata. The stratified HR, is then given by

$$HR_{Stratified} = \frac{\left(\sum_s O_A / \sum_s E_A \right)}{\left(\sum_s O_B / \sum_s E_B \right)} \tag{3.16}$$

$$= \frac{11/9.918939}{5/6.081061} = \frac{1.1090}{0.8222} = 1.35.$$

In this numerical example, the adjusted $HR_{Stratified} = 1.35$ is considerably less than $HR = 1.97$ calculated earlier in Table 3.5. This suggests that there is an imbalance of patients with Stages IIb and III in the respective treatment groups. This has clearly affected the estimated difference between the two treatment groups in a serious way. The corresponding K-M survival curves for the four stage by treatment groups are shown in Figure 3.7.

Table 3.8 Ranked survival times by disease stage and treatment in 30 patients with cervical cancer

	Control A				New therapy B		
Patient number	Stage	Survival time	Survival status	Patient number	Stage	Survival time	Survival status
11	III	90	DEAD	28	III	272	DEAD
15	III	142	DEAD	25	III	362	DEAD
23	III	150	DEAD	16	III	373	DEAD
29	III	269	DEAD	27	III	383+	ALIVE
6	IIb	291	DEAD	7	III	519+	ALIVE
30	IIb	468+	ALIVE	18	III	563+	ALIVE
5	III	680	DEAD	22	III	650+	ALIVE
24	III	837	DEAD	3	III	827	DEAD
26	IIb	890+	ALIVE	13	IIb	919+	ALIVE
2	III	1037	DEAD	21	IIb	978+	ALIVE
14	IIb	1090+	ALIVE	8	IIb	1100+	ALIVE
19	III	1113+	ALIVE	10	IIb	1307	DEAD
20	IIb	1153	DEAD	12	IIb	1360+	ALIVE
17	III	1297	DEAD	1	IIb	1476+	ALIVE
4	IIb	1429	DEAD				
9	IIb	1577+	ALIVE				

By analogy with equation (3.3) the stratified Logrank statistic for comparing treatments is

$$\chi^2_{Stratified} = \frac{\left(\sum_s O_A - \sum_s E_A\right)^2}{\sum_s E_A} + \frac{\left(\sum_s O_B - \sum_s E_B\right)^2}{\sum_s E_B}. \tag{3.17}$$

This also has a χ^2 distribution with $df = 1$ since we are comparing two treatments A and B. We have included the 's', denoting the sum over the strata, here to aid clarity but it is often omitted.

***Example** – stratified Logrank test – patients with cervical cancer of different stages*

For the patients with Stage IIb and III cervical cancer we have, using equation (3.17), for the stratified Logrank test

$$\chi^2_{Stratified} = \frac{(11 - 9.918939)^2}{9.918939} + \frac{(5 - 6.081061)^2}{6.081061} = 0.31.$$

This contrasts with $\chi^2_{Logrank} = 1.649$ derived from the unadjusted Logrank test calculated earlier.

In randomised trials with large numbers of patients it would be unusual to see such a difference in value between the adjusted and unadjusted analyses. However, in non-randomised

Table 3.9 Stratified Logrank test for comparison of treatments *A* with *B* in patients with cervical cancer adjusted for stage of the disease

Patient number	Rank	Survival (days) A	Survival (days) B	—		Dead	Alive	Total	E_{At}	E_{Bt}	V_t
Stage IIb											
6	11	291		A		1	6	7			
				B		0	6	6			
						1	12	13	0.538462	0.461538	0.248520
30	2	468+									
26	3	890+									
13	4		919+								
21	5		978+								
14	6	1090+									
8	7		1100+								
20	8	1153		A		1	2	3			
				B		0	3	3			
						1	5	6	0.500000	0.500000	0.250000
10	9		1307	A		0	2	2			
				B		1	2	3			
						1	4	5	0.400000	0.600000	0.240000
12	10		1360+								
4	11	1429		A		1	1	2			
				B		0	1	1			
						1	2	3	0.666667	0.333333	0.222222
1	12		1476+								
9	13	1577+									
Total						$O_A = 3$ $O_B = 1$ $E_A = 2.105129$ $E_B = 1.894871$ $V = 0.960742$					
Stage III											
11	1	90		A		1	8	9			
				B		0	8	8			
						1	16	17	0.529412	0.470588	0.249135
15	2	142		A		1	7	8			
				B		0	8	8			
						1	15	16	0.500000	0.500000	0.250000
23	3	150		A		1	6	7			
				B		0	8	8			
						1	14	15	0.466667	0.533333	0.248889
29	4	269		A		1	5	6			
				B		0	8	8			
						1	13	14	0.428571	0.571429	0.244899

28	5	272	A	0	5	5				
			B	1	7	8				
				1	12	13	0.384615	0.615385	0.236686	
25	6	362	A	0	5	5				
			B	1	6	7				
				1	11	12	0.416667	0.583333	0.243056	
16	7	373	A	0	5	5				
			B	1	5	6				
				1	10	11	0.454545	0.545455	0.247934	
27	8	383+								
7	9	519+								
18	10	563+								
22	11	650+								
5	12	680	A	1	4	5				
			B	0	1	1				
				1	5	6	0.833333	0.166667	0.138888	
3	13	827	A	0	4	4				
			B	1	0	1				
				1	4	5	0.800000	0.200000	0.160000	
24	14	837	A	1	3	4				
			B	0	0	0				
				1	3	4	1.000000	0.000000	0.000000	
2	15	1037	A	1	2	3				
			B	0	0	0				
				1	2	3	1.000000	0.000000	0.000000	
19	16	113+								
17	17	1297	A	1	0	1				
			B	0	0	0				
				1	0	1	1.000000	0.000000	0.000000	

Total $\quad O_A = 8 \; O_B = 4 \; E_A = 7.813810 \; E_B = 4.186190 \; V = 2.019478$

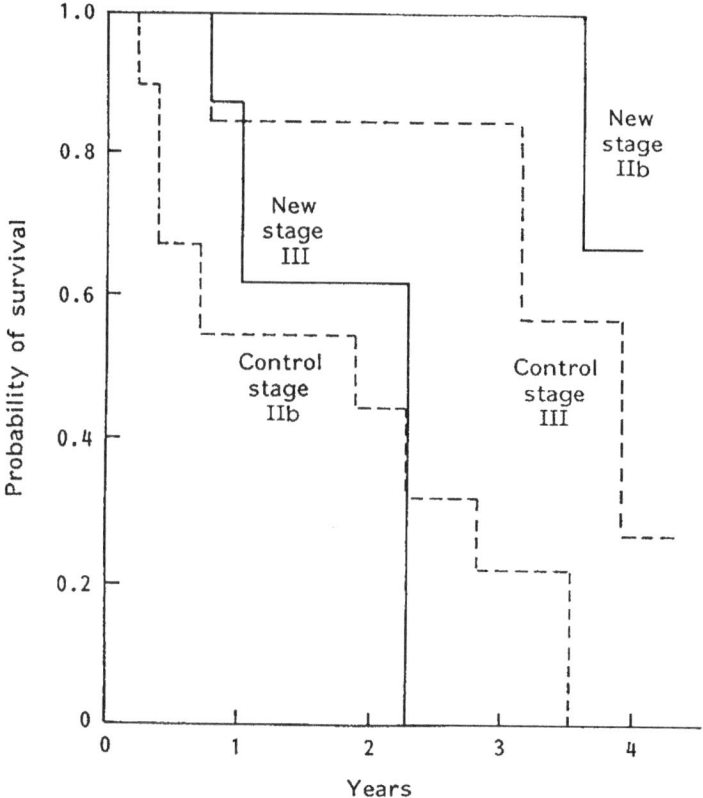

Figure 3.7 Survival for patients with cervical cancer by the four stage by treatment groups

or smaller randomised trials, large differences between adjusted and unadjusted analyses can be expected. In these instances it is very important that adjusted analyses are performed and any consequences on the interpretation of the results reported.

3.5   THREE OR MORE GROUPS

Consider the data for the 30 women with cervical cancer that we have discussed earlier (see Tables 3.1 and 3.2) and whose age at diagnosis is presented by treatment group in Table 3.10. For purposes of illustration we divide these women into three groups according to age, and for convenience label them as young (less than 50), middle aged (50 to less than 60) and senior (60 or more) in an obvious notation of Y, M and S. The corresponding K-M plots are shown in Figure 3.8. In this small data set, the 11 older women (S) fare the best, the nine middle-aged (M) the worst and the youngest 10 women (Y) intermediately.

The Logrank comparison for these three groups (Y, M, S) proceeds in a similar way to the two-group comparison of Tables 3.3 and 3.4. Thus, the patients are first ordered by their survival times, as before, but now in three rows, one for each age group. At each death the data are summarised in a 3×2 contingency table, the first of which is shown in the upper panel of Table 3.11.

Table 3.10 Age, age-group and survival of 30 patients with cervical cancer by treatment group

Control A				New therapy B			
Patient number	Age (years)	Age-group	Survival (days)	Patient number	Age (years)	Age-group	Survival (days)
2	64	S	1037	1	63	S	1476+
4	69	S	1429	3	43	Y	827
5	38	Y	680	7	27	Y	519+
6	53	M	291	8	74	S	1100+
9	61	S	1577+	10	63	S	1307
11	59	M	90	12	39	Y	1360+
14	53	M	1090+	13	70	S	919+
15	56	M	142	16	68	S	373
17	65	S	1297	18	69	S	563+
19	48	Y	1113+	21	73	S	978+
20	45	Y	1153	22	58	M	650+
23	55	M	150	25	55	M	362
24	58	M	837	27	58	M	383+
26	49	Y	890+	28	45	Y	272
29	43	Y	269				
30	42	Y	468+				

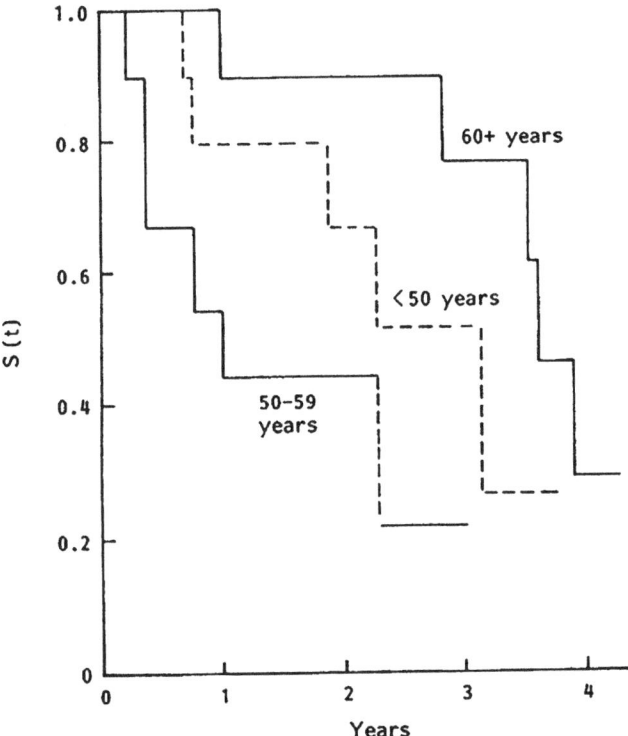

Figure 3.8 Survival curves of women with cervical cancer in three age groups

Table 3.11 Comparison of observed and expected deaths following the first death at 90 days and the general notation used at time t

Time, $t = 90$									
Age-group	Dead	Alive	Total	$O_{Y,90}$	$O_{M,90}$	$O_{S,90}$	$E_{Y,90}$	$E_{M,90}$	$E_{S,90}$
Young	0	10	10						
Middle	1	8	9						
Senior	0	11	11						
Total	1	29	30	0	1	0	0.333333	0.300000	0.366667

Time, t									
Age-group	Dead	Alive	Total	$O_{Y,t}$	$O_{M,t}$	$O_{S,t}$	$E_{Y,t}$	$E_{M,t}$	$E_{S,t}$
Young, Y	a_t	d_t	m_t						
Middle, M	b_t	e_t	n_t						
Senior, S	c_t	f_t	l_t						
Total	r_t	s_t	N_t	a_t	b_t	c_t	$r_t m_t / N_t$	$r_t n_t / N_t$	$r_t l_t / N_t$

The full calculations are summarised in Table 3.12, from which it can be seen that, for example, $n_Y = 10$, $O_Y = 5$ and $E_Y = 4.610203$. The corresponding expression for the Logrank statistic is an extension of equation (3.3) to three groups is

$$\chi^2_{Logrank} = \frac{(O_Y - E_Y)^2}{E_Y} + \frac{(O_M - E_M)^2}{E_M} + \frac{(O_S - E_S)^2}{E_S}.$$

The general expression corresponding to this for g groups is given by

$$\chi^2_{Logrank} = \sum_{j=1}^{g} \frac{(O_j - E_j)^2}{E_j}. \tag{3.18}$$

The calculated value of $\chi^2_{Logrank}$ has to be referred to Table T3, but with the corresponding $df = g - 1$ in this case.

***Example** – Logrank test for three groups – patients with cervical cancer*

Substituting the values from Table 3.12 in equation (3.18) gives $\chi^2_{Logrank} = 7.40$. In this example there are $g = 3$ age groups so we have $df = 2$ and so Table T3 gives p-value $= 0.025$. This suggests some evidence of a survival difference between the three age groups.

In general, for a contingency table with R rows and C columns, the degrees of freedom are given by $df = (R - 1)(C - 1)$. In the above analysis, we are analysing a series of 3×2 contingency tables therefore $R = g = 3$ and $C = 2$ from which we obtain $df = 2$. Such a χ^2 test is termed a test for homogeneity between groups. Using this test we can conclude, for example, that there appear to be larger differences between the three age

Table 3.12 Calculation of the Logrank test for a three-group comparison

Patient number	Rank	Survival (days) Y	M	S		Dead	Alive	Total	E_{Yt}	E_{Mt}	E_{St}
11	1		90		Y	0	10	10	0.333333	0.30000	0.366667
					M	1	8	9			
					S	0	11	11			
						1	29	30			
15	2		142		Y	0	10	10	0.344828	0.275862	0.379310
					M	1	7	8			
					S	0	11	11			
						1	28	29			
23	3		150		Y	0	10	10	0.357143	0.250000	0.392857
					M	1	6	7			
					S	0	11	11			
						1	27	28			
29	4	269			Y	1	9	10	0.346154	0.230769	0.423077
					M	0	6	6			
					S	0	11	11			
						1	26	26			
28	5	272			Y	1	8	9	0.346154	0.230769	0.423077
					M	0	6	6			
					S	0	11	11			
						1	25	26			
6	6		291		Y	0	8	8	0.320000	0.240000	0.440000
					M	1	5	6			
					S	0	11	11			
						1	25	26			
25	7		362		Y	0	8	8	0.333333	0.208333	0.458333
					M	1	4	5			
					S	0	11	11			
						1	23	24			
16	8			373	Y	0	8	8	0.347826	0.173913	0.478261
					M	0	4	4			
					S	1	10	11			
						1	22	23			
27	9		383+								
30	10	468+									
7	11	519+									
18	12		563+								
22	13		650+								

Table 3.12 (Continued)

Patient number	Rank	Survival (days) Y	M	S		Dead	Alive	Total	E_{Yt}	E_{Mt}	E_{St}
5	14	680			Y	1	5	6	0.352941	0.117647	0.529412
					M	0	2	2			
					S	0	9	9			
						1	16	17			
3	15	827			Y	1	4	5	0.312500	0.125000	0.562500
					M	0	2	2			
					S	0	9	9			
						1	15	16			
24	16			837	Y	0	4	4	0.266667	0.133333	0.600000
					M	1	1	2			
					S	0	9	9			
						1	14	15			
26	17		890+								
13	18			919+							
21	19			978+							
2	20			1037	Y	0	3	3	0.272727	0.090909	0.636364
					M	0	1	1			
					S	1	6	7			
						1	10	11			
14	21		1090+								
8	22			1100+							
19	23	1113+									
20	24	1153			Y	1	1	2	0.285714	0.000000	0.714286
					M	0	0	0			
					S	0	5	5			
						1	6	7			
17	25			1297	Y	0	1	1	0.166667	0.000000	0.833333
					M	0	0	0			
					S	1	4	5			
						1	5	6			
10	26			1307	Y	0	1	1	0.200000	0.000000	0.800000
					M	0	0	0			
					S	1	3	4			
						1	4	5			
12	27	1360+									

THREE OR MORE GROUPS

4	28	1429	Y	0	0	0	0.000000	0.000000	1.000000
			M	0	0	0			
			S	1	2	3			
				1	2	3			
				1	2	3			
1	29	1476+							
9	30	1577+							

Totals			$E_Y = 4.610203$	$E_M = 2.367988$	$E_S = 9.021806$
			$O_Y = 5$	$O_M = 6$	$O_S = 5$
			$n_Y = 10$	$n_M = 9$	$n_S = 11$

groups than would be expected by chance alone. However, this test does not identify where the differences occur. This information may be sought in an informal way from Figure 3.9 in this example, or by making further statistical tests using features of the study design.

Example – Logrank test for three score groups – patients with myelodysplastic syndromes

Mufti, Stevens, Oscier et al. (1985) compare patients with myelodysplastic syndromes with respect to three Bournemouth score groupings (0 or 1, 2 or 3, 4) representing the severity of the disease and determined from characteristics at diagnosis. They give $\chi^2_{Logrank} = 37.96$, $df = 2$ and a p-value $= 0.000001$, demonstrating differences in survival in these three groups.

LINEAR TREND

As we have indicated earlier, in patients diagnosed with colon cancer, their subsequent survival time is influenced by stage of disease at diagnosis. Thus, experience tells us that a patient with Dukes' A disease is likely to survive longer than a patient with Dukes' B disease. In turn, a patient with Dukes' B disease is likely to survive longer than one with Dukes' C disease. There is, therefore, a natural ordering of the groups which we can make use of in a test for linear trend. Such a test addresses the specific question of whether prognosis deteriorates with stage, rather than the more general question addressed by the test for homogeneity of whether there are any differences in survival between stages. This test for trend is evolved from the test for trend in a general $G \times 2$ contingency table.

Example – *test for linear trend* – *patients with cervical cancer*

At the beginning of the trial of 30 women with cervical cancer, it may have been suggested that older women have a poorer prognosis than younger women. At the end of the trial a test for a trend in prognosis with age may help us assess the evidence for this hypothesis.

To illustrate the test for trend, consider the last part of Table 3.12, which is extended in Table 3.13. Here the $g(=3)$ age groups are labelled with the value of the variable a_j representing age. In this example, $a_Y = 45, a_M = 55$ and $a_S = 65$ years, where 45, 55 and 65 represent the centres of the three age groups of the 30 women. Alternatively, these can be labelled 0, 1 and 2 merely by subtracting 45 and dividing each by 10. Such a change in the code for the as will usually simplify the arithmetic in what follows. Even more saving on the subsequent arithmetic can be made by further subtracting 1 to obtain the codes $-1, 0, 1$.

Table 3.13   Notation for a test for trend

Age-Group	Age (years)	Coded age	Recoded age	a_j	Deaths O_j	E_j	Difference $d_j = O_j - E_j$
Young, Y	45	1	-1	a_Y	O_Y	E_Y	$O_Y - E_Y$
Middle, M	55	2	0	a_M	O_M	E_M	$O_M - E_M$
Senior, S	65	3	1	a_S	O_S	E_S	$O_S - E_S$

The test for trend involving g groups requires the calculation of the following terms:

$$D_j = a_j d_j = a_j (O_j - E_j), F_j = a_j E_j \text{ and } G_j = a_j^2 E_j \qquad (3.19)$$

for each of the $j = 1, 2, \ldots, g$ groups.

These terms are then summed over the g groups to obtain D, F and G. Similarly, we sum to obtain E, which is equivalent to the total number of deaths across all groups. The test for trend is then given by

$$\chi^2_{Trend} = D^2 / V_{Trend}, \qquad (3.20)$$

where

$$V_{Trend} = G - (F^2 / E).$$

This test is a usual χ^2 test, but has $df = 1$ irrespective of the number of groups g.

We emphasise that one should not test for trend after first inspecting the data (such as that of Figure 3.8) as such 'data snooping' exercises may discourage a formal test of the original (design) hypothesis and encourage the substitution of a data-dependent hypothesis to test in its place. For example, in our problem, after the results are in we may postulate that the disease is likely to be more aggressive during the menopausal stage (the intermediate age group) and we may suggest that it is this, rather than age, which is of major prognostic importance.

Example – test for linear trend – patients with cervical cancer

The calculations for the 30 women with cervical cancer, classified into three age groups, and using the codes -1, 0 and 1, are summarised in Table 3.14. From this table we obtain $V_{Linear} = 13.632 - [(4.412)^2/16.000] = 12.415$ and the test for linear trend gives $\chi^2_{Linear} = (-4.412)^2/12.415 = 1.57$.

Reference to Table T3 with $df = 1$ indicates a p-value > 0.1. However, since $df = 1$, a more precise value can be obtained by referring $\sqrt{1.57} = 1.25$ to Table T1, which gives a p-value $= 0.2113$ or 0.21. Thus, a test for linear trend is not statistically significant, as might have been anticipated by inspection of Figure 3.8, since this suggests that the younger women have an intermediate prognosis. We emphasise again that we are using the data here for 'statistical' illustration and not for drawing conclusions about relative prognosis in patients with cervical cancer.

Table 3.14 Illustration of the calculation of the test for linear trend for the 30 women with cervical cancer

Age group (code, a_j)	Deaths O_j	E_j	d_j	D_j	F_j	G_j
45(-1)	5	4.610	0.390	-0.390	-4.610	4.610
55 (0)	6	2.368	3.632	0.000	0.000	0.000
65 ($+1$)	5	9.022	-4.022	-4.022	9.022	9.022
Total		$E = 16.000$		$D = -4.412$	$F = 4.412$	$G = 13.632$

In this example, we have replaced '*Trend*' in equations (3.20) by '*Linear*' as shorthand for '*Linear Trend*'. The linear part arises from the specific example because we have used equal age differences between the groups.

Example – test for linear trend – changing pregnancy rates with a vaginal ring by bodyweight

The World Health Organization Task Force on Long-acting Systemic Agents for Fertility Regulation (1990) investigated the pregnancy rates associated with the differing body weights of women using a contraceptive vaginal ring. Their results are summarised in Table 3.15. These data give $V_{Linear} = 89.81 - (-12.38)^2/26.00 = 83.92$ and $\chi^2_{Linear} = (24.38)^2/83.92 = 7.08$. Reference to Table T3 with $df = 1$ or Table T1 gives a p-value $= 0.008$.

This suggests a strong linear effect of increasing pregnancy rate with weight at first use of the vaginal ring. The 12-month discontinuation rates for the four weight groups in increasing order are given as 1.8%, 2.6%, 5.3% and 8.2%, respectively, by WHO (1990).

Table 3.15 Observed and expected numbers of pregnancies by weight of women at first use of a vaginal ring (Reproduced from *The Lancet*, **336**, WHO, Task Force on Long-acting Systemic Agents for Fertility Regulation, 955–959, © 1990. Reproduced by permission of Elsevier)

Weight (kg)	a_j	Number of women (n_j)	Number of pregnancies Observed (O_j)	Number of pregnancies Expected (E_j)	$O_j - E_j$	D_j	F_j	G_j
−49	−3	227	3	5.28	−2.28	6.84	−15.84	47.52
50 − 59	−1	425	7	11.33	−4.33	4.33	−11.33	11.33
60 − 69	1	253	10	6.72	3.28	3.28	6.72	6.75
70+	3	100	6	2.69	3.31	9.93	8.07	24.21
Total		1005	26	$E = 26.00$		$D = 24.38$	$F = -12.38$	$G = 89.81$

There is no requirement in the test for trend that the codes (sometimes referred to as weights), a_j, have to be equally spaced. For example, if the Senior women of Table 3.10 were better represented by an age group centred at 70 (rather than 65), then a_S may be set at 70. This would result in codes of either (0, 1 and 2.5), or (−1, 0, 1.5), depending on which code for age is used in the calculation. A different value for χ^2_{Linear} will result, but this is a consequence of the change in the codes and would be expected.

NON-LINEAR TREND

In the preceding section, we have referred to linear trend since, for example, with the 30 women with cervical cancer we were assuming a linear change in prognosis with age as displayed by the use of the codes −1, 0, and +1. However, let us suppose that we had postulated at the beginning of the trial that the menopausal women (the middle age group) might have the worst prognosis. In this situation, one can test for non-linear (quadratic) trend by assigning codes a_j equal to +1, −2, and +1 to the successive age groups. The calculations proceed using equations (3.19) and (3.20) but with the new values for a_j.

***Example** – test for non-linear trend – patients with cervical cancer*

If we apply the weights 1, −2, 1 to the data of Table 3.14 we obtain $E = 16.000$ as before, but $D = -10.896, F = 8.896$ and $G = 23.104$. Therefore $V_{Quadratic} = 23.104 - (8.896)^2/16.000 = 18.1578$. The test for quadratic trend gives $\chi^2_{Quadratic} = (-10.896)^2/18.1578 = 6.54$. Reference to Table T3 with $df = 1$ indicates a p-value <0.02. More precise calculations, using Table T1, give a p-value $= 0.0105$ or 0.01. Thus, a test for quadratic trend indicates, from this illustrative data set, that there is some evidence that menopausal women have poorer survival.

3.6 FACTORIAL DESIGNS

2×2 DESIGN

The basic reason for using a factorial design in a clinical trial or any designed intervention study is that two (or more) types of treatment may be compared simultaneously. Conventionally, the types of treatment are termed factors and the alternatives within each factor the levels. A 2×2 factorial design will have two factors A and B. Each factor has two levels,

Example – 2×2 *factorial design* – *patients treated for pain using transcutaneous nerve stimulation*

Nash, Williams and Machin, (1990) describe a randomised trial of two levels of frequency, F, and two types of stimulation, S, with transcutaneous nerve stimulation (TENS) to relieve pain in patients with chronic pain. The two levels of Factor F are a low frequency of 10 Hz and a high frequency of 100 Hz. The two levels of Factor S are non-continuous (pulse) stimulation and a continuous stimulation. The four treatment options are therefore $(1) =$ low frequency and pulse stimulation, $f =$ high frequency and pulse stimulation, $s =$ low frequency and continuous stimulation and $fs =$ high frequency and continuous stimulation. The investigators recruited 50 patients to each of the four options of the 2×2 design. Their results are summarised in Figure 3.9, which suggests that those patients receiving high-frequency (100 Hz), pulse stimulation TENS treatment may experience the greater benefit.

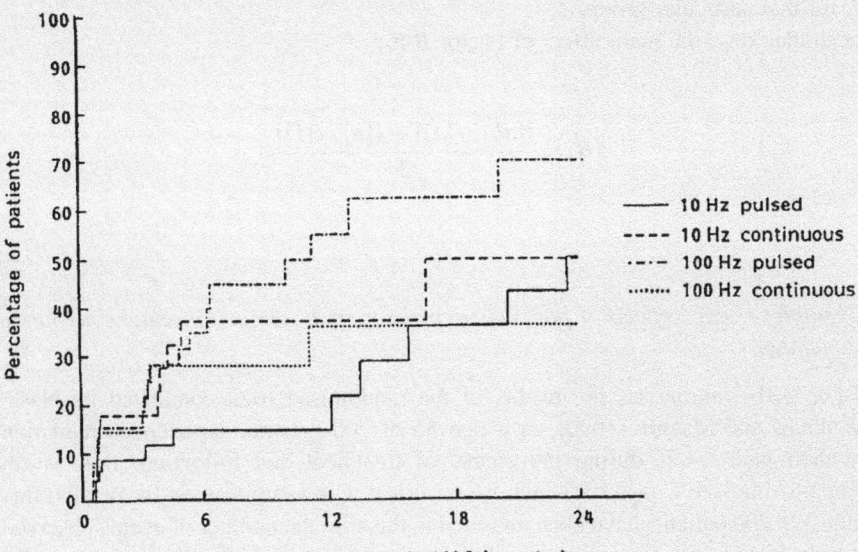

Figure 3.9 Kaplan-Meier estimate of the cumulative percentage of patients achieving a 50% reduction in visual analogue score (VAS) from baseline values for four types of TENS (From Nash, Williams and Machin, 1990. Reproduced by permission of VSP International Science Publishers, an imprint of Brill Academic Publishers)

a first and a second level, denoted *(1)* and *a* for Factor *A* and *(1)* and *b* for Factor *B*. The two factors are combined to give four (2×2) treatment combinations *(1)(1)*, *a(1)*, *(1)b* and *ab*, which are conventionally summarised by *(1)*, *a*, *b* and *ab* respectively. The *(1)* represents the combination treatment of the first level of Factor *A* with the first level of Factor *B*. Combination treatment *a* represents the second level of Factor *A* with the first level of Factor *B*. Combination treatment *b* represents the first level of Factor *A* with the second level of Factor *B*. Finally, combination treatment *ab* represents the second level of Factor *A* with the second level of Factor *B*.

MAIN EFFECTS

In the analysis of a 2×2 factorial design to estimate the main effect of Factor *A*, patients who receive *ab* are compared with those who receive *b*, and patients who receive *a* are compared with those who receive *(1)*. We use the shorthand, main effect of Factor *A*, to represent the difference in effect of the two levels of Factor *A*. The mean of these two comparisons is then taken to obtain a main effect of Factor *A*. This process is expressed as

$$A = \frac{\{[ab] - [b]\} + \{[a] - [1]\}}{2} \tag{3.21}$$

Here the brackets, [.], denote the 'statistical measure' from those patients receiving the particular treatment option. For survival time studies, such a measure will be the corresponding $O - E$ for that particular group.

In a similar way, the main effect of Factor *B* is

$$[B] = \frac{\{[ab] - [a]\} + \{[b] - [1]\}}{2}.$$

***Example** – main effects – patients treated for pain using transcutaneous nerve stimulation*

Table 3.16 summarises the results of the randomised trial, conducted by Nash, Williams and Machin (1990), in which 55 of 200 patients experienced reduction in their pain levels during the course of treatment and follow-up. It is worth emphasising (see Chapter 9 which is concerned with sample sizes, for details) that although 200 patients have been recruited to this trial the number of events observed is only 55 (27.5%). Consequently, the trial does not have high statistical power for the question(s) intended.

The values of $d = (O - E)$ corresponding to the four treatment groups are given in Table 3.16. Combined in the format of equation (3.21), these give the main effect for high versus low frequency treatment as

Table 3.16 Observed and expected numbers of patients who achieved 50% reduction in pain levels (From Nash, Williams and Machin, 1990. Reproduced by permission of VSP International Science Publishers, an imprint of Brill Academic Publishers)

Frequency (Hz)	Stimulation		Number of patients	Number of patients achieving pain relief			
				Observed (O)	Expected (E)	Difference ($O-E$)	Ratio O/E
10	Pulse	(*l*)	50	11	17.3	−6.3	0.63
	Continuous	(*s*)	50	13	11.4	1.6	1.14
100	Pulse	(*f*)	50	19	13.5	5.5	1.41
	Continuous	(*fs*)	50	12	12.8	−0.8	0.94

$$[F] = \frac{\{[fs - s]\} + \{[f - l]\}}{2}$$

$$= \frac{\{(12 - 12.8) - (13 - 11.4)\} + \{(19 - 13.5) - (11 - 17.3)\}}{2} = \frac{9.4}{2} = 4.7.$$

This suggests that the high-frequency TENS achieves more remissions than the low-frequency TENS, since $[F] = 4.7$ is positive.

In more familiar terms, this can be alternatively expressed as a *HR*. This is obtained by summing the observed and expected values for pulse and continuous in Table 3.16 for each frequency. This gives for 10 Hz, $O_{10} = 11 + 13 = 24$, $E_{10} = 17.3 + 11.4 = 28.7$ and for 100 Hz, $O_{100} = 19 + 12 = 31$, $E_{100} = 13.5 + 12.8 = 26.3$. Finally $HR_F = (31/26.3)/(24/28.7) = 1.41$, suggesting a benefit to the high-frequency TENS.

A formal test of significance for the main effect of frequency is a stratified Logrank test of the form described in equation (3.17). This takes the form of comparing the groups *fs* with *s* and *f* with (*l*). It is calculated as

$$\chi_F^2 = \frac{(24 - 28.7)^2}{28.7} + \frac{(31 - 26.3)^2}{26.3} = (4.7)^2 \left(\frac{1}{28.7} + \frac{1}{26.3} \right) = 1.61.$$

It is useful to note that $[F] = 4.7$ appears in the numerator of the expression for χ_F^2. This result is far from statistically significant since use of Table T1 with $z = \sqrt{1.61} = 1.27$ gives a *p*-value $= 0.20$.

In a similar way, the main effect of the type of stimulation is $[S] = \frac{\{[s] - [f]\} + \{[s] - [l]\}}{2} = 0.8$, $HR_S = (25/24.2)/(30/30.8) = 1.06$ and a stratified analysis yields $\chi_S^2 = (30 - 30.8)^2/30.8 + (25 - 24.2)^2/24.2 = 0.05$. This is again far from statistically significant since the corresponding p-value $= 0.83$.

The K-M curves for the Factor F and Factor S comparisons of Nash, Williams and Machin (1990) are shown in the panels of Figure 3.10.

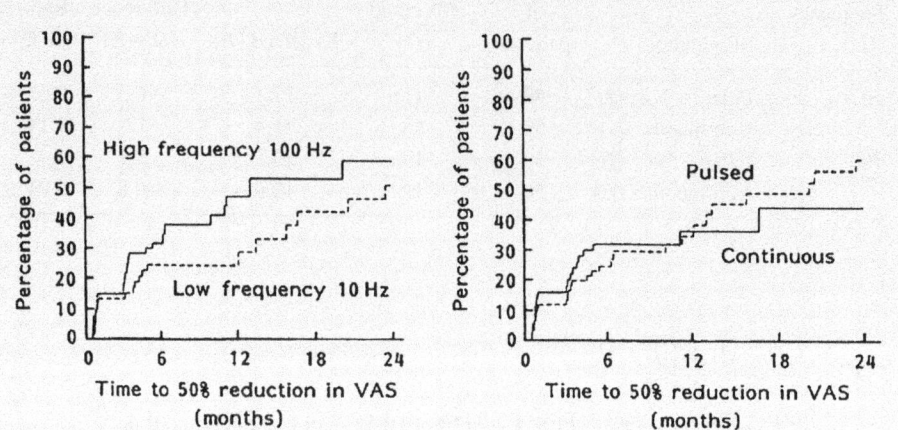

Figure 3.10 Kaplan-Meier estimate of the percentage of patients achieving a 50% reduction in VAS from baseline values for low and high frequency and for pulse and continuous frequency types of TENS (From Nash, Williams and Machin, 1990. Reproduced by permission of VSP International Science Publishers, an imprint of Brill Academic Publishers)

INTERACTION

There is one other important comparison that can be assessed in a factorial design and that is the interaction effect. This is estimated by

$$[AB] = \{[ab] - [a] - [b] + [I]\}/2. \tag{3.22}$$

The interaction effect is aimed at assessing whether the effect of Factor A is similar at the two levels of Factor B. Similarly, because of the symmetry in expression (3.22) between A and B, it also assesses whether the effect of B is similar at the two levels of Factor A. If there is good evidence of an interaction, that is, the effect of A appears to be different at the lower and higher levels of Factor B, then taking the simple average effect, as given in equation (3.21), to be the estimate of the effect of Factor A may be questioned. Emphasis may be placed on the individual effects at the higher and lower levels of Factor B, depending on practical considerations. By symmetry, similar considerations hold for Factor B.

Example – interaction – patients treated for pain using transcutaneous nerve stimulation

For the data of Table 3.16 we have

$$[FS] = \{[fs] - [f] - [s] + [1]\}/2$$
$$= \frac{(12 - 12.8) - (19 - 13.5) - (13 - 11.4) + (11 - 17.3)}{2}$$
$$= \frac{0.8 - 5.5 - 1.6 - 6.3}{2} = \frac{-14.2}{2} = -7.1.$$

In this example, the interaction effect $[FS]$ is larger than either of the main effects $[F]$ or $[S]$. This can be seen from Table 3.16 in that the effect, for example, of pulsed stimulation with 100 Hz is to increase the relief rate ($O/E = 1.41$), but has the opposite effect with 10 Hz ($O/E = 0.63$). Such a differential effect can only be estimated if a factorial design is used for the design.

The corresponding $HR_{FS} = (23/30.1)/(32/24.9) = 0.59$ where $23 = 11 + 12$, $30.1 = 17.3 + 12.8, 32 = 13 + 19$ and $24.9 = 11.4 + 13.5$, from Table 3.16. This suggests that it is better giving either continuous low-frequency (10 Hz) (s) or pulsed high-frequency (100 Hz) (f) as opposed to either pulsed low-frequency (10 Hz) (1) or continuous high-frequency (100 Hz) (fs) TENS. However, some care needs to be taken in drawing such a conclusion from these data, as the number of events observed is small and, therefore, associated CIs will be wide.

A Logrank test for the $[FS]$ interaction with $df = 1$ gives $\chi^2_{FS} = (23 - 30.1)^2/30.1 + (32 - 24.9)^2/24.9 = 3.70$. This is larger than the corresponding values for the main effects and leads, with $z = \sqrt{3.70} = 1.92$, to a p-value $= 0.0549$ which is close to statistical significance

In general the test for interaction will only be sensitive enough to detect relatively large interaction effects and thus care should be taken in assuming a 'non-significant' implies there is no interaction.

Example – 2 × 2 factorial – cumulative risk of myocardial infarction after treatment with aspirin, heparin, neither or both

The cumulative risk of myocardial infarction (MI) and death in the first 30 days during treatment as reported by The RISC Group (1990) is shown in Figure 3.11. The four treatment groups used in this trial were in a 2 × 2 factorial form. This figure suggests a benefit of aspirin and an apparent lack of benefit of heparin either given alone or as an addition to aspirin treatment.

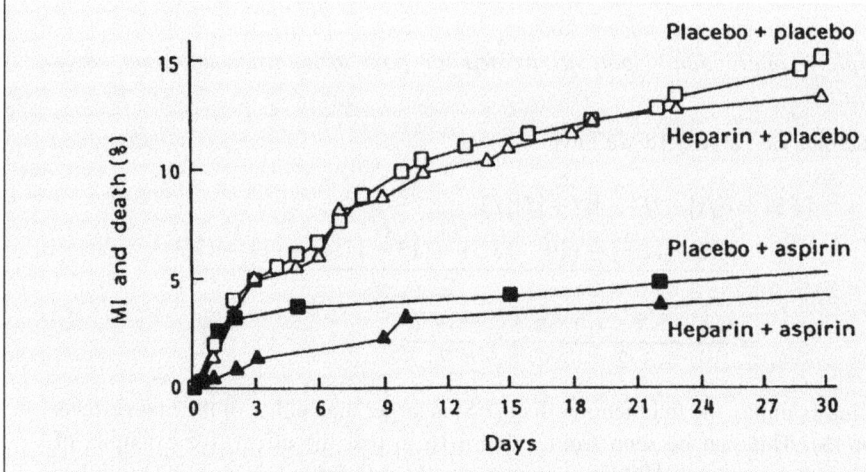

Figure 3.11 Risk of myocardial infarction (MI) and death during treatment with aspirin, heparin, both and none. (Reprinted from *The Lancet*, **336**, the RISC Group, Risk of myocardial infarction and death during treatment with low dose aspirin and intravenous heparin in men with unstable coronary artery disease, 827–830, © 1990, with permission from Elsevier)

When analysing 2×2 factorial designs in which the data are without censoring, it can be shown that the χ_A^2, χ_B^2 and the χ_{AB}^2 each with $df = 1$ sum to the overall χ^2 test for homogeneity with $df = g - 1 = 3$. For technical reasons, associated with summing over tables at different death times t, together with the different numbers of events occurring in each treatment, this is not generally true for survival data. It is usually best to analyse factorial designs using a Cox regression model as described in Chapter 5. This approach avoids technical difficulties that can occur.

3.7   SUMMARISING FOLLOW-UP

We described in Section 2.3 a method of summarising the maturity of the follow-up data for a single patient group. This method can be extended to two or more groups by use of the *K-M* plots of the follow-up curves. These curves can be visually compared to assess any differences and the corresponding median, minimum and maximum follow-up in the groups obtained.

If we return to the situation of comparing two or more survival curves, we usually assume that the censoring mechanisms do not depend on the group. For example, in a randomised clinical trial, it is assumed that patients are just as likely to be lost to follow-up in one treatment group as in the other. In contrast, if one is comparing new patients with a historical series, one might expect, since the new patient set is less mature, a greater proportion of censored data in this group. These censored data are not necessarily lost to follow-up but are made up of subjects that are currently being followed at the time of analysis or census date.

Such imbalances in follow-up can lead to a spurious difference in survival between groups. In the context of a randomised trial any imbalance in follow-up, for whatever reason, is likely to be important. This is particularly the case at an interim analysis when only relatively few events, of the total anticipated by the design, have been observed. Such an imbalance in follow-up between the treatment groups could lead to the spurious conclusion that there is a difference in the survival patterns in the groups. Thus, any survival comparisons between groups, whether final or interim, should always be accompanied by a comparison of the follow-up in the groups being compared. A simple way of doing this is to form the K-M follow-up curves as described in Section 2.3. Nevertheless, such follow-up curves have to be interpreted with care. For example, if in a randomised trial aimed at assessing the difference between two treatments one treatment is considerably more effective in preventing death than the other, we would anticipate a difference in the patterns in the follow-up curves. This occurs even if there is, in truth, no difference in follow-up, simply because the attrition in follow-up will be greater in one treatment arm than the other, as a consequence of the shorter survival times in one group. This problem will not be important if the difference between treatments is relatively small.

At an interim analysis, that is one conducted when either the recruitment or follow-up or both are incomplete, a check for similar follow-up is particularly important, since we could anticipate seeing 'large' differences between groups at such a stage. A simple solution to this difficulty is to exclude those patients who have died and to form follow-up curves just for those patients who are left alive. Minimum, maximum and median follow-up times can then be read from these curves in the usual way. When there are a high proportion of deaths the K-M follow-up curves obtained in this way will obviously be relatively unstable, since these curves include only those patients still alive. However, if a high proportion of deaths have been observed, a comparison of the follow-up in the two groups is probably not so important.

Example – *summarising follow-up* – *patients with non-small cell lung cancer treated with or without adjuvant radiotherapy*

In a trial of the value of postoperative radiotherapy in patients with non-small cell lung cancer, the Medical Research Council Lung Cancer Working Party (1996) randomised 308 patients to receive either surgery followed by radiotherapy (SR) or surgery alone (S). The follow-up curves by allocated treatment group for the 44 patients remaining alive are shown in Figure 3.12. It can be seen that there is no obvious difference between the two groups.

The minimum is given by the time of the first event, the median by the 50th percentile and the maximum by the time of the last event. These are 1, 18 and 36 months, respectively, for the S group and 2, 21 and 36 months for the SR group of patients. These are clearly very similar for both treatment groups.

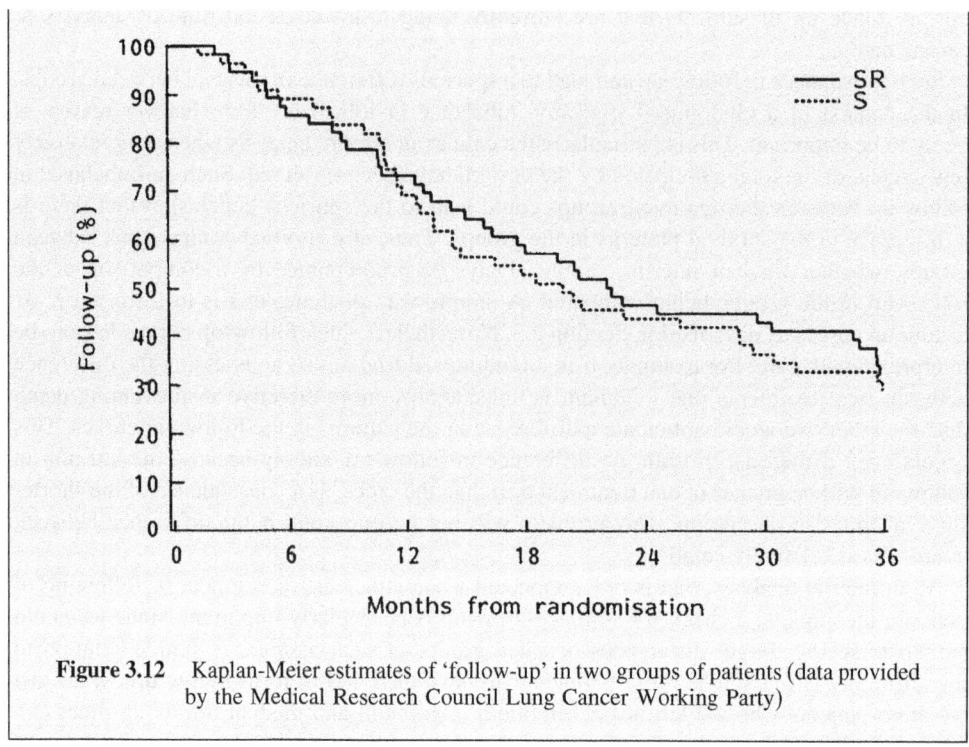

Figure 3.12   Kaplan-Meier estimates of 'follow-up' in two groups of patients (data provided
by the Medical Research Council Lung Cancer Working Party)

In cases where there does appear to be a difference in follow-up curves between groups,
any differences in survival between the two groups should be interpreted with care.

4 Parametric Modelling

Summary

This chapter describes parametric models which are often useful for analysing survival data. We first introduce the Exponential distribution, which can be used when the hazard rate is constant within a particular group of individuals. A graphical technique to help assess the validity of the assumption of a constant hazard rate is presented. The Weibull distribution is described for situations when the hazard rate is not constant but smoothly increasing (may stay the same or increase but never decreases) or decreasing with time. In addition the Log-Normal and the Log-Logistic distributions, which have a hazard rate that initially increases and then declines after reaching a peak, and the even more flexible Generalised Gamma distribution are introduced. The distinction between proportional hazard and accelerated failure time models is made. We show how survival models are used in the context of multiple regression analysis.

4.1 THE EXPONENTIAL DISTRIBUTION

CONSTANT HAZARD RATE

As indicated by equation (2.20) in Section 2.6, there is a relationship between the hazard function, $h(t)$, and the survival function $S(t)$. In fact it is stated there, with a small change in notation, that

$$h(t) = -\frac{d}{dt}[\log S(t)] \tag{4.1}$$

The right-hand side of equation (4.1) is the negative of the differential of the logarithm of $S(t)$ with respect to time t. Suppose we specify that the hazard does not change with time, t; that is, we set

$$h(t) = \lambda, \tag{4.2}$$

where λ is a constant. Then, in this case, it turns out that the survival function, $S(t)$, has the form

$$S(t) = e^{-\lambda t}. \tag{4.3}$$

This is often written $S(t) = \exp(-\lambda t)$ and is termed the survival function of the Exponential distribution. This constant hazard rate is a unique property of the Exponential distribution.

Survival Analysis Second Edition   David Machin, Yin Bun Cheung, Mahesh K.B. Parmar
© 2006 John Wiley & Sons, Ltd   ISBN: 0-470-87040-0

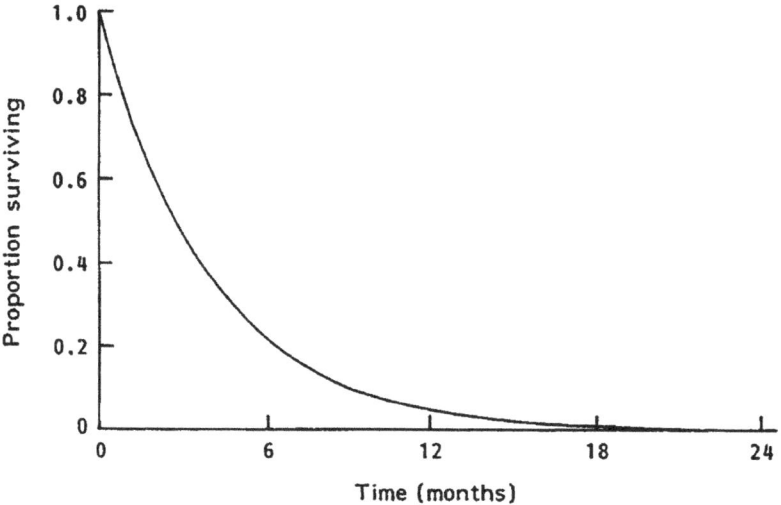

Figure 4.1   The Exponential survival function with a constant hazard $\lambda = 0.25$

The shape of the Exponential survival distribution of equation (4.3) is shown in Figure 4.1 for a particular value of the hazard rate $\lambda = 0.25$ per month. It is clear from this graph that only about 0.2 (20%) of the population remain alive at six months, less than 10% at 12 months, and there are very few survivors beyond 18 months. This is not very surprising since the hazard rate tells us that one-quarter of those alive at a given time will die in the following month.

For a value of the hazard rate $\lambda < 0.25$ the Exponential survival function will lie above that of Figure 4.1 since the death rate is lower; for $\lambda > 0.25$ it will fall below since, in this case, the death rate is higher.

A constant value of the hazard rate implies that the probability of death remains constant as successive days go by. This idea extends to saying that the probability of death in any time interval depends only on the width of the interval. Thus the wider the time interval the greater the probability of death in that interval, but where the interval begins (and ends) has no influence on the death rate.

Example – Exponential distribution – patients with colorectal cancer

Figure 4.2a shows the Exponential survival function fitted to the survival time data of the 24 patients with Dukes' C colorectal cancer used to construct Figure 2.4. It is clear that the Exponential survival function provides a close, but smoothed, summary of the *K-M* survival curve. Since there is a close fit of the Exponential survival function to these data we can conclude that patients with this disease are therefore dying at an approximately constant rate. We can see that, for those patients alive at the beginning of any month, the risk of death within that month appears not to change from that of the preceding month.

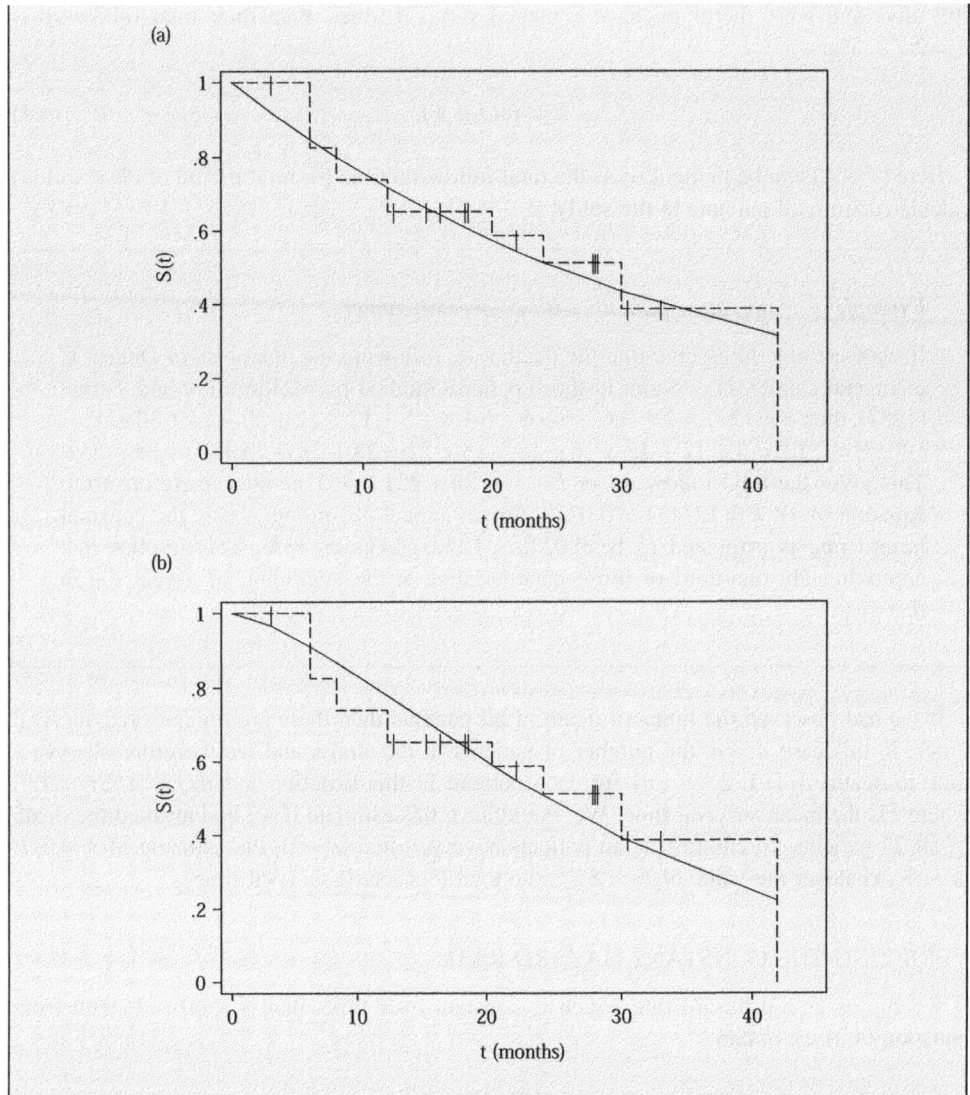

Figure 4.2 (a) Exponential survival distribution with $\lambda = 0.0278$ and (b) Weibull distribution, with $\lambda_{ML} = 0.0319$, $\kappa_{ML} = 1.4294$, fitted to the Dukes' C colorectal cancer data of McIllmurray and Turkie (1987). Reproduced by permission of *British Medical Journal*, **294**, 1260 and **295**, 475

ESTIMATING THE CONSTANT HAZARD RATE

As we have already indicated in Section 2.5, an overall estimate of the hazard rate, λ, is given by the number of deaths observed, d, divided by the total follow-up or exposure time. If t_i represents the individual survival times of the d patients who have died then their total follow-up is $f = \Sigma t_i$, and if T_j^+ represents the individual survival times of the $(n - d)$ patients still alive and who, therefore, have censored survival times, then their total follow-up is $F = \Sigma T_j^+$. Thus

$$\lambda = d/(f + F). \tag{4.4}$$

Here $(f + F)$ can be thought of as the total follow-up time (or total period of observation) calculated from all patients in the study.

Example – *death rate* – *patients with colorectal cancer*

If we were able to assume that the death rate, following the diagnosis of Dukes' C colorectal cancer, is constant in those patients studied by McIllmurray and Turkie (1987), then $d = 12$, $f = \Sigma t_i = 6+6+6+6+8+8+12+12+20+24+30+42 = 180$, $F = \Sigma T_j^+ = 3+12+15+16+18+18+22+28+28+28+30+33 = 251$. This gives the total follow-up as $f + F = 80 + 251 = 431$ months; therefore from equation (4.4), $\lambda = 12/431 = 0.0278$. On an annual (12-month) basis the constant hazard rate is estimated to be $0.0278 \times 12 = 0.3336$ or 33%. This implies that approximately one-third of those patients alive at the beginning of a year die in that year.

If we had observed the times of death of all patients then there are no censored survival times. In this case $d = n$, the number of patients in the study, and we therefore observe a time to death $t_i (i = 1, 2, \ldots, n)$ for each patient. In this situation $\lambda = n/f = n/\Sigma t_i = 1/\bar{t}$, where $\bar{t}$ is the mean survival time. We would have this estimate if we had awaited the death of all 24 patients. In contrast, if no patients have yet died ($d = 0$) the estimate of $\lambda = 0/F$ is zero, whatever the value of $F = \Sigma T_j^+$, the total (censored) survival time.

VERIFYING THE CONSTANT HAZARD RATE

If we can assume a hazard rate which is constant over time, that is, $h(t) = \lambda$, then from equation (4.3) we obtain

$$\log[S(t)] = -\lambda t \tag{4.5}$$

or

$$-\log[S(t)] = \lambda t.$$

Further, if we then take the logarithms of each side of this latter equation we obtain

$$\log\{-\log[S(t)]\} = \log \lambda + \log t. \tag{4.6}$$

This is the form of an equation of a straight line $y = a + bx$, where $y = \log\{-\log[S(t)]\}$ is the left-hand side of equation (4.6). On the right-hand side of the equation, we have $a = \log \lambda$ as the intercept, while $b = 1$ is the slope of the line and $x = \log t$.

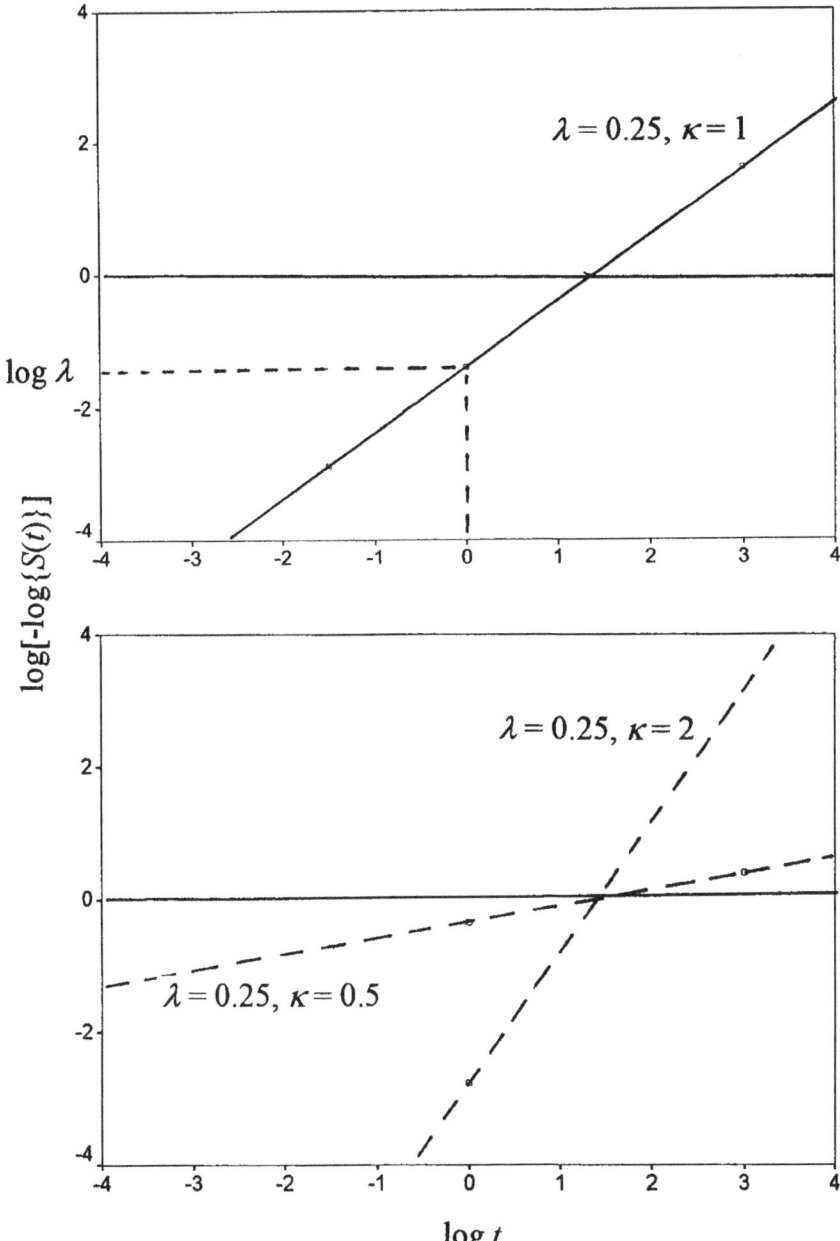

Figure 4.3   Graph of $\log\{-\log[S(t)]\}$ against the logarithm of time, $\log t$, for the Exponential survival distribution with $\lambda = 0.25$ (upper panel) and the Weibull distributions for $\lambda = 0.25$ and $\kappa = 0.5$ and 2 (lower panel)

Note that we have introduced $\log\{-\log[S(t)]\}$ when obtaining a *CI* for $S(t)$ by use of equation (2.14). Furthermore, the quantity $-\log[S(t)]$ is called the 'cumulative hazard', that is, the total hazard cumulated up to time t.

The straight-line form of equation (4.6) is shown in Figure 4.3 for the Exponential survival function with $\lambda = 0.25$. When time $t = 1$, and hence $\log t = 0$, then the right-hand side of equation (4.6) is $\log \lambda$, which is the value on the vertical axis as indicated by the hatched lines in Figure 4.3. In this case $\log \lambda = \log 0.25 = -1.386$.

With a real data example the complementary logarithmic transformation, $\log\{-\log[S(t)]\}$, is plotted against $\log t$, where $S(t)$ is the K-M estimate of the survival function at each successive death time t. If this graph is approximately a straight line then we may assume that there is a constant hazard rate. The intercept of such a graph for time $t = 1(\log t = 0)$ provides an estimate of $\log \lambda$ and hence λ, the constant hazard rate. Systematic departures from a straight line indicate that it is not appropriate to assume λ is constant. In such circumstances the value of the hazard rate depends on t and therefore changes as time passes.

Example – complementary log plot – patients with colorectal cancer

Table 4.1 summarises the calculations necessary for the complementary log plot using the K-M estimates of $S(t)$ from Table 2.2 for the data of McIllmurray and Turkie (1987). It is only possible to calculate the plot at time-points when a death occurs and the value of $S(t)$ changes. The final death at $t = 42$ months with $S(42) = 0.0000$ is omitted since the logarithm of zero is not defined.

There are six points here rather than the 12 which would have occurred if there were no tied observations. These six points are plotted in Figure 4.4. This graph indicates an approximate linear form and hence the assumption of a constant hazard rate seems reasonable for these patients.

Drawing a straight line through the data points (by eye) and extending it downwards to cut the $\log$ (time) axis at zero gives the intercept $\log \lambda = -3.24$ as indicated in Figure 4.4. From this we have $\lambda = \exp(-3.24) = 0.0392 \approx 0.04$.

This contrasts somewhat with the estimator of $\lambda = 0.0278(\approx 0.03)$ given earlier. However, the discrepancy is likely to be caused by drawing the line by eye, as the intercept is far removed from the data points, and there is the presence of both a large proportion of censored observations (50%) and tied observations in these data.

Table 4.1 Calculations necessary for testing for a constant hazard rate using the data of McIllmurray and Turkie, 1987. Data reproduced by permission of *British Medical Journal*, **294**, 1260 and **295**, 475

Survival time, t (months)	$\log t$	K-M Estimate $S(t)$	$\log[S(t)]$	$\log\{-\log[S(t)]\}$
6	1.79	0.8261	−0.1910	−1.66
8	2.08	0.7391	−0.3023	−1.20
12	2.48	0.6522	−0.4274	−0.85
20	3.00	0.5780	−0.5482	−0.60
24	3.18	0.5136	−0.6663	−0.41
30	3.40	0.3852	−0.9540	−0.05
42	3.74	0.0000	−	−

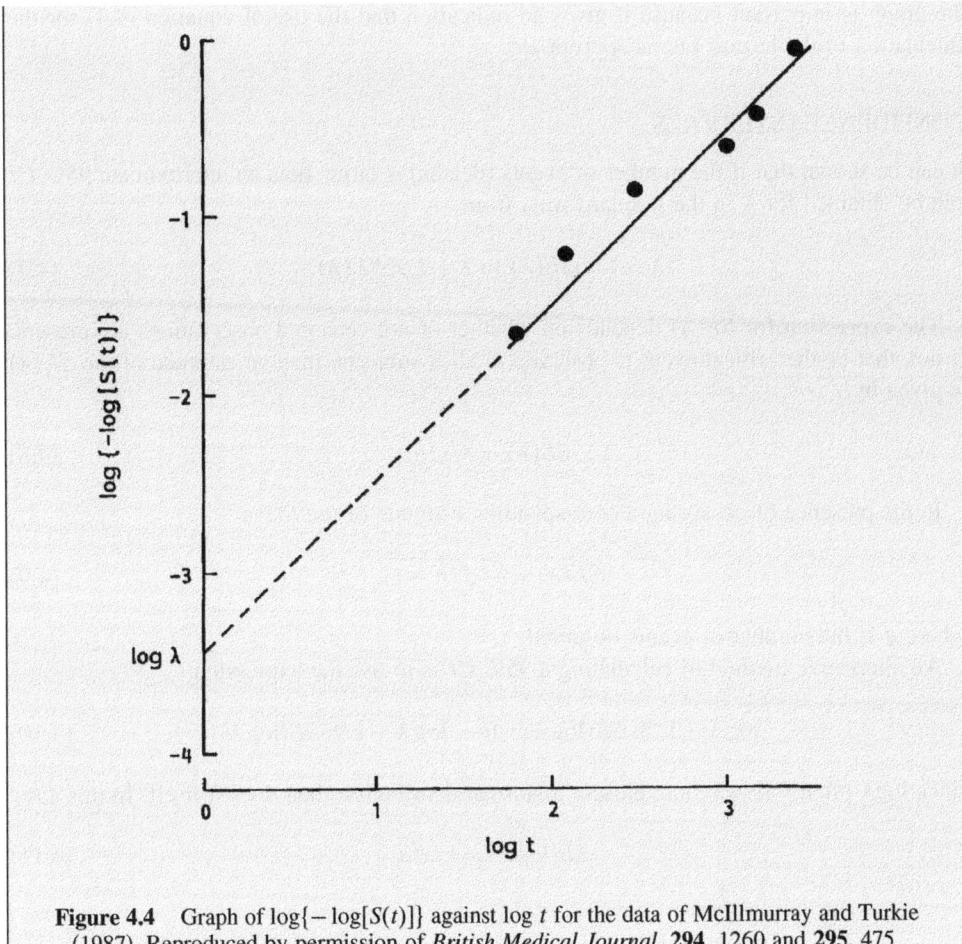

Figure 4.4   Graph of $\log\{-\log[S(t)]\}$ against $\log t$ for the data of McIllmurray and Turkie (1987). Reproduced by permission of *British Medical Journal*, **294**, 1260 and **295**, 475

As we have already noted from equation (4.6) the slope of the fitted line, the multiplier of $\log t$, is unity, and so if the Exponential distribution is appropriate then the slope, b, of Figure 4.4 should be approximately unity also.

In fact, we can estimate b from the graph by calculating the change in y divided by the corresponding change in x. To do this we take any two values for x (say) $x_1 = \log t_1 = 1$ and $x_2 = \log t_2 = 3$ for convenience, with corresponding values $y_1 = -2.46$ and $y_2 = -0.52$ read from the graph. These give

$$b = \frac{y_2 - y_1}{x_2 - x_1} = \frac{-0.52 - (-2.46)}{3 - 1} = \frac{1.94}{2} = 0.97.$$

This is close to unity and gives further support for the use of the Exponential distribution in describing these data.

However, the expression given in equation (4.4) should always be preferred to calculate λ as it makes full use of the censored survival times and the tied observations. Nevertheless, the graph is important because it gives an indication that the use of equation (4.4) for the calculation of the hazard rate is appropriate.

CONFIDENCE INTERVALS

It can be shown that if the number of events (deaths) is large, then an approximate 95% *CI* can be obtained for λ in the standard way, from

$$\lambda - 1.96 SE(\lambda) \text{ to } \lambda + 1.96 SE(\lambda). \tag{4.7}$$

The expression for $SE(\lambda)$ depends on whether or not censored observations are present. If not, that is, the critical event is observed in all n subjects, then an estimate of the $SE(\lambda)$ is given by

$$SE(\lambda) = \lambda/\sqrt{n}. \tag{4.8}$$

In the presence of censoring a corresponding estimate of the *SE* is

$$SE(\lambda) = \lambda/\sqrt{(d-1)}. \tag{4.9}$$

where d is the number of events observed.

An alternative method of calculating a 95% *CI* is to use the expression

$$\log \lambda - 1.96\ SE(\log \lambda) \quad \text{to} \quad \log \lambda + 1.96 SE(\log \lambda) \tag{4.10}$$

since $\log \lambda$ often follows more closely a Normal distribution than does λ itself. In this case

$$SE(\log \lambda) = 1/\sqrt{d}. \tag{4.11}$$

Example – CI for a death rate – patients with colorectal cancer

Applying equation (4.9) to the Dukes' C colorectal cancer data with $d = 12$, $\lambda = 0.0278$ (but remembering that the number of deaths here is quite small) gives $SE(\lambda) = 0.0278/\sqrt{11} = 0.008395$. A 95% CI for λ is therefore $0.0278 - 1.96 \times 0.008395$ to $0.0278 + 1.96 \times 0.008395$ or 0.0113 to 0.0442 per month. On an annual basis this is 14% to 53%, which is extremely wide, as one might expect from such a small study.

Alternatively, substituting $\lambda = 0.0278$ in equation (4.10) gives $\log \lambda = -3.5827$, $SE(\log \lambda) = 1/\sqrt{12} = 0.2887$ and the 95% CI for $\log \lambda$ as $-3.5827 - 1.96 \times 0.2887$ to $-3.5827 + 1.96 \times 0.2887$ or -4.1485 to -3.0169. If we exponentiate both limits of this interval we obtain $\exp(-4.1485) = 0.0158$ to $\exp(-3.0169) = 0.0490$ for the 95% CI for λ. These are very similar to those obtained previously but the CI is no longer symmetric about $\lambda = 0.0278$. It is preferable, however, always to use this latter approach as equation (4.7) can lead, for example, to negative values of the lower confidence limit.

GRAPHICAL COMPARISON OF TWO SURVIVAL CURVES

We have introduced the use of the Logrank test to compare the survival curves of patients with cervical cancers on either a standard therapy A or a new therapy B, the data for which were given in Table 3.8. Figure 4.5 shows the graph of $\log\{-\log[S(t)]\}$ against $\log t$, by therapy allocated, for these same data. Two features can be seen: Firstly, each of the two curves is roughly linear with a slope about 1, suggesting that the Exponential distribution may give a reasonable representation of the survival data for the individual treatment arms. Secondly, the two curves are approximately parallel. In fact, the (hatched) straight lines have been drawn to be parallel and have slope 1, so that deviations from these two assumptions could be graphically revealed. As it happens, the lines fitted by 'eye' under these constraints give a reasonable description of these data. Since the sample size was small, some deviation from linearity and non-parallelism would be expected. If we use h_A and h_B to represent the hazard rates in the two groups then the curves indicate that their ratio, $HR = h_B/h_A$, is approximately constant. This implies that at whatever time, t, we choose to compare the groups this ratio is maintained.

Reading from the intercepts, that is where the curves cross $\log(\text{year}) = 0$, gives $\log h_A \approx -1.0$, $\log h_B \approx -1.7$, leading to $h_A = \exp(-1.0) = 0.37$ and $h_B = \exp(-1.7) = 0.18$ respectively. This indicates that the hazard in group B was approximate half ($0.18/0.37 = 0.49$) that of group A.

A parametric model assumes that the survival data can be described by a particular survival-time distribution, the parameters of which have to be estimated. When the hazard ratio for the groups to be compared is constant over time or is approximately so, this is termed proportional hazards (PH). This PH assumption has an important role in survival analysis.

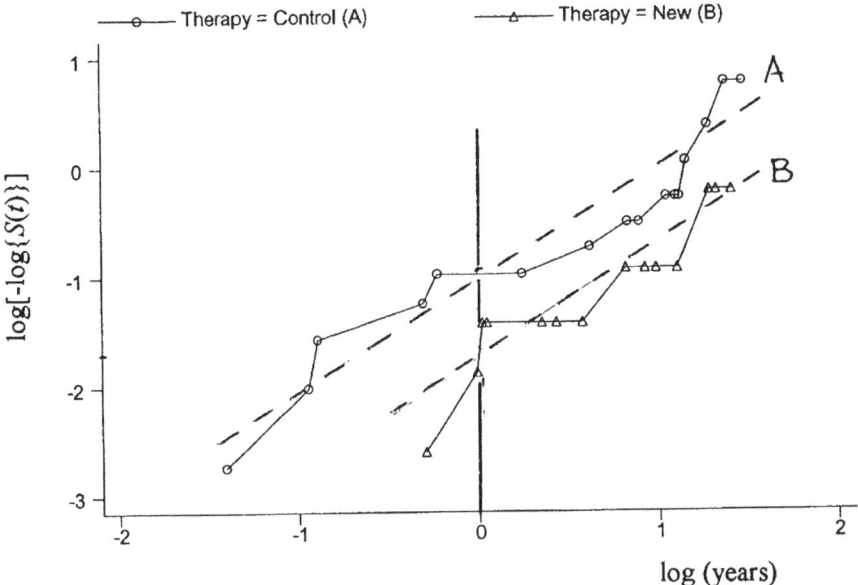

Figure 4.5   Graph of $\log\{-\log[S(t)]\}$ against $\log t$ for two treatment groups for 30 patients recruited to a cervical cancer clinical trial

REGRESSION (OR MODEL BASED) COMPARISON OF TWO SURVIVAL CURVES

Since the $\log\{-\log[S(t)]\}$ plots of Figure 4.5 are (approximately) parallel and therefore suggest the individual hazards from the two groups do not vary with time, then the hazard for group A can be specified by $h_A = \lambda$ while for group B it is $h_B = \lambda \times HR$. [Had they been approximately parallel but did vary with time we would have written, $h_A = \lambda(t)$ and $h_B = \lambda(t) \times HR$.]

On the log scale these two hazards can be combined into one expression or regression model, that is

$$\log(h) = \log\lambda + (\log HR)x. \tag{4.12}$$

Here $x = 0$ for group A and $x = 1$ for group B. This is in the familiar form $y = a + bx$ with the regression coefficient $b = \log HR$. The corresponding survival functions are expressed as

$$S(t) = \exp[-\exp\{\log\lambda + (\log HR)x\} \times t]. \tag{4.13}$$

Estimation of the parameters $\log\lambda$ and $\log HR$ is usually performed using a computer to obtain the maximum likelihood estimates by an iterative or 'trial-and-error' method as described in the technical details Section 4.7.

Example – HR – patients with cervical cancer

Using an Exponential distribution, it is estimated that the $\log HR$ that contrasts the new therapy group (B) in relation to the control group (A) for the patients with cervical cancer is -0.6676 (95% $CI = -1.72$ to 0.39) (see Table 4.2). This gives $HR = \exp(-0.6676) = 0.51$ (95% $CI = 0.18$ to 1.48).

This confirms our observation from the Figure 4.5 that the hazard rate of group B is approximately half that of group A. However, the CI of the HR is quite wide and included the null value of $HR = 1$.

Table 4.2 Parametric proportional hazard modelling of the cervical cancer trial data of Table 3.8 using Exponential and Weibull models

Distribution	Parameter	Estimate	SE	z	p-value	95% CI
Exponential	$\log HR$	-0.6676	0.5394	-1.24	0.216	-1.72 to 0.39
	$\log\lambda$	-1.1367	0.3015	-3.77	0.000	-1.73 to -0.55
	λ	0.3209				
Weibull	$\log HR$	-0.6400	0.5400	-1.19	0.236	-1.70 to 0.42
	$\log\lambda$	-1.4658	0.4262	-3.44	0.001	-2.30 to -0.63
	$\log\kappa$	0.2801	0.2160	1.30	0.195	-0.14 to 0.70
	λ	0.3303				
	κ	1.3233				

> Note that in our earlier calculations in Chapter 3 we expressed the *HR* as the ratio of the hazard of group *A* to that of group *B*, this gave $HR = 1.97$ but $1/1.97 = 0.51$, whereas here we have expressed the *HR* in the inverse sense. The two formats (group *A* compared with group *B* or vice-versa) are clearly equivalent. In this example the numerical estimates given by the two approaches to calculating the *HR*, here and in Chapter 3, are the same.

Parametric models have the ability to simultaneously analyse the effect of more than one independent variable. For the case with ν independent variables, equation (4.12) can be extended to

$$\log(h) = \beta_0 + \beta_1 x_1 + \cdots + \beta_\nu x_\nu, \qquad (4.14)$$

where $\exp(\beta_1), \ldots, \exp(\beta_\nu)$ are hazard ratios for the covariates $x_1, \ldots, x_\nu$. Finally $\exp(\beta_0) = \lambda_0$, corresponds to the hazard of a subject who has a value zero for each independent variable.

If an independent variable is continuous, it is often desirable to centre the values at the mean before analysis so the $\exp(\beta_0)$ has an interpretation of the hazard level of an 'average' person. To estimate the coefficients β_i the maximum likelihood method via computer is used.

***Example** – influence of age at diagnosis – patients with cervical cancer*

Table 3.8 shows the age of the patients in the cervical cancer trial. The mean age at diagnosis is 55, to the nearest integer and so we generate a new variable, $Age_{centre} = Age - 55$. The $\log HR$ estimated from an Exponential model is given in Table 4.3. The analysis suggests that patients on therapy *B* have a hazard reduced by

Table 4.3 Multivariable analysis using parametric proportional hazard (*PH*) and accelerated failure time (*AFT*) models with the Exponential distribution

Model	Independent variable	log *HR*	*SE*	*z*	*p*-value	95% *CI*
Proportional Hazards (*PH*)	Intercept	−1.1431	0.3024	3.780	0.000	−1.74 to −0.55
	Therapy	−0.6344	0.5409	−1.173	0.241	−1.69 to 0.43
	$Age_{centred}$	−0.0131	0.0224	−0.585	0.557	−0.06 to 0.03
	Independent variable	log *TR*	*SE*	*z*	*p*-value	95% *CI*
Accelerated Failure Time (*AFT*)	Intercept	1.1431	0.3024	3.780	0.000	0.55 to 1.74
	Therapy	0.6344	0.5409	1.173	0.241	−0.43 to 1.69
	$Age_{centred}$	0.0131	0.0224	0.585	0.557	−0.03 to 0.06

a factor of $HR = \exp(-0.6344) = 0.53$, and for every year older (at diagnosis) the hazard was reduced by a factor of $\exp(-0.0131) = 0.99$. The value of the HR, here adjusted for the patient age, is little different from that of $HR = 0.51$ obtained from the analysis summarised in the upper portion of Table 4.2. This suggests that, although age may be influential for outcome, the two treatment groups are sufficiently well balanced in age that taking this into account does not change our view of the relative merits of the two treatment options to any degree.

ACCELERATED FAILURE TIME (AFT) MODELS

In studies of mortality, it usually makes sense to think in terms of the hazard and the hazard ratio when making comparisons between groups. In some other situations, it is easier to think in terms of the relative length of time to the event. For instance, Cheung, Yip and Karlberg (2001b) studied the age at which infants achieve the developmental milestones of building a tower of three cubes and independent walking. They considered it more intuitive to estimate and present the effects of covariates in terms of time ratios (TR). A TR less than one implied that the infants achieved the developmental milestones at an earlier age. In other words, the time-to-event is accelerated. The corresponding models are termed Accelerated Failure Time (AFT) models.

It is often said that the life expectancy of a man is seven times that of a dog. According to this statement, we may say that the TR for a man to die is seven (decelerated):

$$\bar{t}_{Man} = TR \times \bar{t}_{Dog} = 7\bar{t}_{Dog}. \tag{4.15}$$

Earlier in this section we have worked out that, for an Exponential distribution, the relation between the hazard rate and mean time-to-event is given by $h(t) = \lambda = 1/\bar{t}$, or equivalently, $\bar{t} = 1/\lambda = 1/h(t)$. Even if there is censoring and hence not all t are observed, we may still use the inverse of the constant hazard to estimate the mean survival time. Substituting this relation into equation (4.15), it can be seen that the ratio of mortality hazard of a man to that of a dog is $1/7$, that is, $HR = 1/TR = 1/7$.

If the log scale is used, then $\log(TR) = \log(7) = 1.9459 = -(-1.9459) = -\log(1/7) = -\log(HR)$. This very simple relation between the $\log(TR)$ and $\log(HR)$ is not a coincidence; this is a characteristic of the Exponential distribution but this is not the case when the hazard changes with time.

The AFT estimates the relation between log expected time-to-event and covariates in the familiar form of a linear regression equation

$$\log(\bar{t}) = \eta_0 + \eta_1 x_1 + \cdots + \eta_k x_k. \tag{4.16}$$

This contrasts with the PH model of equation (4.14), which estimates a linear relation between log hazard and covariates in the form of $\log(h) = \beta_0 + \beta_1 x_1 + \cdots + \beta_k x_k$. However, since

$$\log(\bar{t}) = \log(1/h) = \log(1) - \log(h) = 0 - \log(h) = -\log(h), \tag{4.17}$$

then by substituting equation (4.14) into the right-hand side, and (4.16) into the left-hand side of equation (4.17), it can be seen that the regression coefficients arising from the *PH* and *AFT* models only differ in sign, that is, $\eta_i = -\beta_i$. This highlights the fact the *PH* and *AFT* models are equivalent in the Exponential distribution situation; they are just expressed in different ways. Effectively we are saying that if the risk or hazard *increases* then the average survival time *decreases*.

Now, if the independent variable x_1 is associated with a higher hazard, then β_1 is positive while η_1 is negative, and the expected log survival time is shorter. In the Exponential AFT model $\exp(\eta_1)$ is the time ratio (*TR*). Furthermore, η_0 gives the expected log survival time of subjects whose covariate values are $x_1 = 0$. The *TR*s and 95% CI of the Exponential *AFT* model fitted to the cervical cancer trial data are shown in Table 4.3 and these confirm that for the Exponential distribution the parameter estimates are the same, with just a sign change.

4.2   THE WEIBULL DISTRIBUTION

VARIABLE HAZARD RATE

As we have indicated, the exponential distribution assumes the hazard rate, λ, is constant and does not depend on time. Thus, as time progresses for a particular individual, the risk in successive time intervals remains unchanged. There are, however, circumstances in which we know that this will not be the case. For example, following major surgery, death is more likely to occur in the immediate postoperative period in many situations but then may return to an approximately constant (and lower) level thereafter. In other words, the operative procedure itself brings a risk of death over and above that of the disease itself. There are other situations in which the (instantaneous) hazard could be increasing or decreasing with time. For example, the risk of death to a newborn infant is high in the first days of life; thereafter it rapidly decreases and remains low and approximately constant, until much later in life, when it begins to increase again.

One way of making the hazard depend on time is to modify the Exponential survival function of equation (4.3) in a simple way, as follows:

$$S(t) = \exp\left[-(\lambda t)^\kappa\right] \qquad (4.18)$$

where κ is a constant whose value is greater than zero. This is known as the Weibull distribution. In the particular case of $\kappa = 1$ equation (4.18) becomes equation (4.3), and we have the Exponential distribution again.

Equation (4.18) can be written as $\log[S(t)] = -(\lambda t)^\kappa$, which can be compared with equation (4.5). The hazard function is obtained from this expression by differentiating with respect to t, see equation (4.1), to give

$$h(t) = \kappa\lambda(\lambda t)^{\kappa-1}. \qquad (4.19)$$

This is known as the hazard function for the Weibull distribution and clearly depends on time, since t is included on the right-hand side of the expression.

This hazard function looks somewhat complicated but if we set $\kappa = 1$ in equation (4.19) then $h(t) = 1 \times \lambda(\lambda t)^{1-1} = \lambda(\lambda t)^0 = \lambda$. This is then the constant hazard of the Exponential survival distribution that we have discussed before.

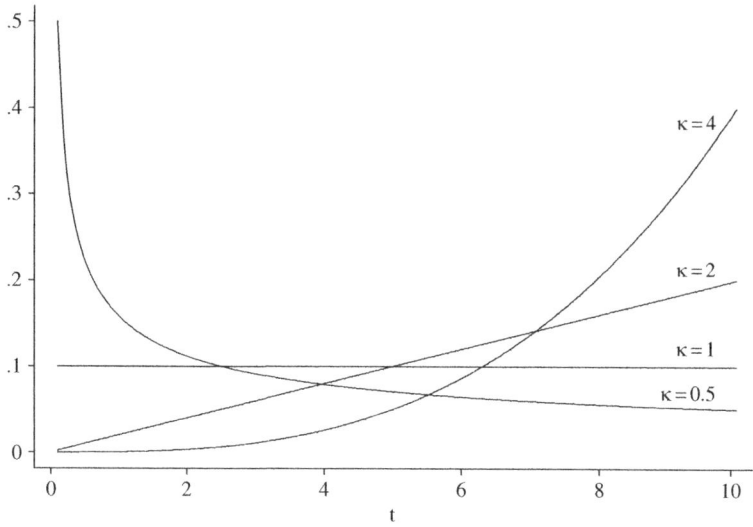

Figure 4.6 Hazard functions of the Weibull distribution with $\lambda = 0.1$ and varying values of κ

Equation (4.19) gives a hazard rate which changes with time and whose shape depends on the value of κ. Some of these shapes are illustrated in Figure 4.6, with a value of $\lambda = 0.1$. For example, with $\kappa = 0.5$, $h(t) = 0.5 \times 0.1 \times (0.1 \times t)^{0.5-1} = 0.1581/\sqrt{t}$, and the hazard rate is at first high, then rapidly falls until $t = 3$, beyond which the fall slows down. If $\kappa = 1$ then the hazard rate is the constant value of the Exponential situation already referred to. For $\kappa = 2$, $h(t) = 2 \times \lambda(\lambda t) = 2\lambda^2 t$ and the hazard rate increases from zero in a linear way with t with slope $2\lambda^2$. For $\kappa = 4$, $h(t) = 4\lambda^4 t^3$ and this hazard rate increases from zero at time $t = 0$.

Such a range of shapes for the possible hazard function makes the Weibull distribution a good choice to describe a variety of survival time problems.

GRAPHICAL METHODS

A graphical test for suitability of the Weibull distribution to describe the data can be derived in a similar way to that for the Exponential distribution. Thus taking logarithms, changing signs and taking logarithms again of equation (4.18), we have

$$\log\{-\log[S(t)]\} = \kappa \log \lambda + \kappa \log t. \tag{4.20}$$

This is the equation for a straight line with respect to $\log t$ and with intercept $a = \kappa \log \lambda$ and slope $b = \kappa$. This expression reduces to equation (4.6) in the situation when $\kappa = 1$.

Hence a plot of $\log\{-\log[S(t)]\}$ against $\log t$ with a particular data set provides a graphical test of the Weibull distribution. If the resulting plot is indeed approximately a straight line with a slope different from unity (the value for the constant hazard Exponential distribution), then this indicates that a Weibull distribution may describe the data sufficiently well.

***Example** – fitting the Weibull distribution – patients with colorectal cancer*

We use the data of McIllmurray and Turkie (1987) plotted in Figure 4.4 for illustration. As noted earlier the plot is approximately linear and we have calculated the slope $b = 0.97$. This provides us with our estimate of $\kappa = b = 0.97$. The intercept at $t = 1$ gives $a = \kappa \log \lambda = -3.24$ and therefore $\log \lambda = -3.24/\kappa = -3.24/0.97 = -3.340$. Finally $\lambda = \exp(-3.340) = 0.0354$. This estimate differs from the graphical estimate of the hazard rate of 0.0278 for the Exponential distribution given earlier.

The estimate of the hazard rate, λ, from this Weibull model is close to that from the Exponential model because κ is close to unity in this example.

ESTIMATING λ AND κ

To obtain the maximum likelihood estimates of λ and κ using the full information available rather than that provided by the graphical method of Figure 4.4, it is necessary to solve quite complicated equations. These equations are

$$W(\kappa) = \frac{\Sigma t_i^\kappa \log t_i + \Sigma T_j^{+\kappa} \log T_j^+}{\Sigma t_i^\kappa + \Sigma T_j^{+\kappa}} - \frac{\Sigma \log t_i}{d} - \frac{1}{\kappa} = 0 \qquad (4.21)$$

and

$$\lambda = \left[d / (\Sigma t_i^\kappa + \Sigma T_j^{+\kappa}) \right]^{1/\kappa}. \qquad (4.22)$$

To solve equation (4.21) for κ involves finding a particular κ which makes $W(\kappa) = 0$. Once κ is obtained, λ is calculated using equation (4.22). One method of solving equation (4.21) is by 'trial-and-error'. For example, we can obtain an estimate of $\kappa = \kappa_G$ from the graphical method just described. We then substitute κ_G in equation (4.21) to obtain $W(\kappa_G)$. If this is zero then our graphical estimate itself is indeed the solution to the equation. More usually $W(\kappa_G) \neq 0$ and we need to choose a second value of κ perhaps a little smaller (or larger) than κ_G and calculate $W(\kappa)$ again. If this is nearer to zero, or perhaps of the opposite sign to the previous value then this may indicate the next value of κ to choose and that the calculations be repeated once more. The same process is repeated with differing values for κ until $W(\kappa) = 0$ is obtained. The corresponding value of κ is then the maximum likelihood solution, κ_{ML}, of equation (4.21). Substituting κ_{ML}, in equation (4.22) then gives the maximum likelihood estimate of λ, or λ_{ML}.

***Example** – estimating the parameters of the Weibull distribution – patients with colorectal cancer*

From the graphical approach of Figure 4.4, we have $\kappa = 0.97$ for the data of McIllmurray and Turkie (1987) and with this value the calculations of

Table 4.4 are required. Substituting the appropriate column totals in equation (4.21) gives

$$W(0.97) = \frac{491.7489 + 715.8394}{166.5359 + 228.4675} - \frac{29.6730}{12} - \frac{1}{0.97}$$
$$= 3.0572 - 2.4728 - 1.0309 = -0.4465.$$

This is clearly not equal to zero and so a different value for κ is required. Table 4.5 gives the value of $W(\kappa)$ for differing values of κ and shows that when $\kappa = 1.4294$, $W(\kappa) = 0$. We then use $\kappa_{ML} = 1.4294$ in equation (4.22) to obtain $\lambda_{ML} = 0.0319$. The final Weibull fit to the Kaplan-Meier survival curve is shown in Figure 4.2(b). This describes the data reasonably well but differs from the Exponential fit of Figure 4.2(a) in that there is a small 'shoulder' in the early part of the curve.

Table 4.4 Summary of calculations to obtain $W(\kappa)$ as a step to obtaining the maximum likelihood estimate of κ for a Weibull distribution beginning with a starting value of $\kappa = 0.97$ obtained from the graphical approach of Figure 4.4

t_i	t_i^κ	$\log t_i$	$t_i^\kappa \log t_i$	T_j^+	$T_j^{+\kappa}$	$\log T_j^+$	$T_j^{+\kappa} \log T_j^+$
6	5.6860	1.7918	10.1879	3	2.9027	1.0986	3.1890
6	5.6860	1.7918	10.1879	12	11.1380	2.4849	27.6768
6	5.6860	1.7918	10.1879	15	13.8296	2.7081	37.4512
6	5.6860	1.7918	10.1879	16	14.7230	2.7726	40.8208
8	7.5162	2.0794	15.6295	18	16.5050	2.8904	47.7055
8	7.5162	2.0794	15.6295	18	16.5050	2.8904	47.7055
12	11.1380	2.4849	27.6768	22	20.0516	3.0910	61.9805
12	11.1380	2.4849	27.6768	28	25.3363	3.3322	84.4258
20	18.2810	2.9957	54.7649	28	25.3363	3.3322	84.4258
24	21.8175	3.1781	69.3372	28	25.3363	3.3322	84.4258
32	28.8400	3.4657	99.9519	30	27.0899	3.4012	92.1381
42	37.5450	3.7377	140.3307	33	29.7138	3.4965	103.8946
Total	166.5359	29.6730	491.7489		228.4675		715.8394

Table 4.5 Summary of the iterative calculations necessary to estimate λ of the Weibull distribution

Iteration	κ	$W(\kappa)$	λ
0	0.97	−0.4465	0.0273
1	1.0	−0.4070	0.0277
2	1.2	−0.1871	0.0301
3	1.4	−0.0211	0.0317
4	1.4294	0.0000	0.0319
5	1.5	0.0478	0.0323

REGRESSION (OR MODEL BASED) COMPARISON OF TWO SURVIVAL CURVES

If the *PH* assumption is valid but the hazard rates within the individual groups to be compared appear to increase or decrease over time, one may consider using the Weibull model. The parameter κ is assumed to be the same for each treatment group, but the hazard functions differ by a constant ratio. To compare groups A and B, therefore, the model has the hazard functions, expressed in a rather complex way, as $h_A(t) = \kappa\lambda(\lambda t)^{\kappa-1} = \kappa(\lambda^\kappa)t^{\kappa-1} = \kappa\exp(\kappa\log\lambda)t^{\kappa-1}$ and $h_B(t) = HR \times h_A(t) = \exp(\log HR) \times \kappa\exp(\kappa\log\lambda)t^{\kappa-1}$. From these the two hazard functions can then be expressed in a single model as:

$$h(t) = \kappa\exp[\kappa\log\lambda + (\log HR)x]t^{\kappa-1}, \tag{4.24}$$

where $x = 0$ represents Group A and $x = 1$ Group B.

The estimation has to be performed by maximum likelihood method with a computer. Since the Weibull distribution requires that κ is always greater than 0, the computer algorithm usually estimates $\log\kappa$ instead of κ itself. This guarantees that the estimate obtained for κ is always greater than 0. One can then exponentiate the estimate of $\log\kappa$ and also the limits of the corresponding 95% CI, to obtain κ and the 95% CI.

Example – *comparing Exponential and Weibull survival distributions* – *patients with colorectal cancer*

Fitting the Weibull distribution to the colorectal cancer trial data gives a $\log HR = -0.6400$. This is very similar to the result when using an Exponential distribution as is shown in Table 4.2. and so the estimates of λ too are very close. The second parameter is estimated by $\kappa = \exp(0.2801) = 1.32$ with 95% CI of $\exp(-0.1433) = 0.87$ to $\exp(0.7034) = 2.02$. This interval includes the null hypothesis value of $\kappa = 1$, and suggests for these data that the extra complexity of the Weibull model provides little advantage over the Exponential model.

Just as for the Exponential model, the Weibull model can be used for performing multi-variable regression. For the case of ν explanatory variables, equation (4.24) becomes

$$h(t) = \kappa\exp[\kappa\log(\lambda) + \beta_1 x_1 + \beta_2 x_2 + \cdots + \beta_\nu x_\nu 1]t^{\kappa-1},$$

where the β's are the $\log HR$s of the ν variables.

ACCELERATED FAILURE TIME (*AFT*) MODELS

The Weibull regression model can also be parameterised as an *AFT* model. For the Weibull model, the relationship between the regression coefficients under the *PH* and *AFT* models is more complicated and involves the parameter κ, in that each $\eta_i = -\beta_i/\kappa$. More details about the relation between the *PH* and *AFT* forms of the Weibull regression model can be found in Collett (2003).

Example – *Weibull and AFT models* – *patients with cervical cancer*

In Table 4.6 we fit the cervical cancer data again but now using the Weibull *PH* and *AFT* models. The first thing to note is that the estimate of κ under both models is precisely the same and, although indicative of $\kappa > 1$, the 95% CI covers the null value of 1. This suggests that this model may be no better than the Exponential regression model. The log *TR* and log *HR* estimated are very similar to those of Table 4.3, which are based on an Exponential distribution.

Table 4.6 Multivariable analysis of therapy adjusted for age using *PH* and *AFT* Weibull models to data from patients with cervical cancer

Model	Independent variable	log *HR*	SE	z	p-value	95% CI
PH	Therapy	−0.6040	0.5401	−1.118	0.263	−1.6627 to 0.4546
	Age$_{Centred}$	−0.0179	0.0226	−0.792	0.429	−0.0623 to 0.0265
	Intercept	−1.5042	0.4297			
	log κ	0.3075	0.2170			−0.1177 to 0.7327
	κ	1.36				0.89 to 2.08
	Independent variable	**log *TR***	**SE**	**z**	**p-value**	**95% CI**
AFT	Therapy	0.4441	0.4126	1.076	0.282	−0.3645 to 1.2528
	Age$_{Centred}$	0.0132	0.0164	0.805	0.422	−0.0190 to 0.0453
	Intercept	1.1060	0.2226			
	log κ	0.3075				−0.1177 to 0.7327
	κ	1.36				0.89 to 2.08

4.3 OTHER ACCELERATED FAILURE TIME (*AFT*) DISTRIBUTIONS

The Exponential and Weibull distributions are special in that they can be parameterised as both *PH* and as *AFT* models. For these two distributions these two forms are equivalent, they are just expressed differently. In contrast we now introduce the log-Normal, Generalised Gamma and the Log-Logistic distributions which are all *AFT* models but they cannot be expressed in terms of *PH* models.

LOG-NORMAL

If the log survival time, log t, follows a Normal distribution with mean μ and SD σ, then the Log-Normal distribution has the following hazard function:

$$h(t) = \frac{\frac{1}{t\sigma\sqrt{2\pi}} \exp\left[-\frac{1}{2}\left(\frac{\log t - \mu}{\sigma}\right)^2\right]}{1 - \Phi\left[\left(\frac{\log t - \mu}{\sigma}\right)\right]}. \tag{4.25}$$

Here Φ is the cumulative Normal distribution function and this corresponds to the area to the left of any point on the z-axis of Figure 1.7. The notation ϕ is used in a similar way in equation (2.18). One can see from equation (4.25) that this is a rather complex expression which prevents expressing log h in a linear form that depends on explanatory variables without involving t. This is why it cannot lead to a *PH* model.

Figure 4.7(a) shows some hazard functions with different combinations of μ (mu) and σ^2 (sigma2). Note that even for the same σ, the ratio of two hazard functions with different μ changes over time, reflecting the non-*PH* feature.

This form of hazard may be useful in certain circumstances as, in contrast to that of the Exponential and Weibull distributions, this hazard function increases initially and then decreases with time. This form of hazard may arise in many clinical and epidemiological

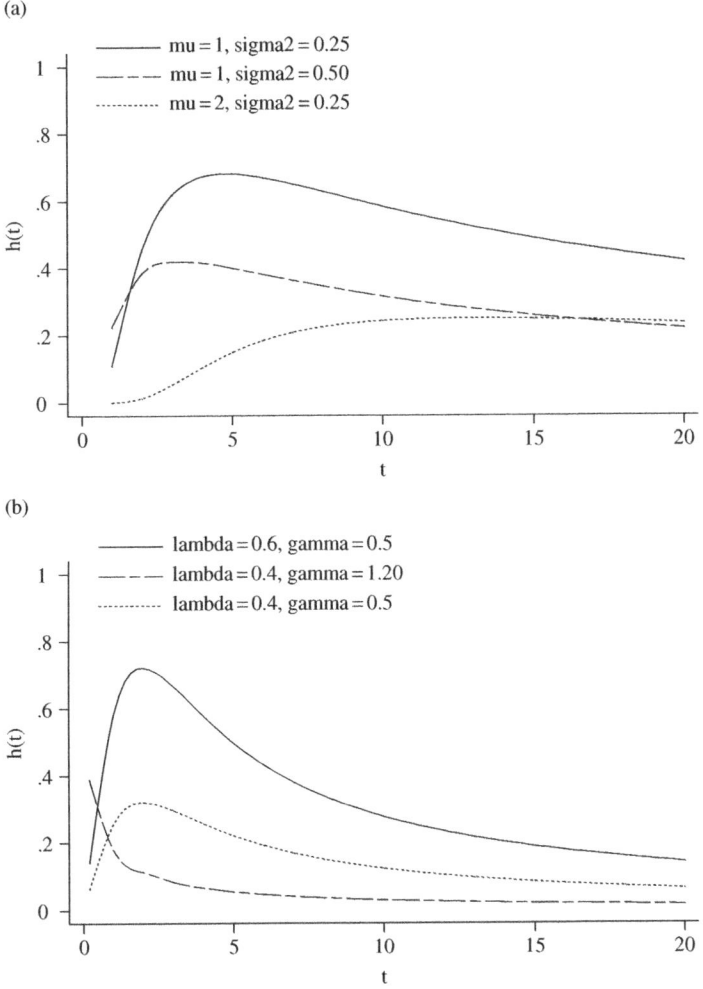

Figure 4.7 Some examples of the (a) Log-Normal and (b) Log-Logistic hazard functions

situations. For example, immediately after surgical removal of a cancer, the risk of tumour recurrence is often small but then may increase for a period but thereafter begins to decline once more. Similarly, in many countries the likelihood of first marriage is small in the neighbourhood of the minimum legal age for marriage, then it increases sharply and reaches a peak amongst the 25 to 30 year age groups, then it slowly declines thereafter.

GENERALISED GAMMA

The Generalised Gamma distribution allows an even wider range of hazard patterns to be modelled. For instance, it may increase smoothly but with an ever-decreasing rate and so eventually approach an asymptote. The flexibility is achieved by having two model-specific distributional parameters, often referred to as a shape parameter and a scale parameter. This shape of hazard function cannot be described by, for example, the Weibull distribution for which the hazard increases without boundary. An important feature of the Generalised Gamma distribution is that the Exponential, Weibull and Log-Normal distributions are each a special case (nested) of this distribution. One can then compare the goodness-of-fit of the Generalised Gamma model with that of its special cases by the *LR* test.

However, it is sometimes difficult to fit as the maximum likelihood estimation procedure may not converge. This is a reason why the Generalised Gamma distribution is not routinely used in place of the Exponential, Weibull and Log-Normal distributions. Furthermore, it is mathematically very complex, and so its algebraic form is omitted here. As with other *AFT* models, this relates log *t* to explanatory variables by the regression equation (4.16).

Example – time ratio(TR) – motor development in infants

In a study of motor development in Pakistani infants, Cheung, Yip and Karlberg (2001b) used a Generalised Gamma multivariable regression model to investigate the relation between the z-score of weight-for-length at birth to the age at independent walking. As size at birth is usually associated with socio-economic status and some other social or clinical variables, multiple regression was needed to adjust for these potential confounders. Having controlled for covariates, a time ratio of $TR = 0.96$ (95% *CI* 0.94 to 0.98) was found. That is, a higher z-score at birth was associated with an earlier achievement of the milestone. Since the mean age that infants started independent walking was about $\bar{y} = 14$ months, the *TR* suggested that an infant with a weight-for-length of 1 z-score above average would start walking at about $TR^1 \times \bar{y} = 0.96^1 \times 14 = 13.44$ months compared to the average. More generally, an infant with a weight-for-length of k z-score units above average would start walking at about $TR^k \times \bar{y} = 0.96^k \times 14$ months.

Example – Generalised Gamma distribution – patients with recurrent nasopharyngeal carcinoma

Poon, Yap, Wong, *et al.* (2004) used non-parametric methods to assess the relation between various clinical characteristics and survival time (in months) in 35 patients with recurrent nasopharyngeal carcinoma who were referred to a tertiary centre. The hazard in half-yearly intervals is estimated using the method described in Section 2.5 and is shown in Figure 4.8. The mortality hazard was initially low. It then climbed and peaked at the interval 18 to 24 months since referral to the centre, from which it started to decline. There was some fluctuation from 30 to 42 months. However, the number of patients at risk at this period was small and so some fluctuation is not surprising. For such a pattern of hazard the Exponential and Weibull distributions are clearly inappropriate. The mean age of the patients was about 45. Twenty four patients had only one recurrence of tumour prior to referral and 11 had more than one prior recurrence (multiple recurrences = 0 and 1, respectively).

The analysis of the survival time in relation to age at diagnosis (centred at the mean) and the presence of multiple recurrences, using a Generalised Gamma model is shown in Table 4.7. The mean log survival time (in months) of a patient with mean age, that is at $Age_{centred} = 0$, and only one recurrence, that is with multiple recurrence = 0, is $2.770 - (0.082 \times 0) - (0.396 \times 0) = 2.770$, giving an expected survival time of $\exp(2.770) = 15.96$ months. The log TR for one-year increase in age is -0.082 and is statistically significant (p-value = 0.002), indicating that older patients had shorter survival time. Under this model, with history of tumour recurrence being the same, a patient, say, 10 years older than the mean age has a log survival time of $2.770 - (0.082 \times 10) - (0.396 \times 0) = 1.950$, or a survival time of only $\exp(1.950) = 7.03$ months.

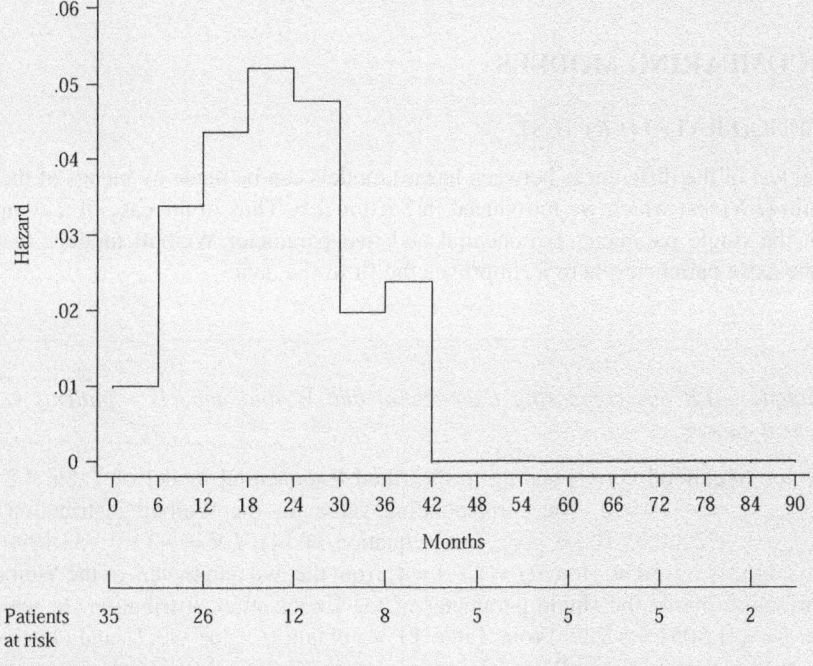

Figure 4.8 Mortality hazards of patients with nasopharyngeal cancer in successive six-month intervals (Data courtesy of Donald Poon, National Cancer Centre, Singapore)

Table 4.7 Multiple regression analysis of survival time of patients with recurrent nasopharyngeal carcinoma using Generalised Gamma model

	log *TR*	*SE*	*z*	*p*-value	95% *CI*
Age (centred at mean)	−0.082	0.026	−3.125	0.002	−0.134 to −0.030
Multiple recurrence	−0.396	0.367	−1.079	0.280	−1.115 to 0.323
Intercept	2.770	0.383			

LOG-LOGISTIC

The Log-Logistic distribution has the following hazard function:

$$h(t) = \frac{\lambda^{\frac{1}{\gamma}} t^{\frac{1}{\gamma}-1}}{\gamma \left[1 + (\lambda t)^{\frac{1}{\gamma}}\right]}. \tag{4.26}$$

The parameter γ (gamma) has a simple effect on the hazard. As illustrated in Figure 4.7b, when it is $\gamma < 1$ the hazard initially increases and then decreases and is quite similar to that of the Log-Normal distribution; while if $\gamma \geq 1$ the hazard decreases continuously. Once more the parameters λ (lambda) and γ are obtained by maximising the log-likelihood.

4.4   COMPARING MODELS

LIKELIHOOD RATIO (*LR*) TEST

A formal test of the differences between hazard models can be made by means of the likelihood ratio (*LR*) test which we introduced in Section 1.6. Thus in the case of a comparison between the single parameter Exponential and two parameter Weibull models, we ask if fitting the extra parameter, here κ, improves the fit to the data.

Example – LR test comparing Exponential and Weibull models – patients with cervical cancer

The log-likelihood corresponding to the fitted Exponential model of Table 4.2 is $L_{Exponential} = -33.1990$. The corresponding value for the Weibull distribution is $L_{Weibull} = -32.4463$. These give, from equation (1.14), $LR = -2 \times [-33.1990 - (-32.4463)] = 1.5054$. Here $df = 2 - 1 = 1$, from the two parameters of the Weibull distribution minus the single parameter of the Exponential distribution. In which case $z = \sqrt{1.5054} = 1.227$. From Table T1 we obtain *p*-value ≈ 0.21 and conclude the more elaborate Weibull model does not fit these data significantly better than the Exponential model.

NESTED MODELS

In the above example, the Exponential model is nested within the Weibull model, that is, it is a special form of the Weibull model with $\kappa = 1$. This 'nesting' allows the comparisons of the likelihoods to be made and hence provides a test of the relative improvement in fit. The Weibull is, in turn, nested within the Generalised Gamma distribution. However, although the two-parameter Log-Normal distribution is nested within the Generalised Gamma distribution, the Exponential distribution is not nested within the Log-Normal distribution. The Log-Logistic distribution is not nested within any of these distributions. Only nested models can be compared using the LR test.

Example – *testing nested models of the Generalised Gamma distribution – patients with recurrent nasopharyngeal carcinoma*

The results of fitting the Generalised Gamma distribution, and the corresponding nested models, to the data of Poon, Yap, Wong *et al.* (2004) from the survival times of 35 patients with recurrent nasopharyngeal carcinoma are given in Table 4.8. The table also includes the corresponding log-likelihoods, L.

The LR test statistic comparing the simplest (Exponential) versus the most complicated (Generalised Gamma) model is $LR = -2 \times [-44.633 - (-39.003)] = 11.260$. Since the Generalised Gamma model has two more parameters than the Exponential, the LR statistic follows the χ^2 distribution with $df = 2$. Referring to Table T3, the corresponding p-value < 0.01 whereas the exact value in Table 4.8 is taken from computer output as p-value $= 0.004$. This suggests that the Generalised Gamma distribution fits the data better than the Exponential distribution.

Similarly, the Generalised Gamma distribution fits the data significantly better than either the Weibull or Log-Normal distributions.

The Log-Logistic model is not nested within the Generalised Gamma distribution and so the LR test cannot be used to compare them.

Table 4.8 The log-likelihoods and likelihood ratio (LR) tests, for comparing alternative models to describe the time to death in patients with recurrent nasopharyngeal carcinoma

Distribution	No of parameters m	Log-likelihood L	Test against the Generalised Gamma distribution LR	df	p-value
Exponential	1	−44.633	$-2 \times [-44.633 - (-39.003)]$ $= 11.260$	2	0.004
Weibull	2	−44.061	$-2 \times [-44.061 - (-39.003)]$ $= 10.116$	1	0.001
Log-Normal	2	−41.073	$-2 \times [-41.073 - (-39.003)]$ $= 4.140$	1	0.042
Generalised Gamma	3	−39.003			
Log-Logistic	2	−40.992	Not nested		

NON-NESTED MODELS

As we have indicated, the *LR* test is not valid for comparing models that are not nested. However, Akaike's Information Criterion (*AIC*) can be used instead. This is defined as:

$$
\begin{aligned}
AIC &= -2 \times (L - \text{the number of parameters fitted in the modelling process}) \\
&= -2 \times (L - k - c)
\end{aligned}
\tag{4.27}
$$

Here k is the number of *HR*s to be estimated, and c is the number of parameters of the chosen survival distribution itself. Thus for a model with a single *HR* to be estimated, $k = 1$ and, if the Weibull model is used, $c = 2$ corresponding to the parameters λ and κ. The *AIC* is a penalisation of the log-likelihood, as the value of L is reduced (and *AIC* increased) according to the complexity of the model fitted. Lower values of the *AIC* suggest a better model. It can be used to compare nested as well as non-nested models.

***Example** – Akaike's Information Criterion (AIC) – patients with recurrent nasopharyngeal carcinoma*

In the example of recurrent nasopharyngeal carcinoma, $k = 2$ as the analysis involved two covariates, hence two *HR*s, and the number parameters for the Exponential distribution is $c = 1$. Therefore for the Exponential distribution the $AIC = -2 \times [-44.633 - 2 - 1)] = 95.266$. Those of the other models are calculated similarly and are given in Table 4.9. Using the *AIC* to compare the five models, we arrive at the same conclusion that the Generalised Gamma model fitted the data better than its special cases. The Log-Normal and Log-Logistic models have similar *AIC*, both showed lower level of goodness-of-fit than the Generalised Gamma but higher than the Exponential and Weibull models. Since the *AIC* of the Log-Normal model is smaller than those of the Exponential and Weibull, we may also conclude that the Log-Normal distribution is better than these two.

Table 4.9 Akaike Information Criterion (*AIC*) in the analysis of the recurrent nasopharyngeal carcinoma data

Distribution	Log-likelihood	k	c	*AIC*
Exponential	−44.633	2	1	95.266
Weibull	−44.061	2	2	96.122
Log-Normal	−41.073	2	2	90.146
Log-Logistic	−40.992	2	2	89.984
Generalised Gamma	−39.003	2	3	88.006

A difficulty in applying the *AIC* is that there are no formal statistical tests to compare different *AIC* values. When two models have very similar *AIC* values, the choice of model may not be clear and supplementary information, such as the Cox-Snell residual defined below, and external knowledge may be needed. For example, comparison with other published results may be required to judge the relative plausibility of the models rather than relying on *AIC* values alone.

4.5   MODEL DIAGNOSTICS

COX-SNELL RESIDUALS

Previously we introduced the complementary logarithmic plot to assess which of the Exponential and Weibull distributions best describes a particular data set. However, this approach only works if all the covariates influencing the hazard to an important extent have been recorded. In practice this is very unlikely.

For instance, suppose there are really two clinical sub-types, each with a different prognosis, within a population but this fact had not been recorded. Further suppose the hazards are constant over time within each clinical sub-type, but $\lambda = 0.1$ for clinical Type I and $\lambda = 0.5$ for clinical Type II. The combined data from the two clinical sub-types representing the whole group will therefore show an average hazard of between 0.1 and 0.5 when the follow-up time is close to $t = 0$.

However, since the Type II patients die more quickly, as time goes by there will gradually be more patients of Type I left in the study. In which case the observed hazard will gravitate away from the average downwards to the rate of 0.1 of the Type I patients. This *changing hazard* argues against an Exponential distribution for the combined data set including both clinical sub-types whereas if these had been identified the Exponential distribution would describe each clinical sub-type (each with its own rate) effectively.

This type of phenomenon makes it important to identify important sub-groups, whenever they exist, and to create plots of $\log\{-\log[S(t)]\}$ separately for each sub-group as appropriate.

However, when there are many sub-groups or some of the important covariates are continuous variables, this method becomes impractical because of the small sample size for each sub-group. In this situation, the Cox-Snell (CS_i) residuals defined as

$$CS_i = -\log[S(t_i|x_i)] \tag{4.28}$$

can be used.

Here each t_i is the survival or censored time for individual i and x_i represents all the covariate values for that subject. The survival probability, $S(t_i|x_i)$, is estimated using all these covariate values in the regression model. The calculations usually require computer software but they are available in major statistical packages such as Stata (StataCorp, 2005)

If the model fits the data well, then the Cox-Snell residuals have an approximately Exponential distribution with parameter $\lambda = 1$. If an observed survival time is censored, so is CS_i. Due to censoring one cannot examine the distribution of CS_i so easily but, in Section 4.1, we have discussed how to examine whether a survival time data follows an Exponential distribution by plotting $\log\{-\log[S(t)]\}$. We can apply exactly the same graphical examination method to study the Cox-Snell residuals by replacing t_i by CS_i. So a plot of $\log\{-\log[S(CS_i)]\}$ against $\log(CS_i)$ would show a linear trend with intercept zero (since $\log \lambda = \log 1 = 0$) and slope 1, that is a 45°-line, if the distribution chosen is appropriate. However, even if the model indeed fits well, some departure from a 45°-line in the left-hand tail is not uncommon as this part of the graph can be influenced by just a small number of observations with small CS_i values.

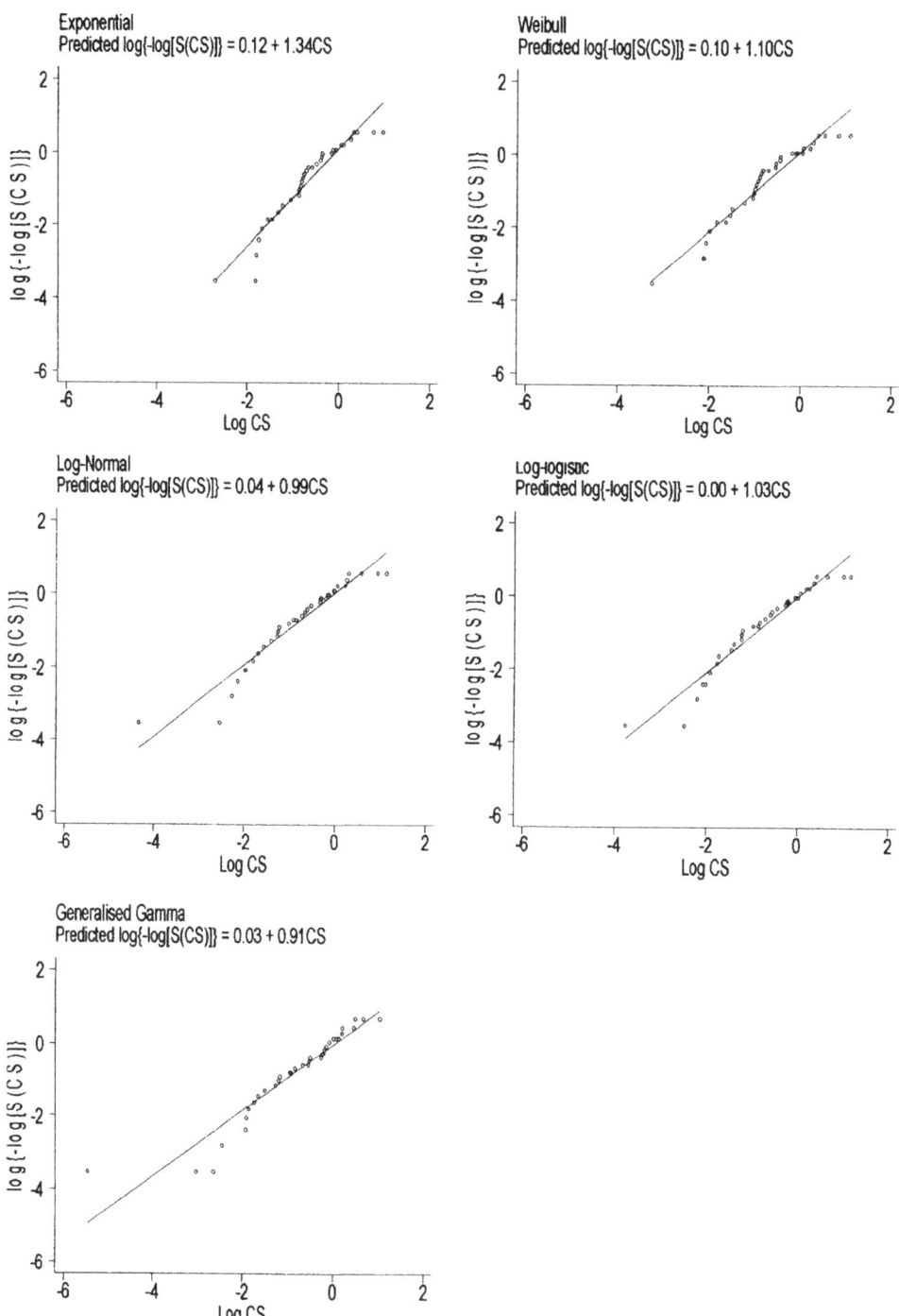

Figure 4.9 Plots of Cox-Snell residuals from five different parametric models, with age and the presence of multiple recurrences as covariates, of patients with recurrent nasopharyngeal carcinoma (Data courtesy of Donald Poon, National Cancer Centre, Singapore)

> ***Example** – Cox-Snell residuals – patients with nasopharyngeal carcinoma*
>
> Figure 4.9 shows the Cox-Snell residual plots of the nasopharyngeal carcinoma using five different distributions and the covariates age and presence of multiple recurrences.
>
> The interpretation is the same as that on Figure 4.4, although here we have fitted a straight line to each set of data points by ordinary least squares regression rather than by eye. The fitted intercept and slope are given at the top of each panel. The data points for the Exponential and Weibull distributions do not seem to follow a straight line closely. Furthermore they have intercepts 0.12 and 0.10 respectively, quite different from zero, and slopes 1.34 and 1.10, quite different from one. The plots for the other three distributions more closely comply with a straight line and the intercepts and slopes are closer to the expected values of zero and one, respectively.
>
> The analysis suggests that the Exponential and Weibull distributions do not describe the data well. Thus distributions that allow the hazard to fluctuate up and down are required.

One difficulty in using the Cox-Snell residuals is that, especially if sample size is small, a small number of data points may depart substantially from a 45°-line and these make it difficult to fit an appropriate straight line. Another is that it is not easy to tell how much deviation is acceptable. So the interpretation is somewhat subjective. For the two reasons combined, in the above example, we conclude that the Exponential and Weibull distributions are inappropriate but we cannot tell which of the remainder are better. This indicates a general problem with Cox-Snell (and other) residuals in that they are helpful in assessing whether a particular model does *not* fit the data well, but are not helpful in assessing whether a model does fit the data adequately.

4.6   MODELLING STRATEGY

It is recognised that some of the parametric models described in this chapter are mathematically complex. Fortunately all can be fitted relatively easily in many of the standard computer packages and when fitted the output is reasonably straightforward to interpret. One recommendation is to start with the easiest of models to fit, in this case the Exponential, without any of the possible covariates you may wish to investigate. This can then be compared with the Weibull fit to the same data by examining: size of κ and associated CI, graphical plots, and the LR test. Should the extra complexity of the Weibull not be justified, return to the Exponential and construct a regression model with the principal covariate. In a randomised controlled trial this would be the model with treatment group alone, beginning this process with the most complex hazard distribution with many regression covariates should be avoided. Once one is familiar with the computer package then these steps may be accelerated but all modelling procedures require careful thought by the investigator concerned – it should not be left to the computer to decide what happens.

In the model building process, if a major covariate is continuous, then to facilitate graphical assessment it may be necessary to 'categorise it'. If this is done, then we recommend more than two groups, and dividing at the tertiles might be a reasonable first start.

Once the model is fitted a plot of $\log\{-\log[S(t)]\}$ or the hazard rates can be made. From these perhaps a few models that look reasonable can be chosen—perhaps in a particular example the Weibull and Log-Normal look potential options but the Exponential distribution does not fit the data well. These models are then fitted with the covariates, and the LR, AIC and Cox-Snell residual plots examined. These will then hopefully lead to a reasonable model choice.

4.7   TECHNICAL DETAILS

MAXIMUM LIKELIHOOD

Rather than denote death times by t_i and censored times by T_j^+ it is often convenient to incorporate these two types of time into one terminology. To do this we can think of each patient, i, having an observed survival time t; which is a death time if an associated variable $\delta_i = 1$ and is censored if $\delta_i = 0$. Thus we can write, for the ith patient, the pair (t_i, δ_i) to describe the survival time and status. This device is often used in statistical packages; thus one (column) variable denotes the survival time and the second (column) the survival status (dead = 1, alive = 0).

If we can assume a constant hazard, then for a patient who has died $\delta_i = 1$ and the probability of death at t_i is (since the distribution of survival times is Exponential) $\lambda e^{-\lambda t_i}$, which is the probability density function value $f(t_i)$ for subject i. If the patient has not died $\delta_i = 0$ then all we can calculate is the probability of survival beyond t_i which is $e^{-\lambda t_i}$, which is the survival function value $S(t_i)$ for the subject. In general, the probability of death at time t_i for patient i, can be written

$$l_i(\lambda) = (\lambda e^{-\lambda t_i})^{\delta_i} (e^{-\lambda t_i})^{1-\delta_i}$$
$$= \lambda^{\delta_i} e^{-\lambda t_i}. \tag{4.29}$$

Equation (4.29) is often termed the likelihood for patient i from which $L_i(\lambda) = \log l_i(\lambda) = \delta_i \log \lambda - \lambda t$. If we differentiate $L_i(\lambda)$ with respect to λ then we obtain

$$\frac{dL_i(\lambda)}{d\lambda} = \left[\frac{\delta_i}{\lambda} - t_i\right], \tag{4.30}$$

and the expression

$$U_i(\lambda) = \frac{\delta_i}{\lambda} - t_i \tag{4.31}$$

is termed the efficient score statistic.

If we calculate U_i, for all n patients and set $\Sigma U_i(\lambda) = 0$ then this leads to $\lambda = \Sigma \delta_i / \Sigma t_i$. This is the form of equation (4.4) with $\Sigma \delta_i$, replaced by the total number of observed deaths, d, and Σt_i replaced by the sum of all the survival times $(f + F)$ whether censored or not. As a consequence, the estimate (4.4) is known as the maximum likelihood estimate of λ.

In the more general multiple regression analysis situation, λ is replaced by $\exp(\beta_0 + \beta_1 x_1 + \cdots + \beta_k x_k)$ in the likelihood. The maximum likelihood estimates of the β's can be obtained by iteratively assigning different values to them until the model log likelihood $L = \Sigma L_i(\lambda) = \Sigma L_i[\exp(\beta_0 + \beta_1 x_1 + \cdots + \beta_k x_k)]$ is maximised.

Further replacing the Exponential distribution form in equation (4.29), by one of the other hazard distributions we have described, the likelihood becomes

$$l_i(\theta) = f(t_i, \theta)^{\delta_i} S(t_i, \theta)^{1-\delta_i}. \tag{4.32}$$

Here θ represents the parameters of the particular survival-time model $f(t, \theta)$, perhaps the Weibull distribution with parameters λ and κ, as well as any β's for the covariates and $S(t, \theta)$ the survival function.

5 Cox's Proportional Hazards Model

Summary

This chapter introduces Cox's proportional hazards regression model, which is used extensively in the analysis of survival data. The use of the model includes assessing treatment effects in studies and in particular adjusting these comparisons for baseline characteristics. A comparison of the method of calculating hazard ratios (HRs) with that derived following the Logrank test of Chapter 3 is made. A further use of these models is to assess variables for prognostic significance for the particular survival type endpoint of concern. In this context the use of both continuous and categorical variables in a model is described. Methods for assessing the proportionality of hazards are included, as are statistical tests for comparing alternative regression models.

5.1 INTRODUCTION

We have described the concept of the hazard rate, or the instantaneous event rate and have said that if the distribution of survival times can be assumed Exponential, then this rate is estimated by the ratio of the number of events observed divided by the total survival time, as given in equation (4.4). One consequence of the assumption of the Exponential distribution of survival times is that the hazard rate, λ, does not vary with time. For example, in a clinical trial, this would imply that the underlying death rate in the first year of patient follow-up equals the death rate in each subsequent year. One example where this would not apply is if there is an excess mortality in the immediate post-surgical period in patients undergoing limb amputation due to possible complications arising from infection. As the postoperative time increases this risk diminishes and consequently so does the risk of death. We have given other examples in Chapter 4. We express this possible lack of a constant value by noting that the hazard rate may depend on follow-up time, t, and we therefore write $\lambda(t)$ in place of λ to reflect this.

A guide to whether or not the hazard rate can be regarded as constant is to plot the complementary log transformation, or $\log\{-\log[S(t)]\}$, against $\log t$, as we have illustrated in Figure 4.4. If the hazard rate does not change with time then the resulting plot will be approximately linear, while departures from linearity indicate that the hazard rate is changing with time.

Survival Analysis Second Edition David Machin, Yin Bun Cheung, Mahesh K.B. Parmar
© 2006 John Wiley & Sons, Ltd ISBN: 0-470-87040-0

Example – complementary log-plot – non-small cell lung cancer

The complementary log plots of two groups of patients with non-small cell lung cancer (NSCLC) are shown in Figure 5.1. One group consists of those patients who presented with NSCLC but without evidence of metastatic disease; the other group comprises those in which metastatic disease was detected. These data are taken from two randomised trials of the Medical Research Council Lung Cancer Working Party (1991, 1992) and include the 304 patients who received the same course of radiotherapy (F2) which was a treatment common to each trial.

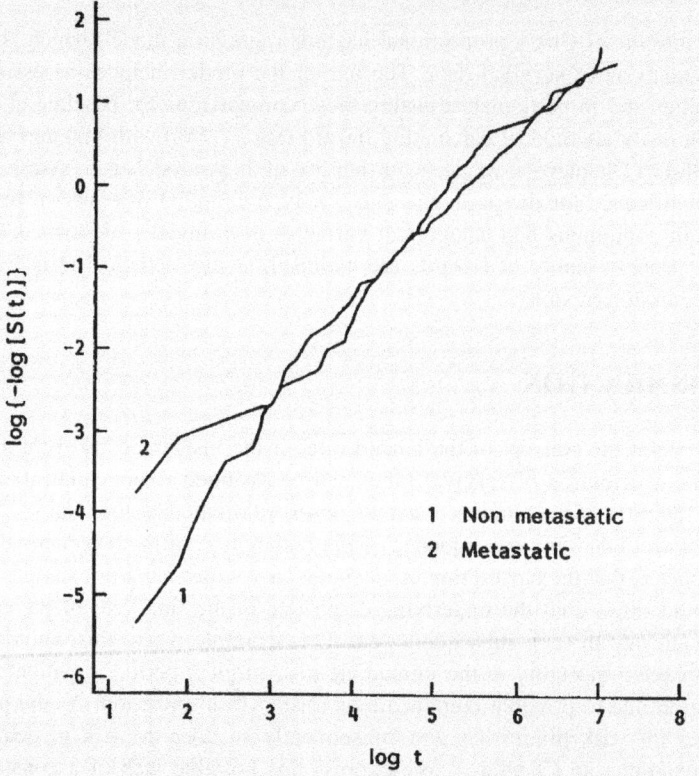

Figure 5.1   Graph of $\log\{-\log[S(t)]\}$ against $\log t$ in patients treated with radiotherapy with metastatic and non-metastatic non-small cell lung cancer (data from Medical Research Council Lung Cancer Working Party, 1991, 1992, reproduced by permission of The Macmillan Press Ltd)

The plots of the hazards for the two groups in Figure 5.1 are approximately linear and overlapping. This suggests that not only is the hazard constant within each group but also that it is similar for both patient groups.

Example – *complementary log plot–small cell lung cancer*

Figure 5.2 shows the complementary log plots for two groups of patients, those with limited and those with extensive disease at diagnosis, with small cell lung cancer (SCLC). These patients all received a combination chemotherapy of etoposide, cyclophosphamide, methotrexate and vincristine (ECMV) for their disease. This was the common treatment arm used in three randomised trials of the Medical Research Council Lung Cancer Working Party (1989a, 1989b, 1993). In total 932 patients presented at diagnosis with either limited or extensive SCLC and were randomised to receive ECMV.

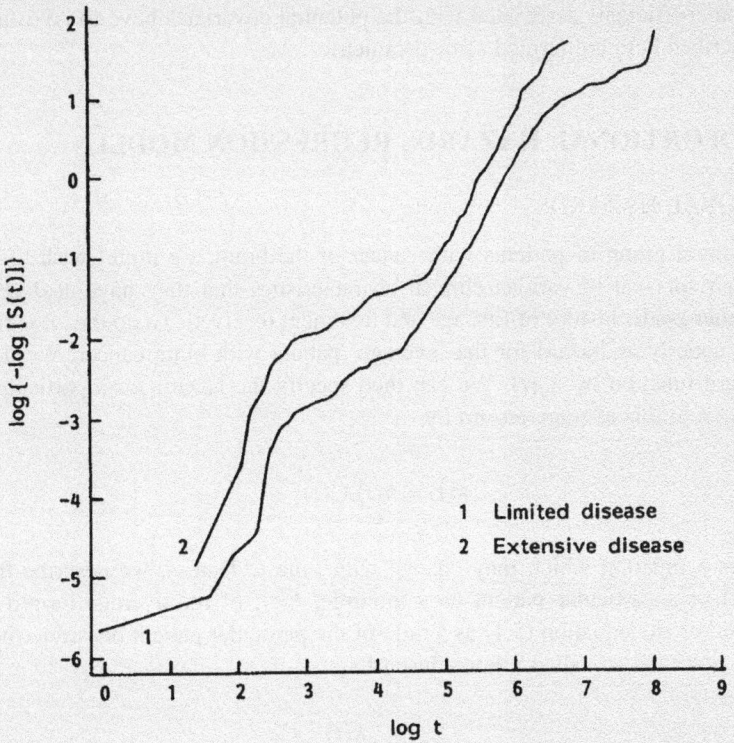

Figure 5.2 Graph of $\log\{-\log[S(t)]\}$ against $\log t$ in patients treated with ECMV chemotherapy with limited and extensive small cell lung cancer (data from Medical Research Council Lung Cancer Working Party, 1989a, 1989b, 1993, reproduced by permission of The Macmillan Press Ltd)

In contrast to the patient groups with NSCLC illustrated in Figure 5.1, the hazard in both the limited and extensive SCLC disease groups of Figure 5.2 appears to vary with time since the two graphs are non-linear. Nevertheless, the two plots appear 'parallel' in that there is an approximately constant vertical distance between them at any given time. In this situation we say that the hazards for the two patient groups are proportional, that is, their ratio remains approximately constant with time. For the patients with NSCLC of Figure 5.1, the hazards are also proportional but with a ratio close to one, because the lines are essentially coincident.

The purpose of this chapter is to relate non-constant hazards, $\lambda(t)$, to variables which may influence their value. Such variables, or covariates, are often those recorded at presentation of the patient for diagnosis or at the time of entry into a study. They may include variables describing the nature of the disease, demographic characteristics of the patient and the treatment received. In contrast to Chapter 4, no assumption with respect to the underlying survival time model is made so parameters, for example λ and κ, do not have to be estimated. Thus the methods are non-parametric in this respect. However, since the parameters, that is, the regression coefficients associated with the potential covariates have to be estimated the methods described here are termed semi-parametric.

5.2   PROPORTIONAL HAZARDS REGRESSION MODEL

PROPORTIONAL HAZARDS

In investigating a group of patients with cancer of the brain, we might wish to relate the length of their survival to various clinical characteristics that they have at diagnosis, for example tumour grade, history of fits, age and treatment received. To do this, it is first useful to define an underlying hazard for the 'average' patient with brain cancer. We denote this average hazard function by $\lambda_0(t)$. We can then specify the hazard for a particular patient, $\lambda(t)$, in relation to this average hazard by

$$\lambda(t) = h(t)\lambda_0(t), \tag{5.1}$$

where $h(t)$ is a function which may change with time t. That is, we describe the hazard function $\lambda(t)$ of a particular patient as a multiple, $h(t)$, of the average hazard function, $\lambda_0(t)$. We can rewrite equation (5.1) as a ratio of the particular patient hazard to the average hazard. This gives the so-called relative hazard as

$$h(t) = \frac{\lambda(t)}{\lambda_0(t)} \tag{5.2}$$

If $h(t)$ does not change with time then we write $h(t) = h$, where h is a constant. In this case, we can write h in place of $h(t)$ in equation (5.1), since the relative hazard no longer depends on t.

Note, however, even when both $\lambda(t)$ and $\lambda_0(t)$ change with time their ratio can remain constant as in Figure 5.2. In this situation, we have proportional hazards (*PH*) as we described in Chapter 4. This implies that at any given time t the hazard rate applying to our particular patient will be h times that of the average patient with this disease. In situations where $h(t) = 1$, for all values of t, then the hazard rate $\lambda(t)$, at a given time t, for any particular patient, does not differ from the average of $\lambda_0(t)$.

We have seen in Chapter 4, when discussing the Exponential and Weibull distributions, that the logarithms of the hazard and of the HR are often used. As a consequence it is convenient to write $h(t) = e^{\beta(t)} = \exp[\beta(t)]$. This implies $\beta(t) = \log h(t)$, so that under PH equation (5.2) can be written as

$$\log[h(t)] = \log h = \log\left[\frac{\lambda(t)}{\lambda_0(t)}\right] = \beta, \tag{5.3}$$

so that both h and β do not depend on time. The estimate of β, denoted b, is obtained from the data of the particular study concerned. The strength of the PH model developed by Cox (1972) is not only that it allows survival data arising from a non-constant hazard rate to be modelled, but it does so without making any assumption about the underlying distribution of the hazards in different groups, except that the hazards in the groups remain proportional over time.

COMPARING TWO GROUPS

Suppose we have patients with brain tumours randomised to receive one of two therapies, standard (control, C) or test (new, N), and we wish to determine whether treatment N improves patient survival.

We write the hazard for those receiving C as

$$\lambda_C(t) = \lambda_0(t), \tag{5.4}$$

which assumes that all patients receiving C have the same underlying hazard $\lambda_0(t)$. If we then assume PH for patients in the two treatment groups, we can write the hazard for those receiving N as

$$\lambda_N(t) = \lambda_0(t)\exp(\beta). \tag{5.5}$$

This is equivalent to saying that the hazard for patients receiving N is a constant, here $\exp(\beta)$, times that of the patients who receive C. The relative hazard or hazard ratio (HR) for patients receiving the respective treatments is the ratio of the hazards given by equations (5.5) and (5.4), respectively. Thus

$$HR = \frac{\lambda_N(t)}{\lambda_C(t)} = \frac{\lambda_0(t)\exp(\beta)}{\lambda_0(t)} \tag{5.6}$$

or

$$HR = \exp(\beta). \tag{5.7}$$

The influence of time on the hazard is summarised in $\lambda_0(t)$ and this is divided out in equation (5.6). As a consequence, the HR is a constant since equation (5.7) does not depend on t. It follows from equation (5.7) that $\log HR = \beta$.

Example – Cox PH regression model – treatment for brain cancer

To illustrate the estimation of β we use the data from patients with brain cancer who were recruited to a randomised trial of the Medical Research Council Working Party on Misonidazole in Gliomas (1983). The patients were treated either by radiotherapy alone (C) or by radiotherapy with the radiosensitiser misonidazole (N). A total of 198 patients received C and 204 received N. For illustration, a portion of the data set is given in Table 5.1.

Using a statistical package gives, for the full data set, the estimate of β for equation (5.7) as $b = -0.0563$, from which $HR = e^b = \exp(-0.0563) = 0.9452$. Such a HR implies a better risk for patients receiving the new therapy since $HR < 1$ and equation (5.6) then implies $\lambda_N(t) < \lambda_C(t)$.

Table 5.1 Survival time and some baseline characteristics for 30 patients with brain cancer receiving radiotherapy alone or radiotherapy plus the radiosensitiser misonidazole (Part data from Medical Research Council Working Party on Misonidazole in Gliomas, 1983 Reproduced by permission of The British Institute of Radiology)

Patient Number	Received misonidazole	Fits before entry	Tumour grade	Age (years)	Survival time(days)	Survival status
1	NO	NO	4	48	1084	ALIVE
2	YES	NO	3	63	22	DEAD
3	YES	NO	4	54	40	DEAD
4	NO	NO	3/4	49	25	DEAD
5	YES	NO	4	44	487	DEAD
6	NO	YES	4	36	696	DEAD
7	YES	NO	3	29	887	ALIVE
8	NO	NO	3	50	336	DEAD
9	NO	NO	4	53	213	ALIVE
10	NO	YES	3	58	361	DEAD
11	YES	NO	3	48	244	DEAD
12	YES	NO	4	49	799	DEAD
13	YES	NO	3/4	60	180	DEAD
14	NO	YES	3	49	488	DEAD
15	NO	NO	4	64	121	DEAD
16	YES	YES	4	61	210	DEAD
17	NO	YES	3	41	575	ALIVE
18	NO	NO	4	58	258	DEAD
19	YES	NO	4	35	273	DEAD
20	YES	NO	3	42	1098	ALIVE
21	YES	YES	3/4	30	819	ALIVE
22	YES	NO	3	66	14	DEAD
23	NO	YES	3	48	734	DEAD
24	YES	YES	4	57	225	DEAD
25	NO	NO	3/4	56	152	DEAD
26	YES	YES	3	43	207	DEAD
27	YES	YES	3	33	943	ALIVE
28	NO	NO	3	39	581	DEAD
29	YES	YES	3/4	48	371	DEAD
30	NO	NO	3	55	85	ALIVE

In addition to the estimate b of β, the computer output provides the associated standard error, $SE(b)$. The test of the null hypothesis of no difference between the control and new treatments is equivalent to testing the hypothesis that $\beta = 0$ in equation (5.7). This in turn is equivalent to testing $HR = 1$ since, in this case, $HR = \exp(\beta) = e^0 = 1$. One method of testing this hypothesis is to calculate the z-statistic equivalent to equation (1.10) which, in this case, is

$$z = b/SE(b). \tag{5.8}$$

We then refer z to Table T1 of the standard Normal distribution to obtain the p-value. Alternatively

$$W = z^2 = [b/SE(b)]^2 \tag{5.9}$$

can be referred to Table T3 of the χ^2 distribution with degrees of freedom, $df = 1$. In this format the test is termed the Wald test and is discussed further in Section 5.6.

Example – Cox PH regression model – treatment for brain cancer

The computer output for the trial of therapies for patients with brain cancer gave $b = -0.0563$ and $SE(b) = 0.1001$. Thus, use of equation (5.8) gives $z = -0.0563/0.1001 = -0.56$. Referring $z = 0.56$ to Table T1 gives a p-value $= 0.5755$. With such a large p-value we would not reject the null hypothesis of equal efficacy of treatments C and N.

In most contexts, it is often appropriate to calculate a confidence interval (CI) rather than merely rely on a test of statistical significance alone. By analogy with equation (3.6) the $100(1 - \alpha)\%$ CI for log HR is given by

$$b - z_{1-\alpha/2}SE(b) \quad \text{to} \quad b + z_{1-\alpha/2}SE(b). \tag{5.10}$$

The CI for the population HR is therefore given by analogy with equation (3.7) by

$$\exp[b - z_{1-\alpha/2}SE(b)] \quad \text{to} \quad \exp[b + z_{1-\alpha/2}SE(b)]. \tag{5.11}$$

Example – Cox PH regression model – treatment for brain cancer

For the patients with brain cancer we have $b = -0.0563$, and $SE(b) = 0.1001$. The corresponding 95% CI is calculated by setting $\alpha = 0.05$ in equation (5.10) to obtain $z_{0.975} = 1.9600$ from Table T2 and hence $\exp[-0.0563 - (1.9600 \times 0.1001)] =$

0.78 to $\exp[-0.0563 + (1.9600 \times 0.1001)] = 1.15$. This 95% CI contains the null hypothesis value, $HR = 1$ (or equivalently $\beta = 0$), of no treatment difference. Nevertheless there still remains some uncertainty about the true efficacy of the treatments as expressed by the HR. For example, both $HR = 0.8$ indicating benefit to N, and $HR = 1.1$ suggesting the reverse to be the case, are both consistent with the 95% CI obtained.

REGRESSION MODELS

Single explanatory variable

We can combine both equations (5.4) and (5.5) into a single expression, or regression model, by introducing the indicator variable x for treatment received, and writing

$$\lambda(t) = \lambda_o(t) \exp(\beta x). \qquad (5.12)$$

Here we set $x = 0$ or $x = 1$ to represent control therapy C and the new treatment N, respectively. Finally, we can write equation (5.12) even more compactly, as

$$T : h(x) = \exp(\beta x). \qquad (5.13)$$

Thus $h(x = 0) = 1$, $h(x = 1) = \exp(\beta)$ and, when comparing the two treatment groups, $HR = h(1)/h(0) = \exp(\beta)$ also.

This expression again emphasises that in PH circumstances the HR does not depend on t. In this format equation (5.13) is termed the Cox PH regression model. The variable x helps to describe or model the variation in the relative hazard and we have to estimate the parameter β with the data.

We use the notation T here to denote the model which is examining the influence of treatment. The null hypothesis of no treatment difference is expressed as $\beta = 0$ in (5.13), in which case $HR = h(1)/h(0) - 1$.

Example – Cox and Logrank estimates of HR – treatment for brain cancer

The estimate of $HR = 0.9452$ in the above calculation, using the Cox model for the full brain cancer patient data corresponding to Table 5.1, is very close to the estimate given by the use of equation (3.5), following the Logrank test. In our example the latter gives $HR_{Logrank} = (O_N/E_N)/(O_C/E_C) = (204/209.61)/(198/193.39) = 0.9456$. The expected number of deaths, E_C and E_N, are obtained from computer output. This estimate differs from the Cox estimate only in the final decimal place.

One important problem is to identify potential prognostic importance of variables: for example, whether individuals with brain cancer, having had no experience of fits before diagnosis, have a different survival than patients who have experienced fits. For this purpose, we can use the same formulation for the Cox model as for when comparing two treatments. In this case, the equivalent expression to equation (5.13) is

$$F : h(x_F) = \exp(\beta_F x_F) \qquad (5.14)$$

where $x_F = 0$ if the patient has had no fits before diagnosis and $x_F = 1$ if the patient has experienced fits. We denote the model as F and the regression parameter to be estimated is β_F. We are ignoring the possible influence of other variables here. We can write the hazard ratio (HR_F) as the ratio of the relative hazard in those who have experienced a fit compared to the relative hazard in those that have not. Thus

$$HR_F = \frac{h(x_F = 1)}{h(x_F = 0)} = \frac{h(1)}{h(0)} = \exp(\beta_F).$$

Example – prognosis – patients with brain cancer

For the patients with brain cancer, the estimate of β_F is $b_F = -0.3925$ with $SE(b_F) = 0.1159$. This gives an estimate of $HR_F = \exp(-0.3925) = 0.6754$. This is less than 1, indicating, perhaps somewhat counter intuitively, that patients with a history of fits have a better prognosis than those who have not. The clinical explanation for this is that a history of fits in the patient tends to suggest that the brain tumour has been present for some time and hence is slow growing and, therefore, not so aggressive. This contrasts with tumours in patients with no such history whose tumours may be rapidly growing and hence bring a poor prognosis.

As before, the null hypothesis of no difference between the two groups is considered by testing whether $\beta_F = 0$. A formal test of this null hypothesis using equation (5.8) gives, $z = 3.39$, which from Table T1 gives a p-value < 0.0020. Computer output gives this more precisely as p-value $= 0.0007$. Thus there is strong evidence that the parameter $\beta_F \neq 0$ and that a previous history of fits does imply improved survival.

Example – Cox PH regression model – factors influencing recovery from stroke

Mayo, Korner-Bitensky and Becker (1991) use the Cox *PH* model to investigate factors influencing recovery time from stroke to full and independent sitting function in 45 post-stroke victims who were not self-sitting immediately following their stroke. One factor they considered that was likely to influence patient recovery was the degree of perceptual impairment, which they categorised in binary form as none-to-mild or moderate-to-severe. They observed a $HR = 0.26$ with a 95% CI 0.10 to 0.66 and concluded from this that those with the least degree of perceptual impairment recovered more quickly. This HR corresponds to $b = -1.35$ and $SE(b) = 0.48$, giving $z = -1.35/0.48 = -2.8$ and p-value $= 0.0051$.

One advantage of PH models over the Logrank test is that they can be used with continuous variables. We illustrate this use to assess the importance of actual age (rather than age-group) in the prognosis of patients with brain cancer of Table 5.1. For the purpose of this example we ignore the possible influence of a history of fits, tumour grade and treatment received, on survival in these patients. By analogy with equations (5.13) and (5.14) we can specify the Cox model taking account of age as

$$A : h(Age) = \exp(\beta_A A), \tag{5.15}$$

where A is the age of the patient and β_A is the corresponding regression coefficient.

Example – *Cox PH regression model* – *age as a prognostic factor in brain cancer*

If this model is fitted to the brain cancer data, then $b_A = 0.0320$ and $SE(b_A) = 0.0049$ and it follows that $HR = \exp(b_A) = \exp(0.0320) = 1.033$. This is the HR for any one age as compared to the year previous. The corresponding test statistic is $z = 0.0320/0.0049 = 6.53$ with an associated p-value < 0.001, obtained by reference to Table T2. This suggests that age is a very clear predictor of survival.

If we wish to compare the survival experience of two patients, of ages A_1 and A_2 respectively, then, from (5.15), we have $h(Age = A_1) = \exp(\beta_A A_1)$ and $h(Age = A_2) = \exp(\beta_A A_2)$. The ratio of these is

$$HR = \frac{h(Age = A_1)}{h(Age = A_2)} = \frac{\exp(\beta_A A_1)}{\exp(\beta_A A_2)} = \exp[\beta_A(A_1 - A_2)]. \tag{5.16}$$

Thus, the HR depends only on the difference in age, $(A_1 - A_2)$, of the two patients under consideration.

> **Example** – *Cox PH regression model – age as a prognostic factor in brain cancer*
>
> A patient aged 50(A_1), compared to one aged 40(A_2), will have an estimated hazard ratio $HR = \exp[b_A(50 - 40)] = \exp(0.0320 \times 10) = 1.3771$. This suggests very strongly that the older patient has the much greater risk of death once diagnosed with this disease. Since the patients differ in age by 10 years we note that $1.3771 = 1.033^{10}$.

As we noted in Chapter 4, for technical reasons it is quite usual in the case of continuous variables, to write the Cox model (5.15) with *Age* expressed $Age_{Centred}$ where this implies, for example, a difference from the mean age of the patients under consideration but this can be any convenient value near the mean, perhaps 50 or 55 in this case. Thus, we write the relative hazard as

$$A : h(Age) = \exp[\beta_A(A - \bar{A})] \tag{5.17}$$

where $\bar{A}$ is the mean age of the patients. A quick check with $A_1 - \bar{A}$ and $A_2 - \bar{A}$ replacing A_1 and A_2 in equation (5.16) shows that this change does not affect the final estimate of the HR for the two patients since $(A_1 - \bar{A}) - (A_2 - \bar{A}) = A_1 - A_2$.

> **Example** – *Cox PH regression model – age as a prognostic factor in brain cancer*
>
> For the brain cancer analysis above, the mean age of the patients is $\bar{A} = 52.3$ years and $b_A = 0.0320$; thus the model described by equation (5.17) is
>
> $$A : h(Age) = \exp[0.0320(Age - 52.3)].$$
>
> This model can be written as $h(Age) = \exp(0.0320 Age) \times \exp[0.0320 \times (-52.3)]$ or $h(Age) = 0.1876 \exp(0.0320 Age)$.
>
> For an individual of age 40, that is, 12.3 years below the mean $h(40) = 0.1876 \exp(0.0320 \times 40) = 0.1876 \exp(1.28) = 0.6747$. This means that a 40-year old person's mortality hazard is $(1 - 0.6747) = 0.3253$ or 33% lower than that of a person with an average age.
>
> This calculation gives the same results as setting $b_A = 0.0320$ in place of β_A together with $A_1 = 40$ and $\bar{A} = 52.3$ directly in equation (5.17).
>
> Similarly, for a patient aged 50, we have $h(50) = 0.1876 \exp(0.0320 \times 50) = 0.1876 \exp(1.60) = 0.9292$. Finally this gives $HR = h(50)/h(40) = 0.9292/0.6747 = 1.3772$. This is the value we had obtained previously for the HR except for rounding error in the fourth decimal place.

Using the form of the Cox model presented in equation (5.17), we can now state that an individual of average age has $h(Age) = 1$, since for this patient $(A - \bar{A}) = 0$. We can now also see that since the estimate of $b_A = 0.0320$ is positive, individuals below the mean age have a decreased hazard. This is because $(A - \bar{A})$ is negative for such a patient, hence $b_A(A - \bar{A})$ is negative and the exponential of a negative quantity gives a $HR < 1$. For individuals whose age is above the mean of the group the hazard is increased. Here $(A - \bar{A})$ is positive, hence $b_A(A - \bar{A})$ is also positive and the exponential of a positive quantity gives a $HR > 1$.

Two explanatory variables

As already indicated, it is well known in patients with brain cancer that a history of fits prior to diagnosis is of prognostic importance. In fact having had previous fits may be more of a determinant of subsequent patient survival than the form of treatment given. In the situation, where more than one variable may influence survival, here treatment as well as their history of fits, we can extend the Cox model in the usual way. Thus to assess the influence (if any) of both treatment and history of fits, we combine equations (5.13) and (5.14) into a single model containing the two variables, as

$$T + F : h(x_T, x_F) = \exp(\beta_T x_T + \beta_F x_F). \tag{5.18}$$

We note that model (5.18) for $T + F$ is merely the product of equations (5.13), with x replaced by x_T, and (5.14) which are the models for T and F, respectively. Alternatively, equation (5.18) can be expressed as

$$\log h(x_T, x_F) = \beta_T x_T + \beta_F x_F. \tag{5.19}$$

Using this model, there are now four groups of patients. For those who receive radiotherapy alone (control) and have had no history of fits $(x_T = 0, x_F = 0)$ and so $h(0, 0) = \exp(0) = 1$. This implies that the hazard for this particular group (control treatment who have had no history of fits) is equal to the underlying or baseline hazard, $\lambda_0(t)$. We therefore regard this as the baseline group against which we compare the other three patient groups. The choice of which group is to be used as the baseline usually depends on which is most convenient in the context of the example being considered. Those patients who receive the new therapy and have had no history of fits have $(x_T = 1, x_F = 0)$, giving $h(1, 0) = \exp(\beta_T)$. Those who receive the control treatment but have experienced fits have $(x_T = 0, x_F = 1)$ with $h(0, 1) = \exp(\beta_F)$ and finally those who receive the new therapy and who also have experienced fits have $(x_T = 1, x_F = 1)$, with $h(1, 1) = \exp(\beta_T + \beta_F)$.

It is worth noting that the ratios

$$\frac{h(1, 1)}{h(0, 1)} = \frac{\exp(\beta_T + \beta_F)}{\exp(\beta_F)} = \exp(\beta_T + \beta_F - \beta_F) = \exp(\beta_T) = HR_T$$

and

$$\frac{h(1, 0)}{h(0, 0)} = \frac{\exp(\beta_T)}{\exp(0)} = \exp(\beta_T - 0) = \exp(\beta_T) = HR_T$$

both have the same value, which is the HR for the treatment comparison. This implies that the treatment effect, which is measured by the size of β_T, is assumed to be the same, both for patients who have had a history of fits prior to diagnosis and for those patients who have had no such history.

Similarly,

$$\frac{h(1,1)}{h(1,0)} = \frac{\exp(\beta_T + \beta_F)}{\exp(\beta_T)} = \exp(\beta_F) = HR_F$$

and

$$\frac{h(0,1)}{h(0,0)} = \frac{\exp(\beta_F)}{\exp(0)} = \exp(\beta_F) = HR_F.$$

These imply that with this model the effect on survival of having or not having a history of fits is the same, irrespective of the treatment received.

Example – Cox PH regression model – history of fits and treatment in brain cancer

The K-M estimates of the survival curves of the four treatment by history of fits groups of patients with brain tumours are shown in Figure 5.3(a, b). They are given in two panels to aid clarity of presentation as there is some overlap in the four curves in the early months following the date of randomisation. Figure 5.3(a), which shows the survival curves by treatment group for those patients with no history of fits, suggests, if anything, a slight advantage to those receiving misonidazole. In contrast, Figure 5.3(b), which shows the survival curves by treatment group for those patients with a history of fits, suggests, if anything, a slight disadvantage to those receiving misonidazole. If this were truly the case then the assumption that the treatment effect, β_T, is constant in both history of fit groups of patients would not hold.

For this trial, the analysis suggests the absence of any real difference between treatments so that in reality we suspect $\beta_T = 0$. This means that the small differences indicated by Figures 5.3(a, b) are likely to be random. The Cox model of equation (5.18) fitted to these data gives the regression coefficients summarised in Table 5.2. The estimate $b_T = -0.0486$ for the treatment comparison, with corresponding $HR_T = \exp(-0.0486) = 0.9526$. This is only very slightly changed from $b = -0.0563$ with corresponding $HR_T = \exp(-0.0563) = 0.9452$, given earlier. The latter was derived from the Cox model for T without information on fits included. There will be circumstances when more major changes to the estimate of the HR will occur, for example, if the proportions of patients having a history of 'fits' and 'no fits' differed markedly in the two treatment groups. Then if, by chance, one of the treatments is given to substantially more patients of good prognosis then it may, as a consequence, *appear* to be the better treatment, since good-prognosis patients survive longer in any event.

For the presence of history of fits, the $HR_F = \exp(-0.3913) = 0.6762$. This represents a substantially reduced risk of death in those who have experienced fits as compared to those who have not. For history of fits, $z = -0.3913/0.1159 = -3.38$ and use of Table T1 gives a p-value < 0.002. This suggests, as we have already observed that patients with a history of fits do indeed have a better prognosis than those with no history of fits. More extensive tables of the Normal distribution give the p-value $= 0.0007$.

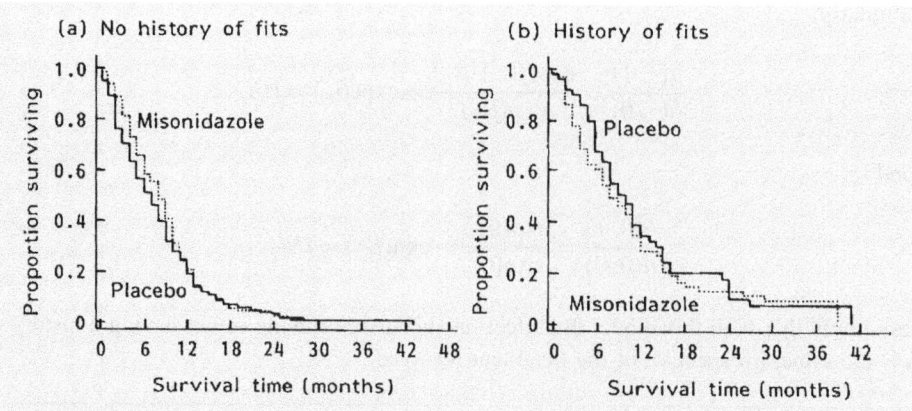

Figure 5.3 Survival in patients with brain cancer by prior history of fits and allocated treatment group (From Medical Research Council Working Party on Misonidazole in Gliomas, 1983. Reproduced by permission of The British Institute of Radiology)

Table 5.2 Cox proportional hazards model fitted to treatments and to history of fits in the patients with brain cancer (From Medical Research Council Working Party on Misonidazole in Gliomas, 1983. Reproduced by permission of The British Institute of Radiology)

Variable	Coefficient	Estimate (b)	HR $= e^b$	$SE(b)$	$z = b/SE(b)$	p-value
Treatment	β_T	−0.0486	0.9526	0.1001	−0.4854	0.6274
History of fits	β_F	−0.3913	0.6762	0.1159	−3.3767	0.0007

More than two explanatory variables

The Cox model can be extended to include more than two variables. Thus, the influence of age (x_A) on the survival of patients with brain cancer could be added to the model describing the effect of treatment (x_T) and history of fits (x_F). In this case the relative hazard for the extended model is

$$T + F + A : h(x_T, x_F, x_A) = \exp(\beta_T x_T + \beta_F x_F + \beta_A x_A) \qquad (5.20)$$

Here x_A is a continuous variable whilst x_T and x_F are binary. To ease presentation and description we have written x_A rather than $(x_A - \bar{x}_A)$ here although we have used the centred value in the actual calculations given below.

Example – Cox PH regression model – history of fits, age and treatment in brain cancer

Fitting the three-variable model of equation (5.20) to the data from the patients with brain cancer gives the results summarised in Table 5.3. This shows that both history of fits and age, even when both are included in the same model, appear to influence survival, although there are smaller values for both the treatment and history of fits regression coefficients, as compared to those of Table 5.2.

Table 5.3 Cox's model incorporating treatment, stage and age in 417 brain cancer patients (From Medical Research Council Working Party on Misonidazole in Gliomas, 1983. Reproduced by permission of The British Institute of Radiology)

Variable	Coefficient	Estimate (b)	$HR = e^b$	$SE(b)$	$z = b/SE(b)$	p-value
Treatment	β_T	−0.0326	0.9680	0.1001	−0.3251	0.7451
Fits	β_F	−0.2729	0.7612	0.1169	−2.3339	0.0196
Age	β_A	0.0303	1.0308	0.0049	6.1395	< 0.0001

Categorical variables

We have discussed earlier how to include a binary variable, such as treatment group or history of fits, into the Cox model. Suppose, however, that we are concerned with assessing the influence of tumour grade (see Table 5.1). There are three tumour grade groups: those patients of definitely Grade 3, those of definitely Grade 4 and an intermediate group of Grade 3/4. In such cases, we ask the basic question as to whether or not tumour grade is influential on prognosis.

One way of doing this is to fit a Cox model using so-called dummy variables to describe the variable Grade. These are also known as indicator variables. We first create, in our case two, dummy variables as follows:

$g_1 = 1$ intermediate Grade 3/4 patient
$g_1 = 0$ not an intermediate Grade 3/4 patient
$g_2 = 1$ Grade 4 patient
$g_2 = 0$ not a Grade 4 patient

In this way the three grade groups correspond to different pairs of values of (g_1, g_2) in the following way. The pair, $g_1 = 0$ and $g_2 = 0$, define Grade 3 patients since the values of g indicate neither an intermediate Grade 3/4 patient nor a Grade 4 patient. Similarly, the pair, $g_1 = 1$ and $g_2 = 0$, define intermediate Grade 3/4 patients and finally the pair, $g_1 = 0$ and $g_2 = 1$, define Grade 4 patients.

The Cox model for Grade, ignoring all other potential variables, is then written as

$$G : \log h = \gamma_1 g_1 + \gamma_2 g_2. \tag{5.21}$$

This model is then fitted to the data in the same way as earlier models. In this model there are two regression coefficients, γ_1 and γ_2, to estimate. These are both concerned with grade. In general, if a categorical variable has g categories then $g - 1$ dummy variables need to be created for the corresponding terms in a Cox model and consequently $g - 1$ regression coefficients have to be estimated. Note, to ensure a correct model is used, all $g - 1$ dummy variables need to be included in the model at the same time.

Example – Cox PH regression model – prognostic factors in breast cancer

A Cox regression model was used by Fisher, Anderson, Fisher *et al.* (1991) to assess the relative influence of 11 potential prognostic variables in 914 patients with breast cancer. The authors reduce the number of variables to the five shown in Table 5.4 by rejecting those variables for which the associated χ^2, analogous to equation (5.9), gave a test statistic yielding a p-value >0.2. Each of the remaining variables—age, nodal status, nuclear grade, tumour type and tumour size-had a p-value <0.2, in fact all were <0.02. As a consequence, the *HR*s quoted for these variables have associated 95% *CI*s which do not include $HR = 1$.

If we focus on the analysis of tumour type in Table 5.4 and ignore the remainder of the table, then the results are highlighted in Table 5.5. The model for the corresponding relative hazard is therefore

$$TT : \log h(g_1, g_2) = 0.492 g_1 + 0.758 g_2.$$

Thus, when the tumour type is Good, $g_1 = g_2 = 0, \log h = 0$ and this provides the baseline group. Similarly, when the tumour type is Intermediate, $g_1 = 1, g_2 = 0$ and $\log h = 0.492$. Finally, when the tumour type is Poor, $g_1 = 0, g_2 = 1$ and $\log h = 0.758$. The corresponding *HR*s, expressed as relative to Good tumour type are therefore, $\exp(0.492) = 1.64$ and $\exp(0.758) = 2.13$ for Intermediate and Poor tumour types, respectively.

Table 5.4 Cox model to determine predictors of time to development of distant disease in patients with breast cancer (Reprinted from *The Lancet*, **338**, Fisher, Anderson, Fisher *et al.*, Significance of ipsilateral breast tumour recurrence after lumpectomy, 327–331, © 1991, with permission from Elsevier)

Variable	b	$SE(b)$	χ^2	p-value	HR	95% CI
Age (years)						
<50	0				1	
>50	0.268	0.113	5.77	0.016	1.31	1.05 to 1.63
Nodal status						
Negative	0				1	
Positive	0.402	0.111	12.99	0.0003	1.49	1.20 to 1.86
Nuclear grade						
Good	0				1	
Poor	0.405	0.117	11.98	0.0005	1.50	1.19 to 1.89
Tumour type						
Good	0				1	
Intermediate	0.492	0.217	5.75	0.017	1.64	1.07 to 2.50
Poor	0.758	0.224	13.33	0.0003	2.13	1.38 to 3.31
Maximum pathologically tumour size						
<2 cm	0				1	
≥ 2 cm	0.274	0.111	6.06	0.014	1.32	1.06 to 1.63

Table 5.5 Cox model assessing the influence of tumour type on time to development of distant metastases in patients with breast cancer (part of Table 5.4)

Tumour type (TT)	Dummy variable, g_1	Dummy variable, g_2	Regression coefficient, (b)	$SE(b)$	HR
Good	0	0	0	–	1
Intermediate	1	0	0.492	0.217	1.64
Poor	0	1	0.758	0.224	2.13

In many circumstances, the categorical variables can be placed on a numeric scale. Suppose, for example, since the categories of tumour type (Good, Intermediate, Poor) are clearly ordered, they may be included in a Cox model with the single associated variable g taking values 0, 1 and 2. This approach assumes a linear trend in prognosis as tumour type changes, since biological differences between tumour types have now been given equal numerical steps of unity. Such an approach is equivalent to describing the change in regression coefficients in Table 5.5 by the broken line in Figure 5.4. Here the relationship

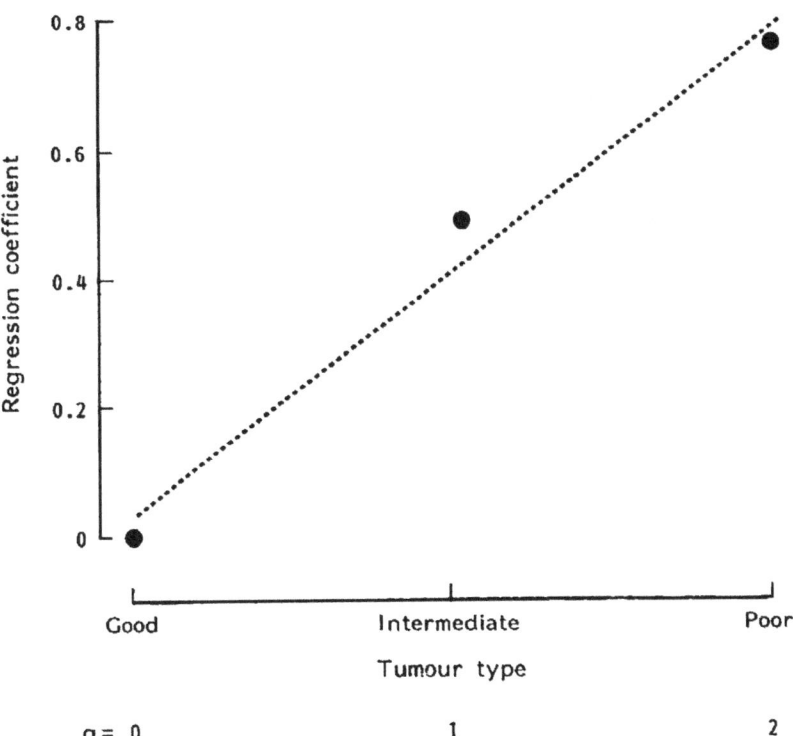

Figure 5.4 Linear relationship between tumour type and time to development of distant metastases in patients with breast cancer (data taken from Table 5.4)

is summarised by one regression coefficient which is the slope of the line. If a linear relationship can be assumed then this model provides a very powerful test of this trend. The final model, however, is of the same form as equation (5.15) which is for a continuous variable. Thus, a numerically ordered categorical variable is treated in a similar way to a continuous variable in the modelling process.

A question often arises as to whether a continuous variable should or should not be transformed into a categorical variable for analysis. For example, is it better to 'categorise' the variable age into three separate categories say, less than 50 (Young), 50–59 (Middle Aged) and 60 or more (Senior), as we did in Section 3.5, or to leave it as a continuous variable in a Cox model?

The answer often lies in the use to be made of the prognostic factor, on the prior information available and the shape of the underlying relationship. If prior information tells us that the prognosis gradually changes with increasing age and we want to know how important a prognostic factor age is, then we may want to employ age as a continuous variable in the modelling process. In doing this, we are assuming that the effect of age is approximately linearly related to prognosis. If, however, age is acting, say, as a surrogate for menopausal status in women with a particular disease, then categories of $-44, 45-54, 55+$ may then be thought of as 'definitely' premenopausal, perimenopausal and 'definitely' postmenopausal. In such circumstances, it is this categorisation that is thought to be more important than age itself.

If we are not sure of the relationship between the variable age and survival, or want to use the prognostic factor 'age' in practice, then transforming the variable into categories may be helpful. Inevitably this involves some subjectivity and may lead to some loss of information. If such a categorisation is made, then to minimise assumptions about the form of the relationship between age and survival, it is then appropriate to include age as a series of dummy variables, and to use the equivalent of equation (5.21) with age (Young, Middle Aged, Senior) in place of Tumour Type (Good, Intermediate, Poor) of Table 5.5.

In making a continuous variable discrete, a number of decisions have to be made. First, we must decide how, and in what number, the categories should be made. Although this depends on the context, we recommend no more than five categories and that three is usually sufficient. Second, the boundaries for these categories need to be considered carefully. These should be decided in such a way as to make divisions at numerically simple values, ensure sufficient numbers in each category and, most importantly, make clinical sense. For example, the age divisions described above are centred about the mean age of 52.3 years using the category Middle Aged for those patients aged 45 to 54 inclusively, with numerically convenient boundaries. As already indicated, this division makes biological sense. A final check of the data should verify that sufficient patients, of the order of 25%, say, are included in each group. Often it is useful to choose boundaries that are the same as those used by others working in a similar context, since we might wish to make comparisons with these related studies.

It is important to stress that we do not recommend the so-called 'optimal cut-point' approach. This involves first ranking the variable under consideration, then (in its most extreme form) going though this ranking (say from the smallest to the largest) systematically and splitting the data in two after every observation. For each of these splits a Cox regression model is fitted and that split which provides the lowest p-value is taken as the cut-point for the explanatory variable.

Other aspects of this problem are discussed in Section 6.5.

Multivariable models

The number of variables that can be added to the Cox model is, in theory, without end. Thus, in general, we have a v-variable regression model for the relative hazard, of the form

$$h(x_1, x_2, \ldots, x_v) = \exp(\beta_1 x_1 + \beta_2 x_2 + \cdots + \beta_v x_v). \qquad (5.22)$$

Now although the number of variables we can add is without limit, there are practical constraints since estimates have to be obtained for the regression coefficients. Thus, for example, we cannot include more variables in a model than the number of events available for the analysis.

***Example** – Cox PH regression model – factors influencing recovery of sperm production*

Meng, Zhu, Chen *et al.* (1988) investigated factors influencing the recovery of sperm production following cessation of gossypol treatment in 46 Chinese males. The factors considered were serum follicle-stimulating hormone (FSH), serum luteinising hormone (LH), serum testosterone, total acid phosphatase, age, weight, duration of gossypol treatment and testicular volume. Their final model includes three variables: duration of gossypol treatment (G), corrected testicular volume (V) and FSH (F). Since both duration of gossypol treatment and FSH have rather skew distributions a log scale was chosen for these variables. The estimated model is

$$G + V + F : \log h = -0.313[\log \text{ duration of gossypol (years)} - 1.15]$$
$$+0.075\,[\text{corrected testicular volume (ml)} - 29.1] - 0.0578\,[\log \text{FSH (IU/ml)} - 1.73].$$

Where 1.15, 29.1 and 1.73 are the mean values of the respective variables included in the model. Further, $\exp(-0.313) = 0.73$, $\exp(0.075) = 1.08$ and $\exp(-0.0578) = 0.94$ give the corresponding *HR* for a unit change in each variable.

They fit three variables to data in which only 20 events (recovery of sperm production) are observed. Such a limited number of events would suggest that considerable uncertainty is likely to remain about the true values of the respective *HRs*.

COX (SEMI-PARAMETRIC) OR PARAMETRIC MODEL?

We have seen that regression models are an integral part of the Cox modelling process and, in Chapter 4, that they are also relevant to situations where the parametric Exponential, Weibull and other survival distributions are used. In some circumstances the choice of whether to use Cox or one of the parametric forms for the regression model will be based on considerations related to *PH*. If, for example, the hazards are not proportional then this may rule out the Cox approach. When the hazards are clearly proportional then a choice between the Cox and Exponential might be made in terms of ease of interpretation of the final model. For instance, if one wants to know the effect of a treatment in terms of its impact on the duration of the time-to-event (instead of the hazard), an *AFT* model may be preferred as it gives the results as a time ratio. When the evidence for or against *PH* is unclear then Cox and a parametric model may be used and the results compared to guide the ultimate choice.

The Cox model has become a 'standard' approach in many modelling situations, largely because it seems to work well in practice. This seems to imply that many variables can be transformed to show approximate *PH* as, for example, we saw in examining the factors affecting sperm production above with the log transformation. It also implies that the model is reasonably robust to modest departures from *PH*. As a consequence in considering potential models, the Cox model should always be considered as an option.

Example *– comparison of Cox and the Weibull – development of asthmatic symptoms*

A comparison of the Cox *PH*s model and a Weibull model both including covariates is given by Samuelson and Kongerud (1994). They describe a study of workers in seven Norwegian aluminium plants in which information on the time to develop asthmatic symptoms in more than 1000 new employees is collected. The two models arising from their analyses are summarised in Table 5.6. From these it is very clear that the results obtained with each model are very similar and so the Cox model may be chosen as it involves fewer parameters.

Table 5.6 A comparison of Weibull and Cox models for the time to develop asthmatic symptoms in workers from seven Norwegian aluminium plants (From Samuelson and Kongerud, 1994 with permission)

Variable	Weibull b(SE)	Cox b(SE)
Age	−0.25(0.16)	−0.29(0.17)
Sex ($M = 1, F = 0$)	−0.40(0.30)	−0.40(0.27)
Allergy ($Y = 1, N = 0$)	0.07(0.37)	0.07(0.35)
Asthma in family ($Y = 1, N = 0$)	0.39(0.26)	0.39(0.24)
Previous exposure ($Y = 1, N = 0$)	0.60(0.24)	0.60(0.23)
Never smoker	0	0
Ex-smoker	1.43(0.66)	1.42(0.55)
Light smoker	0.55(0.28)	0.55(0.27)
Heavy smoker	1.04(0.31)	1.01(0.27)
Soederberg oven	0	0
Prebake oven	0.40(0.26)	0.42(0.27)
Rotation	0.93(0.32)	0.94(0.31)
Low fluoride	0	0
Fluoride not classified	0.72(0.31)	0.75(0.29)
Medium fluoride	1.37(0.39)	1.36(0.38)
High fluoride	2.28(0.47)	2.25(0.48)

5.3   INTERACTIONS

THE 2×2 FACTORIAL DESIGN

In randomised control clinical trials and many other types of study it is possible, in appropriate circumstances, to pose two or more questions simultaneously.

Example – 2×2 *factorial design* – *treatment for colorectal cancer*

In the AXIS trial described by Gray, James, Mossman *et al.* (1991), in patients with colorectal cancer, there were two basic questions. One is the value of radiotherapy, and the second the value of postoperative hepatic infusion of fluorouracil, in prolonging survival in these patients. In brief, there are four treatments corresponding to the two factors: infusion (*I*) and radiotherapy (*R*). These four treatments are summarised in Table 5.7.

Table 5.7   Model for a 2×2 factorial design of the AXIS trial examining the value of radiotherapy and infusion of fluorouracil in patients with colorectal cancer

			Binary Variable	
Treatment options		Model	x_I	x_R
No radiotherapy and No Infusion	(*I*)	Null	0	0
No radiotherapy with Infusion	*I*	Infusion	1	0
Radiotherapy but No Infusion	*R*	Radiotherapy	0	1
Radiotherapy with Infusion	*I + R*	Infusion and Radiotherapy	1	1

The use of (*I*), *I*, *R* and *I + R* notation for models has been introduced, and the analysis of such a 2×2 factorial design using the Logrank test described, in Section 3.6. An alternative approach is by means of the following Cox model, using an analogy with equations (5.18) and (5.21), which is

$$I^*R : h(x_I, x_R) = \exp(\beta_I x_I + \beta_R x_R + \beta_{IR} x_I x_R). \qquad (5.23)$$

Equation (5.23) gives, for the various combinations of values of x_I and x_R of Table 5.7, the following hazard ratios:

Null model	(*I*) :	$h(0,0) = 1$	
Infusion only	*I* :	$h(1,0) = \exp(\beta_I)$	
Radiotherapy only	*R* :	$h(0,1) = \exp(\beta_R)$	(5.24)
Infusion and Radiotherapy	*I + R + I.R* :	$h(1,1) = \exp(\beta_I + \beta_R + \beta_{IR})$	

The regression coefficient β_{IR} in the *I + R + I.R* part of the model emphasises the possibility of some interaction (*I.R*) between the two treatment types in their effect on survival when both treatment types are given simultaneously. This would imply that the effect of, say, the infusion would depend on whether or not radiotherapy was given. If no interaction is present then $\beta_{IR} = 0$ and the model reduces to a main effects model only. That is, the two treatments act independently of each other. This model is

$$I + R : h = \exp(\beta_I + \beta_R) \tag{5.25}$$

The model of equations (5.24) can also be expressed in a convenient shorthand as I^*R and this format is often used in statistical texts and computer package manuals.

Example *– 2 × 2 factorial design – prevention of myocardial infarction in unstable coronary artery disease*

In an example previously presented in Figure 3.11, the cumulative risk of myocardial infarction (MI) and death in the first 30 days during treatment in men with unstable coronary artery disease is reported by The RISC Group (1990). The four treatment combinations used in the trial were a 2 × 2 factorial arrangement of placebo (*I*), aspirin (*a*), heparin (*h*) and aspirin with heparin (*ah*). This figure suggests a benefit of aspirin with a reduction in 30-day morbidity of about 10% compared to placebo. It also suggests lack of efficacy of heparin given either alone or in combination with aspirin treatment, which implies little evidence of the presence of an interaction between aspirin and heparin, so that a model *A + H* analogous to equation (5.25) is likely to be appropriate.

OTHER DESIGNS

As is indicated by equation (5.23), the interaction term in a model is obtained by using a regression coefficient, β_{IR}, with a multiplication term involving $x_I x_R$ from the binary variables concerned. However, the application of equations, like (5.23) above, is not restricted to the analysis of designed experiments involving only two factors with two levels. It can be extended to more complex designs, and also to applications when the variables under consideration do not include a variable for treatment.

Example *– interaction – history of fits and grade of disease in brain cancer*

It is of some interest to see in the example of patients with brain cancer whether there is any interaction between history of fits (*F*) and grade of the disease (*G*). For example, does the influence of grade on prognosis differ between those patients with a history of fits and those without? Here, for simplicity, tumour grade, which is a categorical variable with $g = 3$ values, is now treated as a binary variable with values $x_G = 0$ for both Grade 3 and Grade 3/4 tumours and $x_G = 1$ for Grade 4 tumours. There are now only $g=2$ categories for grade and, thus, only one regression coefficient to be estimated. The corresponding overall model is

$$F^*G = F + G + F.G : h = \exp(\beta_F x_F + \beta_G x_G + \beta_{IR} x_F x_G)$$

The results of fitting this model including the interaction term and the main effects model without the interaction term, which essentially assumes $\beta_{FG} = 0$, are summarised in Table 5.8.

It can be seen from Table 5.8 that the regression coefficient for the interaction term, $b_{FG} = -0.0488$, is not large and has an associated $SE(b_{FG}) = 0.1183$. These give $z = -0.0488/0.1183 = -0.41$ and from Table T1 a p-value $= 0.6818$. This then implies that we have little evidence of an interaction between history of fits and tumour grade. As a consequence, we use the main effects model, that is, $F + G : h = -0.3924 x_F + 0.0144 x_G$ to describe these data.

Table 5.8 Test for interaction between a history of fits and tumour grade in 417 patients with brain cancer (From Medical Research Council Working Party on Misonidazole in Gliomas, 1983. Reproduced by permission of The British Institute of Radiology)

	Model				
	Main effects only $F+G$			Including interaction term $F^*G = F + G + F.G$	
Coefficient	Regression Coefficient	SE		Regression coefficient	SE
Fits β_F	−0.3924	0.1159		−0.3379	0.1748
Grade β_G	0.0144	0.0518		0.0269	0.0601
Interaction β_{FG}	–	–		−0.0488	0.1183
LR		11.69		11.86	

We should note that omitting the interaction term from the model changes the estimates of the regression coefficients corresponding to β_F and β_G. This is because the estimate $b_{FG} = -0.0488$ does not equal zero, although we suspect the corresponding parameter β_{FG} is equal to zero.

***Example** – test for interaction – history of fits and grade of disease in brain cancer*

To test for the interaction term, using the LR values of Table 5.8, we calculate $LR_{F+G+F.G} - LR_{F+G} = 11.86 - 11.69 = 0.17$ and so $\sqrt{0.17} = 0.41$. This corresponds exactly to the $z = -0.41$ that we obtained earlier for the test of the interaction term. More details of the LR test are given in Section 5.6

If the interaction term of Table 5.8 had been statistically significant then we would have retained the model F^*G, rather than the main effects only model $F + G$. In such a circumstance the final model is therefore

$$F^*G : h = \exp(-0.3379x_F + 0.0269x_G - 0.0488x_F x_G).$$

The four patient groups are defined by the combinations of x_F and x_G, which are (0, 0), (0, 1), (1, 0) and (1, 1) respectively. Thus, the relative hazards are $h(0, 0) = \exp(0) = 1$, which is the baseline relative hazard, $h(0, 1) = \exp(0.0269) = 1.0272$, $h(1, 0) = \exp(-0.3379) = 0.7133$ and finally, $h(1, 1) = \exp(-0.3379 + 0.0269 - 0.0488) = \exp(-0.3598) = 0.6978$. These then give the ratios $h(1, 1)/h(1, 0) = 0.6978/0.7133 = 0.9783$, which estimates the effect of tumour grade in those patients without a history of fits. Similarly, $h(0, 1)/h(0, 0) = 1.0272/1 = 1.0272$ estimates the effect of tumour grade in those patients with a history of fits.

These two ratios measuring the effect of tumour grade on prognosis are not exactly equal. In our example, however, the regression coefficient for the interaction term is very small and so has little effect. Consequently, the two estimates of the *HR* for grade, 0.9783 and 1.0272, for absence and presence of history of fits groups respectively, are approximately equal with a value close to one. Thus, they can be combined into one estimate which is obtained from fitting model $F + G$. However, in the presence of an important interaction, we would have to interpret the final model with some care.

We should introduce a word of caution here, in that the test for interaction typically has very low power to detect what might be considered realistic interactions, and thus we may be led to conclude that there is 'no evidence' of an interaction, despite the fact that an interaction may in truth be present. A small indication that we cannot perhaps conclude simply that there is no interaction is if the estimates of the main effects change markedly between the main effects only and interaction models. We note that this may be the case in the history of fits and grade interaction of Table 5.8. In spite of such potential clues, however, the decision about whether an interaction is present in clinical studies depends as much on biological and clinical considerations as statistical ones.

5.4 STRATIFIED ANALYSIS

It is possible to perform an analysis adjusting a treatment effect for imbalances in important prognostic factors either by using a stratified Logrank test (see Section 3.4) or by means of a Cox model. It may be argued that the stratified analysis is easier to explain to non-statisticians and thus it is preferable. However, a stratified Logrank test cannot deal with continuous variables without first making a categorisation into groups. In addition, if there are many would-be variables that influence outcome, there is a danger that there will be no patients or events in one of the intervention groups as they may become very small. In these circumstances, the Logrank approach becomes tedious and potentially difficult. However, the stratified Logrank test, unlike the Cox model, does not require *PH*. Whichever procedure is to be used, it is good practice to specify this before the analysis is performed and to report this in any subsequent publication.

Example – Cox model and stratified Logrank test – treatment for brain cancer stratified by history of fits

For the patients with brain cancer, the stratified Logrank test takes the format summarised in Table 5.9. Thus, for example, for the patients receiving control therapy with no history of fits, the observed and expected number of deaths $O_C = 153$, $E_C = 130.07$ and $O_C - E_C = 19.93$. For those who have experienced fits, the corresponding $O_C = 45$, $E_C = 62.32$ and $O_C - E_C = 45 - 62.32 = -17.32$.

The estimate of the stratified Logrank HR for the treatment comparison is obtained using equation (3.16) as

$$HR_{Stratified} = \frac{[(146+58)/(137.15+72.47)]}{[(153+45)/(130.07+62.32)]} = \frac{[204/209.62]}{[198/192.39]} = 0.9456 \text{ or } 0.95.$$

This is equal to that obtained from the Cox model of Table 5.2 and suggests a marginal benefit of misonidazole as an addition to radiotherapy.

Table 5.9 Logrank survival comparison by history of fits and treatment in patients with brain cancer (From Medical Research Council Working Party on Misonidazole in Gliomas, 1983. Reproduced by permission of The British Institute of Radiology)

			Number of deaths			
Treatment	Fits	Number of patients	Observed (O)	Expected (E)	(O/E)	HR
Control	No	156	153	130.07	1.18	1
Misonidazole	No	148	146	137.15	1.06	0.8983
Control	Yes	49	45	62.32	0.72	0.6102
Misonidazole	Yes	64	58	72.47	0.80	0.6780
Totals		417	402	402.01		

Example – Cox model and stratified Logrank test – treatment for brain cancer stratified by age

A total of 443 eligible patients with Grade 3 or 4 malignant glioma were randomised after surgery into a Medical Research Council Brain Tumour Working Party trial (Bleehen and Stenning, 1991) comparing 45 Gy radiotherapy given in 20 fractions over four weeks, with 60 Gy given in 30 fractions over six weeks. Using a 1:2 randomisation in favour of the higher dose, 144 patients were allocated to receive 45 Gy and 299 were allocated to receive 60 Gy. A Logrank analysis of the survival data gave $\chi^2_{Logrank} = 4.06$, $df = 1$, p-value $= 0.04$ and a $HR = 0.81$ in favour of 60 Gy, with a reported 95% CI 0.66 to 0.99.

Table 5.10   Age distribution of patients with brain cancer by treatment allocated (From Medical Research Council Brain Tumour Working Party, Bleehen and Stenning, 1991, with permission from the Macmillan Press, Ltd)

Age (years)	Percentage of patients allocated treatment	
	45 Gy	60 Gy
18-39	15	16
40-49	24	18
50-59	27	36
60-73	34	30
Total (%)	100	100
Number of patients	144	299

However, as the authors of the report point out, this Logrank analysis may underestimate the true benefit of the higher dose of radiotherapy because of a chance unfavourable age distribution in the high dose group. The age distribution of patients in the two treatment groups is summarised in Table 5.10. Although the age distribution does not appear markedly unbalanced, an adjusted analysis was performed, in which age and treatment allocated were included in a Cox proportional hazards model. In this model, age was included as a continuous variable, because it is known that increasing age is associated with poorer prognosis in this disease.

The model led to a $HR = 0.75$ in favour of 60 Gy and a 95% CI 0.61 to 0.92 with an associated p-value $= 0.007$. Thus, this adjusted analysis gave a somewhat larger treatment difference, and a more definitive statement, than those using the unadjusted Logrank statistic. This illustrates an important practical consideration, that only a small imbalance in an important prognostic factor can influence the conclusions drawn, even from reasonably large patient groups.

Other factors known to affect prognosis, such as clinical performance status, history of fits and extent of neurosurgery, were well balanced between the two treatment groups. Adjustment for these factors, in addition to age, did not alter the estimate of the treatment effect substantially from $HR = 0.75$.

5.5   ASSESSING PROPORTIONALITY OF HAZARDS

Complementary Log Plot

It is important that the PH assumption holds for valid interpretation of regression coefficients in a Cox model. A graphical check on the proportionality is provided by a complementary log plot over several values or grouped values of a variable, as has been indicated in Figures 5.1 and 5.2. The different values of the variables, presence or not of metastatic disease and limited or extensive disease in our examples, are reflected in separate lines in the complementary log plot.

The survival function corresponding to the proportional hazards model of equation (5.12) can be expressed as

$$S(t; x) = S(t; x_0)^{\exp(\beta x)} \tag{5.26}$$

where x and x_0 are values of the explanatory variables. In particular x_0 is the value of the variable in the baseline group. The x's are included here to emphasise their possible influence on survival. From equation (5.26) we have

$$\log\{-\log[S(t; x)]\}) = \log\{-\log[S(t; x_0)]\} + \beta x. \tag{5.27}$$

As a consequence, a complementary log plot, which is a plot of the left-hand side of equation (5.27), against $\log t$ will give separate curves depending on the number of different values of the variable x. This is because the right-hand side of equation (5.27) has a part which varies with t, which is distinct from the part which varies with x. Any changes in the x term cause a step vertically up or down in the plot. The size of the step depends on the importance of the variable on prognosis.

If there are several variables, say, v in all, then βx is replaced in equation (5.27) by $\beta_1 x_1 + \beta_2 x_2 + \cdots + \beta_v x_v$. The corresponding plot will then have the possibility of many distinct curves.

Example – complementary log plots – history of fits and treatment for brain cancer

A check on the proportional hazards of the four treatment by history of fits graphs is provided by the complementary log plots of Figure 5.5. The parallel lines indicate approximately proportional hazards in the four patient groups. The differences in the lines suggest a relatively major difference in prognosis for those with and without a history of fits. In contrast the effect of treatment appears minimal.

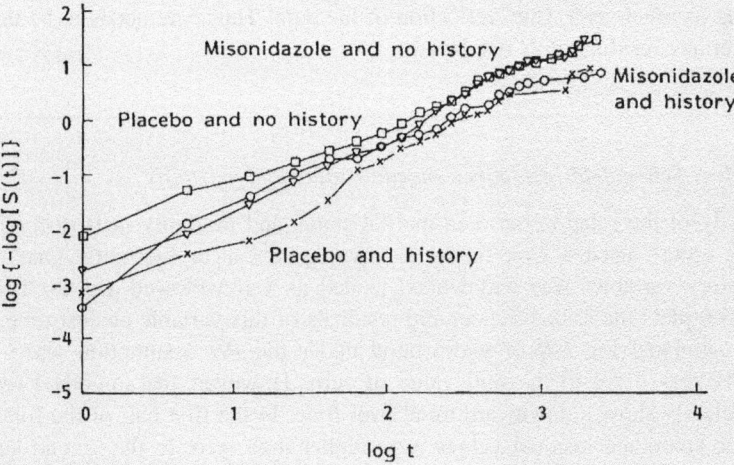

Figure 5.5   Complementary log plot against $\log t$ for each of the four treatment by history of fits groups of patients with brain tumours

SCHOENFELD RESIDUALS

If an explanatory variable is continuous or there are many categorical variables, the complementary log plot is difficult to implement. In such situations, the Schoenfeld (1982) residuals, or the scaled version described in Therneau and Grambsch (2000), are particularly useful for the assessment of the *PH* assumption. The references included in this section are quite technical in nature but are included here for completeness.

A Schoenfeld residual SCH_{kj} can be calculated for each explanatory variable x_k and each non-censored observation j, whose failure time is denoted by t_j, by

$$SCH_{kj} = x_{kj} - E(x_{kj}|R_j), \tag{5.28}$$

where R_j is the set of observations at risk of failure at the time subject j fails, while $E(x_{kj}|R_j)$ is the expected value of x_k for subject j estimated based on the log *HR*s from a Cox model. The SCH_{kj} sum to zero over all and should scatter around zero if the model is correct. A systematic trend in SCH_{kj} in relation to time, or the rank order of time, indicates non-*PH*. If in a time interval the average values of the residuals tend to be positive, the true log *HR* in this interval is higher than estimated, and vice versa.

The scaled residuals behave in much the same manner as SCH_{kj}, but they have a mean value equal to log *HR*, estimated assuming *PH*, and their smoothed average values can be interpreted as estimates of the time-varying log *HR*.

The validity of the *PH* assumption can be assessed graphically, or by performing regression analysis of the (scaled or non-scaled) residuals in relation to time or the rank order of time. A significant regression coefficient indicates that the true log *HR* changes over time. Major statistical packages have built-in functions to calculate the two residuals, as well as facilities to make the scatter plots and smoothing procedures to summarise the trend in the plotted data. However, as we indicated in Chapter 4, although it may be usual to study residuals the plots may be difficult to interpret and any patterns observed may be a consequence of the censoring as much as a 'true' reflection of the data. Thus care needs to be taken not to over-interpret any residual plots displayed.

Example – Schoenfeld residuals – marital status and mortality

In a study of the relation between marital status and mortality in British women, Cheung (2000) used a Cox model to investigate cancer mortality. One of the explanatory variables was widowhood, coded as 1 if widowed and 0 otherwise. Figure 5.6 plots the scaled Schoenfeld residuals of this variable against time.

The estimated log *HR* of widowhood under the *PH* assumption was −0.09, which is very close to the null value of zero. However, the smoothed residual values clearly show a downward trend over time. In the first half of the follow-up time, the smoothed residual values were higher than zero. In the second half the residuals tended to fall below zero. This pattern suggested that in the short-run widowhood was more hazardous than expected, while in the long-run it appeared to be 'protective' against cancer mortality. The latter was thought to be an artefact due to a limitation in the research design.

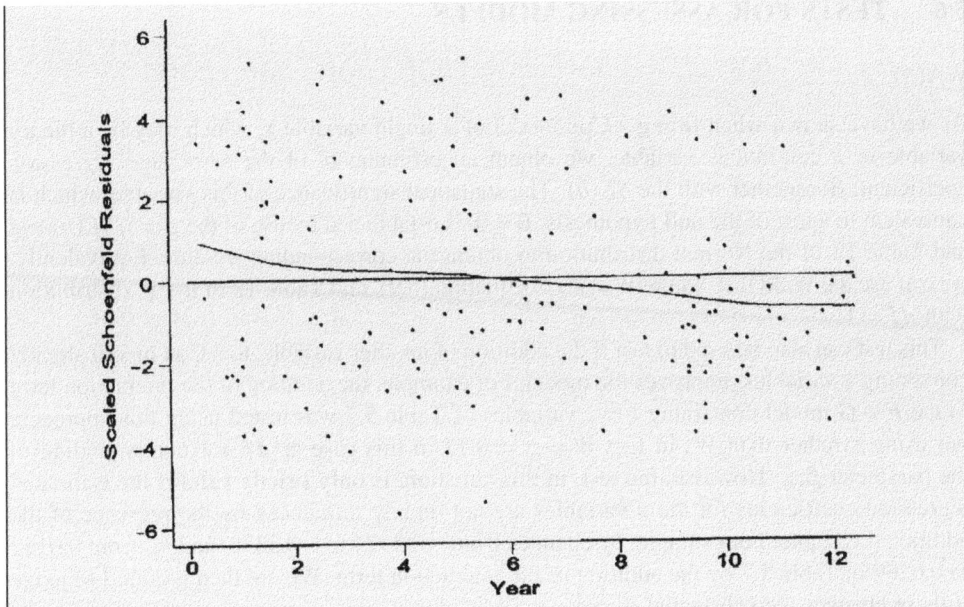

Figure 5.6 Scaled Schoenfeld residuals for the effect of widowhood on cancer mortality plotted against survival time in years. A horizontal reference line at zero and a smoothed fit to these data is included (from Cheung, 2000).

WHAT IF THE PROPORTIONAL HAZARDS ASSUMPTION IS WRONG?

If the *PH* assumption is not valid in the data, one may use 'time-varying covariates' in the Cox model to capture the non-*PH*. This is the topic for Chapter 7. However, the violation of this assumption is not necessarily unacceptable. To assume *PH* is essentially to estimate the effect of an independent variable averaged over time and ignore the possibility that the effect may vary over time. A simple model based on the assumption of *PH* is sometimes preferable to a more 'correct' but complex model if the added complexity does not identify features of scientific or clinical significance.

Example – non-PH – marital status and mortality

In the widowhood example of Cheung (2000), the time-dependent hazard ratio changed from hazardous to seemingly protective. Such a change over time is likely to be of great interest were it to be firmly established. In contrast, were the true $HR = 2$ in the early period of the follow-up, but then steadily declined to (say) 1.5 such a feature may not be of great clinical importance. In such cases one may prefer a simple although *less correct PH* model

5.6   TESTS FOR ASSESSING MODELS

WALD

As we have shown when fitting a Cox model of a single variable x, which may be a binary variable or a continuous variable, we obtain an estimate, b, of the associated regression coefficient, β, together with the $SE(b)$. The statistical significance of this variable, which is equivalent to a test of the null hypothesis, $\beta = 0$, is established by use of the $z = b/SE(b)$ test and Table T1 of the Normal distribution to obtain the corresponding p-value. Equivalently, we can use the Wald test, where $W = z^2$, of equation (5.9), and Table T3 of the χ^2 distribution with $df = 1$.

This test can also be used to test if the addition of another variable, to a Cox model already containing v variables, improves the model. For example, the addition of the interaction term to the $F + G$ model containing $v = 2$ variables of Table 5.7 was tested using this approach, but using z rather than W. In fact $W = z^2 = 0.17$ in this case as $df = 1$ corresponding to the parameter β_{FG}. However, the test, in this situation, is only strictly valid if the estimated regression coefficients for the v variables are not unduly influenced by the presence of the additional variable. For example, b_F changes from -0.3924 to -0.3379, and b_G from 0.0144 to 0.0269 in Table 5.7 by the addition of the interaction term. We are then required to judge if these changes are substantial or not.

LIKELIHOOD RATIO

A more general test than the Wald test, and one which can cope both with categorical variables of more than two levels and with adding several variables simultaneously to a Cox model, is the LR test which we referred to in Section 1.6.

A loose definition of the likelihood is that it is the probability of the observed data being 'represented' by a particular model. To illustrate this test, we first define the null model which, in the terminology of the Cox model, specifies that no variable influences survival. When the variable is treatment, this is equivalent to setting $\beta = 0$ in equation (5.5) to imply $\lambda_N(t) = \lambda_C(t) = \lambda_o(t)$, or that, irrespective of treatment, all patients have the same hazard $\lambda_o(t)$. The likelihood for this model is denoted as ℓ_0 where ℓ denotes likelihood and the zero, 0, represents the fact that all the regression coefficients are set as zero.

In contrast, the likelihood of the model which contains v different regression coefficients is written as ℓ_v and the regression coefficients are estimated by the method of maximum likelihood. The larger ℓ_v is relative to ℓ_0, the better the model explains, or fits, the observed data.

The fit of each model can be tested using the LR as defined by

$$LR = -2\log(\ell_0/\ell_a) = -2(L_0 - L_a) \tag{5.29}$$

where $L_v = \log \ell_v$ and $L_0 = \log \ell_0$. This is in the same form as equation (1.14) with the suffix v replacing suffix a. We can think of the Cox model containing v variables as the alternative hypothesis and that containing no variables as the null hypothesis.

Under the hypothesis of no difference in the two models, that is, where including the variables in the Cox model does not help to explain the survival data any more satisfactorily than the null model with no variables, the LR of equation (5.29) has a χ^2 distribution with $df = v$.

> **Example – LR – patients with brain cancer**
>
> We noted in Table 5.8 that $LR = 11.69$ for the main effects model $F + G$ which, under the null hypothesis or model (1), has a χ^2 distribution with $df = v = 2$ degrees of freedom. Use of Table T3 with $df = 2$ suggests a corresponding p-value between 0.01 and 0.001, since 11.69 is between the tabular values of 9.21 and 13.82. More detailed tables of the χ^2 distribution give a p-value $= 0.005$. From this we conclude that the main effects model is an improvement over the null model.

To assess the relative fit of two models, one with $(v + k)$ regression coefficients and the other with the fewer v regression coefficients, we can use the statistic

$$LR_k = LR_{v+k} - LR_v. \tag{5.30}$$

This statistic also has a χ^2 distribution, but with $df = (v + k) - v = k$. The null hypothesis here is that there is no improvement in the fit of the model, by including the extra k coefficients.

> **Example – test for interaction – patients with brain cancer**
>
> To test for the interaction term, using the LR values of Table 5.8, we used $LR_{F+G+F.G} = 11.86$ and $LR_{F+G} = 11.69$. In the notation of equation (5.30) these are LR_3 and LR_2 respectively and for the χ^2 test the $df = 3 - 2 = 1$. We then consider whether $LR_3 - LR_2 = 11.86 - 11.69 = 0.17$ could plausibly have come from a χ^2 distribution with $df = 1$ against the null hypothesis that the interaction model is not an improvement on the main effects model. Use of Table T1 with $z = \sqrt{0.17} = 0.41$ gives the p-value $= 0.68$. From this we conclude that the interaction model is not an improvement over the main effects model, and hence that there is no convincing evidence for its presence.

5.7   TECHNICAL DETAILS

PARTIAL LIKELIHOOD

Although the Cox regression model is often referred to as the *PH* model, its uniqueness actually lies in the estimation method used, which is called maximum partial likelihood (*PL*), rather than the *PH* assumption itself. After all, the Exponential and Weibull models are also *PH* models.

Suppose in a two-group clinical trial n patients are recruited and their individual survival or censoring times are $t_1, t_2, \ldots, t_n$ which are then ranked to become $t_{(1)}, t_{(2)}, \ldots, t_{(n)}$ as for calculating the *K-M* estimate. Each patient will have received, for example, either the control, C, or new treatment T, coded $x = 0$ or 1 respectively so that a Logrank test comparing groups can be made.

Table 5.11   Illustration of the components required for calculating the partial likelihood (PL)

Rank order	Survival time	Indicator variable for censoring,	Indicator variable for at risk status, $y_{(i)}$	
i	$t_{(i)}$	$\delta_{(i)}$	At $t = 10$	At $t = 12$
1	10	1	1	0
2	10+	0	1	0
3	12	1	1	1
4	13	1	1	1
...	...	...	...	...

Table 5.11 shows, in a hypothetical clinical trial data set, the first few $t_{(i)}$ together with the values of a corresponding indicator variable $\delta_{(i)}$ which takes the value 1 if the time is a death time, and 0 if the time is censored. Further we set $y_{(i)} = 1$ if the subject i is at risk at time $t_{(i)}$, otherwise $y_{(i)} = 0$. Typically prior to the first death all $y_{(i)} = 1$, while just before the last observation all but $y_{(n)}$ will be 0.

The first death in the trial occurs to subject $i = 1$ at day $t_{(1)} = 10$ since randomisation. The corresponding component of the PL contributed by this death is

$$PL_1 = \frac{y_{(1)} \times \lambda_0(10) \times e^{\beta x_1}}{y_{(1)} \times \lambda_0(10) \times e^{\beta x_1} + y_{(2)} \times \lambda_0(10) \times e^{\beta x_2} + \cdots + y_{(n)} \times \lambda_0(10) \times e^{\beta x_n}}. \tag{5.31}$$

Here the numerator is evaluated for patient $i = 1$ who dies at $t = 10$ days while x_1 is the treatment assigned to this patient. We note in equation (5.31) that the term $\lambda_0(10)$, the baseline hazard at $t = 10$, divides out from this expression. Hence no assumption about the form of the hazard rate is required.

The next death occurs in Subject three at $t_{(3)} = 12$ days, Subject one (who has already died) and Subject two (who is censored at day 10+) are no longer at risk and so $y_{(1)} = y_{(2)} = 0$, while $y_{(3)} = \ldots = y_{(n)} = 1$ in PL_3. For the censored Subject two, $PL_2 = 1$ as will be the case for all censored observations.

The censored and uncensored observations can be included in the equivalent of equation (5.31) for all subjects by expressing each PL_i as

$$PL_i = \left[\frac{y_{(i)} \times e^{\beta x_1}}{y_{(1)} \times e^{\beta x_1} + y_{(2)} \times e^{\beta x_2} + \cdots + y_{(n)} \times e^{\beta x_n}} \right]^{\delta_{(i)}}. \tag{5.32}$$

For a censored observation at $t_{(i)}$, $\delta_i = 0$ and hence $PL_i = 1$.

The final PL is the product of all these n terms is $PL = PL_1 \times PL_2 \times \cdots \times PL_n$ that is

$$PL = \prod_{i=1}^{N} \left[\frac{y_{(i)} \times e^{\beta x_1}}{y_{(1)} \times e^{\beta x_1} + y_{(2)} \times e^{\beta x_2} + \cdots + y_{(n)} \times e^{\beta x_n}} \right]^{\delta_{(i)}}. \tag{5.33}$$

The PL has two very useful characteristics. Firstly, as already noted, the term representing the baseline hazard at time t, $\lambda_0(t)$, is present in both the numerator and denominator and therefore divides itself out of the expression. Thus, unlike for considering parametric models, one does not need to specify the form of the hazard function. Secondly, the 'at-risk' indicator $y_{(i)}$ makes it easy to handle complex situations such as delayed entry or gaps in exposure time which are features of some epidemiological studies involving survival times described in Chapter 7.

TIED DATA

The *PL* of equation (5.32) is strictly valid if there are no tied failure times. That is, no more than one failure takes place at the same time. Otherwise, there is a problem in determining which $y_{(i)}$ should be set to 0 or 1. In the presence of ties, the *PL* is given by one of the so-called *exact* methods but these require a great deal of computation time and so approximations are often used. The corresponding sections of the computer reference manuals usually provide details.

6 Selecting Variables within a Cox Model

Summary

A major reason for using the Cox model instead of the Logrank test is that the former easily allows for multivariable analysis. An important issue is how to decide on which variables are to be included in a Cox model. We discuss two main reasons for using multivariable analysis and highlight their relevance to the choice of variable selection methods. We categorise the potential explanatory variables as those fundamental to the research design, those that are known to influence outcome or confound relations, and other variables of uncertain influence; their effect only being known after the analysis stage is complete. The strategies for variable selection of forced-entry, significance tests and change in estimates of hazard ratios are each illustrated.

6.1   INTRODUCTION

As discussed in Section 5.2, one merit of the Cox model is that it can include many explanatory variables in a single model. However, it is subject to the practical constraints imposed by the type of data available for analysis. Furthermore, inclusion of unnecessary variables in a model reduces efficiency, as reflected in larger SEs, wider CIs, and larger p-values. A model with fewer explanatory variables is usually termed 'parsimonious' and is preferred, provided that it sufficiently serves the specific research purposes.

Although by no means exhaustive, there are two major purposes of using multivariable analysis. Firstly, a study may have a key explanatory variable whose relation with the time-to-event of interest may be confounded by some other variables (covariates) of known influence and/or others of as yet unquantified influence. Therefore a multivariable Cox model is required to adjust for these potential confounders so that the effect of the key explanatory variables is correctly estimated. For instance, one may want to study the impact of widowhood on mortality. Clearly widowhood is related to age, which in turn is related to mortality and therefore can confound the estimated HR for widowhood. Hence to obtain the relevant estimate for the HR, we may have to adjust for age and possibly some other potential confounders. Secondly, some studies may wish to explore the associations between various potential predictors of the outcome although there may be no key explanatory variables pre-specified in the study plan. One example is the development of prognostic indices for situations where clinical teams may want to identify variables that predict a poor outcome so that they can develop treatment plans according to the prognosis. The development of prognostic indices is a major area of statistical application in medicine and is discussed in more detail in Chapter 8. The two main purposes for multivariable analysis are not mutually exclusive within a single study, but there usually is a main focus on one of these. Thus it is

Survival Analysis Second Edition   David Machin, Yin Bun Cheung, Mahesh K.B. Parmar
© 2006 John Wiley & Sons, Ltd   ISBN: 0-470-87040-0

important to clarify what is one's main purpose and then choose a variable selection method accordingly.

Knowledge and assumptions concerning the impact of explanatory variables also affects the choice of selection method. A multivariable model can contain many variables of essentially three types, design variables (D), variables knowingly influential (K), and finally unknown, exploratory or query variables of uncertain influence (Q). By an influential *variable* we mean either (a) a *variable* which confounds the association between the 'key explanatory variable' and the 'survival outcome', or (b) a *variable* which is predictive of the 'survival outcome'. These two senses of influence correspond to the two major research purposes mentioned previously.

Most studies are designed with a specific objective to estimate the effect of one or more key explanatory variables. For example, in clinical trials, such a variable is the intervention allocated to patients. We call this a D variable as it clearly plays a key role in the research design. In some clinical trials subjects are first stratified into different groups and randomisation to the intervention is then made within each of these strata separately. The use of this device implies that the stratification factors are an influential (K variable) with respect to survival outcome otherwise there is no need to stratify. As this variable is now a feature of the design, one can consider this a D variable.

K variables are those known or assumed to be influential either from the researchers' own experience or from the published literature. Thus in a study of the effect of widowhood on mortality, age is clearly a K variable because of its role as a confounder. To develop a prognostic index for cancer patients' survival, 'performance status' is usually a K variable because it usually predicts survival. Finally, there are many variables whose influence we do not know and yet want to assess. We call these the Q variables.

We can express the three types of explanatory variables in one Cox model in an obvious format by:

$$\log h = \beta_D D + \beta_K K + \beta_Q Q. \tag{6.1}$$

A model for a particular situation can have any of these components singly or in any combination.

We discuss three approaches of variable selection, namely, 'forced-entry', 'significance-testing' and 'change-in-estimates'. The choice of method certainly depends on the particular situation and no method is always superior. However, experience suggests that quite often some methods can be recommended as preferable in certain situations. These are shown in Table 6.1 but we emphasise that these are not definitive guidelines. The choice is more uncertain in situations where the research purpose is to 'explore' associations or 'identify' predictors. Furthermore, some studies use 'readily available' data to identify associations and predictors so there may not be any D or K variables included.

Table 6.1 Likely approaches to variable selection in Cox regression modelling according to the type(s) of variables under consideration

Research purpose	Design (D)	Known (K)	Query (Q)
Adjust for confounding	Forced-entry	Forced-entry	Change-in-estimate
Explore associations and/or identify predictors			Significance-tests

6.2   FORCED-ENTRY

DESIGN VARIABLES

Forced-entry refers to including variables in a model according to the research design or prior opinion. The key explanatory variable that motivates a study, for example, the randomly allocated interventions in a clinical trial, is a D variable that should be forced entered into a model and the corresponding estimate of the HR should be reported. Even if this variable turns out to give a non-statistically significant HR almost exactly equal to unity, the researchers (and funding agencies and readers) would still want to know this estimate. As we have indicated, sometimes a stratified randomisation schedule is used in the design of a clinical trial. In which case, the stratification variable(s) used in the stratified randomisation should also be forced into the model as a D variable.

***Example** – design variables – randomised trial for prevention of acute rejection in renal transplant*

In the trial conducted by Remuzzi, Lesti, Gotti *et al.* (2004) 336 patients receiving a renal transplant were randomised within each site to receive either mycophenolate mofetil (*MM*) or azathioprine (*Az*) for prevention of acute rejection. The primary endpoint was defined as the time to an occurrence of acute rejection episodes (clinically diagnosed). The authors state: "The hazard ratio for the primary endpoint and its 95% *CI* was calculated by a Cox's regression model, which included site as a covariate". The authors quote the risk reduction on *MM* compared to *Az* as 13.7% (95% *CI* 25.7 to 40.7%).

ADJUSTMENT FOR CONFOUNDERS

Some variables are known to be influential in their ability to confound the key association of interest. Age in the studies of marital status is one example. It is recommended that these variables are forced entered into the Cox model. Even if for peculiar reasons, such as the play of chance arising from random sampling, these variables turn out to be totally unrelated to the outcome and/or the key explanatory variables, it is still recommended to keep them in the model (as forced-entries) and to report the key HR concerned adjusted for these covariates. This is to prove beyond reasonable doubt that the key HR is properly estimated. In epidemiological studies quite often some Q variables are also adjusted for as confounders in this manner.

The seemingly higher mortality among unmarried people may be explained by the possibility that unhealthy people are less likely to be married to begin with. As such, it is important to adjust for health status in studies of the effect of marital status on mortality. Self-assessed health status is known to be predictive of mortality. But not much is known whether it is related to marital status. So, from the confounding point of view, self-reported health is a Q variable instead of a K variable. Nonetheless, it is often adjusted for by forced-entry in order to prove the marital status effect beyond reasonable doubt.

Example *– forced-entry – marital status and mortality*

In a study of the relation between survival and marital status of British women, Cheung (2000) used forced-entry in a Cox model to adjust for age and self-assessed health. Similarly in a study of widowed and married elderly people in the United States, Korenman, Goldman and Fu (1997) also adjusted for age and self-assessed health as two forced-entry variables.

Marital status and widowhood are the *D* variables in these epidemiological investigations; age is a *K* variable, while self-reported health is a *Q* variable.

In the Cheung study the *HR*s for different categories of self-assessed health were reported alongside the *HR*s for different marital status. In contrast, Korenman and colleagues did not report the *HR*s for self-assessed health and other covariates. The authors merely reported in the text, and in table footnotes, which covariates were used for adjustment purposes.

It is a quite common and acceptable practice not to report the *HR*s for the *K* and *Q* variables if the purpose of including them is only to help with getting the correct estimate(s) for the *D* variable(s).

LOSS OF EFFICIENCY

The use of forced-entry may end up including some or even many variables that are statistically 'unnecessary' in the Cox model. This reduces efficiency. Loosely speaking, including one statistically unnecessary explanatory variable in the model is like reducing the sample size (strictly the planned number of events to be observed) by one event. Unless the sample size is small, say less than 50 observed events, and the number of unnecessary variables is large, say more than 10, the use of forced-entry will not pose a big loss in efficiency. Nevertheless, it does highlight that one needs to be cautious in applying the forced-entry method and judicious in choosing the variables for forced-entry. A careful review of the potential mechanisms concerned and a thorough review of the literature are usually required as a preparation for the choice of the forced-entry variables.

6.3   SIGNIFICANCE TESTS

The use of significance tests is very common in medical research. Many computer packages have built-in functions to perform automated selection of variables based on this strategy. Unfortunately this strategy is also very commonly misused and Sections 6.5 and 6.6 include discussion of some of the associated problems. Nevertheless, this strategy is useful in the exploration of associations and in the development of prognostic indices. This strategy may be implemented in a step-up or a step-down manner. Basically, it tests for association between explanatory variables and the outcome and then includes only those variables that are statistically significant.

We use the patients of the standard (control) group of brain cancer patients who received radiotherapy alone for their disease, described in Chapter 5, and the data set was partly reproduced in Table 5.1 to illustrate this strategy. Again, for illustration purposes, we assume that there are only three potential variables: history of fits (F) tumour grade (G) and age (A) recorded at diagnosis, and these are all Q type variables. Again for simplicity, we ignore the possibility of any interaction terms between any of the variables. For discussion purposes, we shall regard all three variables as binary history of fits (No, Yes), grade (3 and 3/4, 4), age (less than 50, 50+). Suppose the data did not arise from a randomised clinical trial, but merely recorded some characteristics of patients with brain cancer. In this situation, the object of the study may be to identify, by means of a Cox model, which if any of these recorded charac-teristics are important in predicting the subsequent prognosis of patients. Once determined, knowledge of these characteristics and the associated prognosis may help in the counselling of future patients with brain cancer and may also influence the choice of therapy for them. For example, advice and/or treatment may differ between those with good and bad prognosis. For the purpose of developing a prognostic index, we see the variables as Q variables here.

For the three variables of interest, the eight possible proportional hazards models are summarised in Table 6.2. We use a shorthand description of these eight models. One standard way is to refer to the null model as model (1), and the remaining models using the full capital letter of the variable names involved; here F, G and A, as we did previously in Section 3.6. A single letter on its own depicts the one-variable model which consists of that variable alone. Thus, model F includes history of fits, but no other variables. In an obvious notation, model $F + G$ includes history of fits and grade, while model $A + F$ includes age and history of fits. The model $F + G + A$ includes all three variables. The order in which we place F, G or A in any model with this notation is not important. The βs within each model of Table 6.2 are the regression coefficients and the x's the values of the associated, potentially prognostic for survival, variables.

The eight Cox models have each been fitted to the data from the control patients with brain cancer who received radiotherapy alone, the majority of whom had died at the time of analysis. The details of the fitted models are given in Table 6.3.

We now have to choose which of these models best describes our data. For example, should we choose model F rather than model $F + G + A$? We might be tempted to do so, since F has fewer terms and is, therefore, simpler than $F + G + A$. However, we may then be

Table 6.2 Possible Cox models for three potentially prognostic variables (history of fits, grade and age) for patients with a brain cancer

Model	Notation	Equation for log h
Null	(1)	1
One-variable		
History of Fits	F	$\beta_F x_F$
Grade	G	$\beta_G x_G$
Age	A	$\beta_A x_A$
Two-variable		
History of Fits and Grade	$F + G$	$\beta_F x_F + \beta_G x_G$
Grade and Age	$G + A$	$\beta_G x_G + \beta_A x_A$
Age and History of Fits	$A + F$	$\beta_A x_A + \beta_F x_F$
Three-variable		
History of Fits, Grade and Age	$F + G + A$	$\beta_F x_F + \beta_G x_G + \beta_A x_A$

Table 6.3 Cox models, using the three binary factors: history of fits, grade and age fitted to survival data from patients with brain cancer receiving radiotherapy alone for their disease (From Medical Research Council Working Party on Misonidazole in Gliomas, 1983. Reproduced by permission of The British Institute of Radiology)

		No-variables	One-variable			Two-variables			Three-variables
Variables		(1)	F	G	A	F+G	G+A	A+F	F+G+A
History + Fits									
(No, Yes)	b	—	−0.4840	—	—	−0.4875	—	−0.4647	−0.4684
	SE (b)	—	0.1715	—	—	0.1718	—	0.1720	0.1730
	HR	—	0.6163	—	—	0.6142	—	0.6284	0.6260
	W	—	7.97	—	—	8.05	—	7.30	7.33
	p-value	—	0.0048	—	—	0.0046	—	0.0069	0.0068
Grade									
(3 and 3/4, 4)	b	—	—	0.0321	—	0.0552	−0.0142	—	0.0300
	SE (b)	—	—	0.1436	—	0.1439	0.1441	—	0.1446
	HR	—	—	1.0327	—	1.0568	0.9859	—	1.0304
	W	—	—	0.05	—	0.15	0.01	—	0.04
	p-value	—	—	0.8228	—	0.7011	0.9212	—	0.8357
Age (years)									
(<50, ≥50)	b	—	—	—	0.6633	—	0.6645	0.6528	0.6513
	SE (b)	—	—	—	0.1569	—	0.1574	0.1575	0.1577
	HR	—	—	—	1.9411	—	1.9434	1.9209	1.9181
	W	—	—	—	17.88	—	17.83	17.17	17.07
	p-value	—	—	—	<0.0001	—	<0.0001	<0.0001	<0.0001
	log ℓ	−880.38	−876.07	−880.36	−870.95	−876.00	−870.94	−867.01	−866.99
	−2 log ℓ	1760.76	1752.14	1760.71	1741.89	1751.99	1741.88	1734.02	1733.98
	LR		8.62	0.05	18.87	8.77	18.88	26.74	26.78
	p-value		0.0033	0.8231	<0.0001	0.012	<0.0001	<0.0001	<0.0001

concerned that we have excluded possibly useful information from factors G and A, which may be of importance in determining outcome. In this context we assume that if a variable has little or no prognostic consequence as indicated by a statistically insignificant HR, we would not want it in our model.

We now describe several approaches to help us make the final choice.

STEP-UP SELECTION

The step-up selection approach begins with simple models that include only one statistically significant explanatory variable, and then adds one variable at a time to the current model. At each step the approach needs to assess whether a particular model reduces the unexplained variation by a significant amount. To do this we need to assess whether it increases the likelihood, ℓ, by a significant amount, or equivalently reduces $-2 \log \ell$ by a significant amount, as we have indicated in Section 5.6. A variable is kept in the model only if it is statistically significant.

We begin by comparing the fit of model F of Table 6.3 with that of the null model (1), we calculate, using equations similar to (5.29) and (5.30), the likelihood ratio or LR as

$$
\begin{aligned}
LR_{F,(1)} &= -2[\log \ell_{(1)} - \log \ell_F] \\
&= -2[L_{(1)} - L_F] \\
&= 2[L_F - L_{(1)}].
\end{aligned} \tag{6.2}
$$

We note a change in the notation from that adopted earlier in equations (5.29) and (5.30) in that the subscripts to L used here are the models under consideration rather than their df. In this case, we use bold case for the subscript to distinguish from the df used earlier, where we use a standard font for the subscript. We also note that we have attached a description of the models being compared as a subscript to the LR of the left-hand side of equation (6.2). This is done for ease of presentation.

The number of df for each model is the number of observed events, O, minus the number of regression coefficients included in the model. Thus, for the model F, there are $v = 1$ regression coefficients fitted, the observed number of deaths, $O = 198$, and hence $df = O - v = 198 - 1 = 197$. In a similar way, the df for the null model, (1), are $198 - 0 = 198$. This is because no regression coefficients are estimated. The degrees of freedom for $LR_{F,(1)}$ are, therefore, the difference between these two sets, that is, $df = 198 - 197 = 1$.

This is, in fact, the difference in the number of parameters in model F, which is one, and the number of parameters in model (1), which is 0. Thus, under the null hypothesis that fitting the model F does not explain any more of the variation in the data than the null model, $LR_{F,(1)}$ has a χ^2 distribution with $df = 1$.

The rule for calculating the df for the comparison of two models, by subtracting the number of parameters fitted in the two models, is a general one, provided the models are nested. As we have discussed in Section 4.4, two models are nested if the model with the larger number of variables includes, amongst these variables, all the variables of the smaller model. Thus, for example, model A is nested in model $F + G + A$, but it is not nested in model $F + G$.

If we wished to compare the model $F + G$ with the model F, then we would calculate the corresponding LR statistic, which is

$$
LR_{F+G,F} = LR_{F+G,(1)} - LR_{F,(1)}. \tag{6.3}
$$

162

SELECTING VARIABLES WITHIN A COX MODEL

We can generalise equation (6.3) and state that in order to obtain the LR statistic for comparing two models, we subtract the two LR statistics obtained by comparing each of the models in turn with the null model. Under the null hypothesis, that the larger model does not reduce the variation in the data, as compared to the nested model containing fewer terms, the LR statistic again follows a χ^2 distribution. The df are equal to the difference in the number of parameters contained in the two models, as indicated earlier.

Example – LR test – patients with brain tumours

Returning to the data for the patients with brain tumours, the LR statistics comparing each model with the null model are included in the last row of Table 6.3 and are also shown in the second column of Table 6.4.

We also calculate the difference between the LR statistics for the two-variable models, using the equivalent of equation (6.3). In this way we obtain the LR statistic for each of the three comparisons of the two-variable and corresponding nested one-variable models. Thus, comparing model $F + G$ with individual models F and G in turn gives $LR_{F+G,F} = 8.77 - 8.62 = 0.15$ and $LR_{F+G,G} = 8.77 - 0.05 = 8.72$ respectively. In a similar way, model $F + G + A$ is compared to each of the three two-variable models. In this case, all three models are nested within model $F + G + A$. All nine LR statistics are given in the main body of Table 6.4.

Finally, we note that the LRs for the models F, G and A are close, but not always exactly equal, to the comparable W statistic of Table 6.3. This will usually be the case. Once all the relevant LRs are calculated, the variable selection procedure is then applied as follows.

Table 6.4 Likelihood ratio (LR) statistics and degrees of freedom (df) for all possible models, including history of fits, tumour grade and age for patients with brain cancer (From Medical Research Council Working Party for Misonidazole in Gliomas, 1983. Reproduced by permission of The British Institute of Radiology)

			LR statistics			
	LR contrasting with the null		Two-variables			Three-variables
Model	model	df	$F+G$	$G+A$	$A+F$	$F+G+A$
(1)	–	198	–	–	–	–
(F)	8.62	197	0.15	–	18.12	–
(G)	0.05	197	8.72	18.83	–	–
A	18.87	197	–	0.01	7.87	–
F + G	8.77	196	–	–	–	18.01
G + A	18.88	196	–	–	–	7.90
A + F	26.74	196	–	–	–	0.04
F + G + A	26.78	195	–	–	–

Step I

From Table 6.4, we see that fitting model A gives a $LR_{A,(I)} = 18.87$ against the null model
(I) with no variables in it. This has a χ^2 distribution with $df = 1$ and, thus, from Table T3
we have a p-value < 0.0005. This is considerably less than 0.05, the conventional level
for statistical significance, and suggests that an improvement over the null model would
be achieved by including age. If we consider the other models with just one variable, then
for model F we have $LR_{F,(I)} = 8.62$, $df = 1$, which has, from Table T3, a p-value <0.01.
Similarly, model G gives $LR_{G,(I)} = 0.05$, again with $df = 1$ and a p-value >0.2, which in
this case is larger than 0.05. By analogy with the situation of the W test, exact values for
these p-values can be obtained by referring $\sqrt{LR}$ to Table T1, since $df = 1$. This gives for
models F and G exact p-values of 0.0044 and 0.8228, respectively. These are both larger
than that for model A and thus our best model at Step I is model A.

Step II

For the second step, we calculate the LRs corresponding to the differences between models
A and $A + F$ and between models A and $G + A$. These are indicated in Table 6.4 and
give $LR_{A+F,A} = 26.74 - 18.87 = 7.87$ and $LR_{A+G,A} = 18.88 - 18.87 = 0.01$, which each have
$df = 1$. The corresponding p-values are 0.0050 and 0.92, respectively. These suggest that,
whereas adding F to the Step I model of A alone 'improves the fit' and therefore gives a
better model, adding G does not improve the model. Our Step II model is therefore $A + F$.

Step III

The final step is to calculate the LR between model $F + G + A$ and model $A + F$. This is
given in Table 6.3 by $LR_{F+G+A,A+F} = 26.78 - 26.74 = 0.04$, with corresponding p-value =
0.84. This comparison implies that grade does not reduce the unexplained variation significantly and so does not add any further information. The 'best' and final model for our data
is thus $A + F$. Therefore, the variables Age and History of fits are to be included in the
multivariable model but Grade is not.

STEP-DOWN SELECTION

Step I

In contrast to the step-up procedures, which start with the null model (I), the step-down
procedure starts with the full model $F + G + A$ fitted to the data. Thus, from the final column
of Table 6.3, we begin with

$$F + G + A : \log h = -0.4684x_F + 0.0300x_G + 0.6513x_A. \tag{6.4}$$

We now check if this model is an improvement over the null model, by considering the
LR statistic $LR_{F+G+A,(I)} = 26.78$ of Tables 6.3 (final column) or 6.4 (second column). Under
the null hypothesis, that this model containing all three variables is no improvement over
the null model containing no variables, the LR statistic has a χ^2 distribution with $df = 3$,
which is equal to the number of parameters in model $F + G + A$. Reference to Table T3
with $LR_{F+G+A,(I)} = 26.78$, $df = 3$, gives a p-value <0.0005. Thus, there is evidence that this
model is an improvement over the null model. Our Step I model is therefore $F + G + A$.

If the p-value had not been statistically significant, then we would have adopted the model containing no variables, that is, model (1). The selection procedure would have then been terminated at Step I.

Step II

The next step checks if any one of the variables contained in the full model can be removed from the model without serious loss of fit. Thus, we calculate the corresponding LR statistics by comparing the three-variable model $F + G + A$ with each of the two-variable models $F + G$, $A + F$ and $G + A$ in turn. The smallest of these three LR statistics, provided it is not statistically significant at a predefined significance level, would indicate that the corresponding variable should be dropped from the full model. The argument here is that if the likelihood is not changed much by omitting a particular variable, then we would prefer to describe the data using a model containing as few variables as possible.

In our example, the respective LRs are $LR_{F+G+A,F+G} = 26.78 - 8.77 = 18.01$, $LR_{F+G+A,A+F} = 26.78 - 26.74 = 0.04$ and $LR_{F+G+A,G+A} = 26.78 - 18.88 = 7.90$. These are included in the final column of Table 6.4. The smallest of these is $LR_{F+G+A,A+F} = 0.04$, with $df = 3 - 2 = 1$. This gives a p-value $= 0.84$, which is much larger than the conventional level of significance of 0.05. Thus, exclusion of G from the model is not regarded as removing much information. As a consequence, we remove G from the Step I model to give model $A + F$ as our Step II model.

Had all three LR statistics considered here been statistically significant, we would have retained the full model $F + G + A$ and gone no further in the (de)selection process.

Step III

The next step is to compare model $A + F$ with the nested single variable models A and F separately to obtain $LR_{A+F,F} = 26.74 - 8.62 = 18.12$ and $LR_{A+F,A} = 26.74 - 18.87 = 7.87$, both of which have $df = 1$. The corresponding p-values obtained by use of Table T3 are <0.0005 and <0.01. Thus, these p-values are considerably less than 0.05 for both comparisons. This indicates that if we omit either of these variables from the Step II model we may seriously affect the fit of the model. Our final model, therefore, remains as

$$A + F : \log h = 0.6528 x_A - 0.4647 x_F. \tag{6.5}$$

This is the same final model as that resulting from the step-up procedure.

ALL POSSIBLE COMBINATIONS

A third option for selecting models is to compare the null model (1) with every other possible model and to calculate the corresponding LR statistics against this null model. These LRs were given in the second column of Table 6.4, but are reproduced in Table 6.5 for convenience, together with their associated degrees of freedom and exact p-values. As before, the values of the LR statistics are compared with a χ^2 distribution, using the appropriate df. The exact p-values corresponding to $df = 2$ and $df = 3$ were obtained as part of the output of a statistical package used for fitting the Cox models and not from Table T3.

Table 6.5 Likelihood ratio (LR) statistics and degrees of freedom (df) of all possible models compared to the null model for the survival data from patients receiving radiotherapy treatment for their brain cancer (From Medical Research Council Working Party on Misonidazole in Gliomas, 1983. Reproduced by permission of The British Institute of Radiology)

Model	Model df	LR	$LR\ df$	p-value
F	197	8.62	1	0.0033
G	197	0.05	1	0.8231
A	197	18.87	1	0.000014
$F+G$	196	8.77	2	0.01246
$G+A$	196	18.88	2	0.000079
$A+F$	196	26.74	2	0.0000016
$F+G+A$	195	26.78	3	0.0000066

Quite simply, we choose the best model from the seven models of Table 6.5 as that with the smallest associated p-value. This gives the same model as before, that is, $A+F$ with p-value $= 0.0000016$. If none of the p-values in Table 6.5 had been <0.05, then this all combinations method would suggest model (1) for our data set.

6.4 CHANGE IN ESTIMATES

CONFOUNDING OF PRACTICAL IMPORTANCE

The statistical significance of a variable in associating with the outcome is only one of the many factors that determine whether it can confound the effect of a key explanatory, type D, variable. The significance-test strategy may not be successful in selecting confounders and when the purpose is to obtain a suitable estimate of the HR for a key variable, the change-in-estimate strategy can be more useful. This approach compares the crude estimate, HR_{Crude}, for the key explanatory variable obtained from the Cox model

$$\log h = \beta_D D \qquad (6.6)$$

with the adjusted estimate, $HR_{Adjusted}$, obtained from the more general model that includes K and/or Q variables described in equation (6.1). If the ratio of the two estimates, $HR_{Crude}/HR_{Adjusted}$ is larger than C or smaller than $1/C$, the change in estimate is considered *practically* or *clinically* important and the extra variables added are kept in the multivariable Cox model. The constant C reflects the researchers' judgement of what constitutes an unacceptable level of confounding that must therefore be adjusted for. The value $C = 1.1$, giving $1/C = 0.9$, has been recommended by Maldonado and Greenland (1993).

STEPWISE SELECTION

Like the significance-test method, the change-in-estimate method can include K and/or Q variables in equation (6.6) in a step-up or step-down manner. There is a long history of studying the relation between age and survival in cancer patients because cancers found at a younger age may be biologically more aggressive than those found in older age. For illustration, we examine the brain cancer data again, considering age as a D variable and

Table 6.6 Change, using a step-down selection approach, in estimates of the *HR* for age according to the Cox model chosen for patients with brain cancer

Step	Model	HR_{Crude}	$HR_{Crude}/HR_{Adjusted}$
I	$G + A$	$\exp(0.6645) = 1.9435$	$1.9435/1.9180 = 1.0133$
	$A + F$	$\exp(0.6528) = 1.9209$	$1.9209/1.9180 = 1.0015$
II	A	$\exp(0.6633) = 1.9412$	$1.9412/1.9209 = 1.0106$

using $C = 1.1$ and a step-down approach. From Table 6.3 the $HR_{Adjusted}$ is $\exp(0.6513) = 1.9180$ in the model $F + G + A$. Some of the information in Table 6.3 is reproduced in Table 6.6 for convenience. If F is excluded, the $HR_{Crude} = 1.9435$ and the ratio of crude to adjusted estimates is 1.0133. This lies between 0.9 and 1.1, indicating only a small change in estimate if F is removed. Excluding G gives an even smaller change in estimate, as the ratio is 1.0015. Since excluding G only makes an unimportant change in estimate, and this change is smaller than that made by excluding F, the variable Grade can be excluded. In step II, the $HR_{Adjusted} = 1.9209$ is to be taken from the model $A + F$ while $HR_{Crude} = 1.9412$ is to be taken from model A. The corresponding ratio of crude to adjusted estimate is 1.0106. This is again within the interval 0.9 to 1.1. Thus, for the purpose of ascertaining the effect of age on survival, the simplest model A is preferred. This differs from the result based on the significance-test strategy, which recommended the model $A + F$. From the viewpoint of estimating the age effect and considering history of fits as a potential confounder, that the latter has a significant relation with survival is not relevant.

6.5   'SPECIAL' VARIABLES

CATEGORICAL

As we have indicated for categorical variables of g levels, it is often necessary to create $g - 1$ dummy variables for use in a Cox model. Some caution must also be exercised if one is incorporating a categorical variable of three (or more) levels into an automatic selection procedure. Thus, in the illustrative example of this chapter, if we were to include a factor G with the three brain tumour grade categories recorded as 3, 3/4 and 4, then we need to specify two dummy variables in the associated model. We do this in the way we described in equation (5.22). In this situation, we must constrain the selection procedure always to consider the pair of dummy variables together. If grade is not predictive of prognosis, then both dummy variables would be excluded from the model. Alternatively if grade is predictive, then both dummy variables are retained in the model. In some statistical packages all that is necessary to ensure this is to declare that the variable is categorical with g groups. The program then creates the dummy variables automatically and, most importantly, will either include or not include, as appropriate, all dummy variables for that categorical variable in any model.

CONTINUOUS

Although we have treated age as a binary categorical variable in this chapter, this is not always desirable as, in general, some information is lost by so doing. In addition, if a reduction of a continuous variable to a binary variable is made, then this implies a discrete jump from 1 to $\exp(\beta)$ in the hazard at the breakpoint, for example at a patient's 50th birthday. This step-up, or step-down, of the hazard at the cut-point is unlikely to be realistic in practice, as one might expect a smooth transition of the hazard with changing values rather than an abrupt change.

In general, we would prefer to model variables such as weight and age as continuous variables if possible, as in equation (5.15). However, such models also have their problems, as they imply (in their usual form at least) that the effect of the variable is linear over the whole range of possible values from, for example, the youngest patient with a brain tumour to the oldest. This may not always be the case. One method of checking for linearity is to divide age, at the preliminary stage of analysis, into $g \geq 3$ categories and to fit a model containing these dummy variables. If a plot of the resulting Cox $(g - 1)$ regression coefficients against the corresponding age category—a similar plot to that of Figure 5.4—is approximately linear, then we may assume that the influence of age may also be regarded as linear for our continuous model.

On the other hand, if such a graph does indicate some non-linearity, but the change in hazard is smooth from category to category, then one model that could be used to describe such a pattern is

$$A^*A : \log h_{A^*A} = \beta_A A + \beta_{AA} A^2. \tag{6.7}$$

The model is denoted here by A^*A as an abbreviation for $A + A \cdot A$. In mathematical terms, equation (6.7) is the equation of a parabola, or more usually termed a quadratic, since it contains a squared (in age) term. The model enables us to try to describe data with a smooth 'bend' in one direction. Formally, we check the extra fit provided by this model over the linear model of equation (5.15), by testing the null hypothesis, $\beta_{AA} = 0$. The procedure is the same as that for comparing any two nested models, which we described earlier. Thus, we calculate $LR_{A^*A,A}$ and this has a χ^2 distribution with $df = 1$. The latter is because equation (6.7) contains two parameters β_A and β_{AA}, while equation (5.15) has only one parameter, β_A. Hence, $df = 2 - 1 = 1$.

There is a distinction, however, between this situation and that when we are deciding, for example, between models $A + F$ and models A or F individually. In the latter case, model A or model F is nested within the full model and both are candidates to replace $A + F$. In contrast, in the situation when testing for linearity, there is only one alternative to A^*A, and that is model A, which is nested within it. It is useful to check if this is the selection procedure adopted by the computer package being used for the analysis. Some packages define a new variable, say $U = A^2$, then fit the model $A + U$, without any regard to the basic structure of equation (6.7). In this formulation model U alone is regarded as one of the possibilities for the final model. This is an inappropriate procedure.

Example – dummy variables – patients with end-stage renal disease

Umen and Le (1986) described a study investigating survival of patients with end-stage renal disease. They derive models including age, presence or absence of arteriosclerotic heart disease (ASHD), cerebrovascular accident (CVA), cancer (CA) and chronic obstructive pulmonary disease (COPD) for non-diabetic patients in their study, but find a model including age alone as appropriate for diabetic patients.

Their models, derived by considering a larger group of models containing up to 16 potentially prognostic variables, are summarised in Table 6.7. To determine which variables to include, they screened each variable individually and in combination with others, and then eliminated those variables that failed to generate a p-value ≤ 0.1. Using those variables remaining after this initial screen, they used a step-wise forward selection process to achieve the final models.

In both models, age is regarded as a three-group categorical variable (≤ 45, $46 - 60$, and ≥ 61) requiring two dummy variables in the modelling process. In the patients who do not have diabetes, a comparison of those patients aged ≤ 45 years with the oldest patients of 61 or more years, used as the reference group, gives $HR = \exp(-1.576) = 0.21$. This indicates a much-reduced risk of death for the younger group of patients. In those patients with diabetes, the same comparison between the youngest and oldest age groups gives $HR = \exp(-0.676) = 0.51$. This also provides evidence of a reduced risk, but is not of the magnitude of that observed in those without diabetes. This suggests that there may be an interaction between the presence or absence of diabetes and age.

The HRs associated with ASHD, CVA, CA and COPD are all greater than unity. The presence of any of these indicates an increased risk of death for non-diabetic patients with end-stage renal cancer. These same variables were not found to influence survival amongst the diabetic patients.

Table 6.7 Cox regression models for survival in end-stage renal disease for patients with and without diabetes (From Umen and Le, 1986 with permission from John Wiley & Sons, Ltd)

	Non-diabetic patients			Diabetic patients		
	Regression coefficient	SE	HR	Regression coefficient	SE	HR
Age (≤ 45)	−1.576	0.402	0.21	−0.676	0.307	0.51
(46–60)	−0.644	0.238	0.53	−0.569	0.313	0.57
ASHD	0.424	0.178	1.53	–	–	–
CVA	0.741	0.254	2.10	–	–	–
CA	0.441	0.212	1.55	–	–	–
COPD	0.452	0.199	1.57	–	–	–

We note that the quadratic equation (6.7) is also termed a polynomial of order 2. It can be extended to a polynomial of any power of age by, for example

$$\log h_v = \beta_1 A + \beta_2 A^2 + \cdots + \beta_{v-1} A^{v-1} + \beta_v A^v. \tag{6.8}$$

Such an equation has v regression coefficients, $\beta_1, \beta_2, \ldots, \beta_v$, and is termed a polynomial in age of order v. This model can be fitted to an appropriate data set and nested models of order less than v compared, using the LR test that we have described.

However, if linearity is not the case, then creation of categories (at least three are advised) to reflect the shape of the relationship is recommended in preference to attempting to describe the precise detail of the non-linear relationship. Although in certain circumstances, a transformation of the basic variable may achieve the desired linearity of which log x is the most useful.

Example – *investigating linearity – patients with colorectal cancer*

Chung, Eu, Machin *et al.* (1998) investigated whether young age was an adverse prognostic factor for survival in patients with colorectal cancer. In general colorectal death rates increase with age (as is the case for many cancers) and so if young age (≤ 39 years) is indeed indicative of a worse prognosis then the age-specific death rates would be U-shaped when plotted against decade. This was indeed the case, with those aged 40–59 of lowest risk whilst those ≤ 39 were at a similar risk to those aged 60–79.

As a consequence, for age an unordered categorical variable was created of the age decades for the modelling process. This despite the fact that the underlying variable was continuous and hence the successive categories had a natural order. Had ordered categories been used in the modelling process, this is then equivalent to coding them as 0, 1, 2, etc and this would then be regarded as numerical data. If the model is then fitted with this variable, it will take a linear form which, in this situation, is not appropriate. Using the unordered categories allows the shape of the underlying relationship to be examined without imposing an algebraic form such as the quadratic referred to earlier.

As we have indicated, one difficulty with categorising continuous variables is the fact that, once created, there is an implicit assumption that there is a step change in risk at a boundary between adjacent categories. Sometimes boundaries are chosen by investigating a range of options and then choosing that which 'magnifies' the difference between adjacent categories. As Altman, Lausen, Sauerbrei and Schumacher (1994) point out, such devices, known as 'optimal cut-points' can lead to an over-optimistic view of the prognostic variable in question. If a dichotomy is to be chosen, then one common method is to take the cut at the median value of the explanatory variable. However, there is no guarantee that the risk in terms of ultimate survival time will divide along these same lines so this somewhat arbitrary method is not recommended. Since the purpose of categorising the variable is to better investigate the 'shape' of the associated risk, a minimum number of three categories is required for this, and a maximum of five would seem reasonable.

INTERACTIONS

Suppose we were investigating the possible interaction between patient age *(A)* and history of fits *(F)* on survival of patients with brain cancer. In this investigation, we conjecture that the survival advantage of those with a history of fits, as opposed to those who do not have a history, may not be of the same magnitude in the two patient age groups (< 50 and ≥ 50 years). Thus, the prognostic influence of history of fits may be dependent on the age of the patient at diagnosis. We may wish to test this conjecture by means of a Cox model.

We will assume here that both A and F are important for our model. We could test for the presence of an interaction by fitting model $A*F$, that is, model $A + F + A.F$, to the data and comparing it with model $A + F$. It is then necessary to calculate $LR_{A*F, A+F}$, which will have a χ^2 distribution with $df = 1$.

In formal terms we have, by analogy with equation (5.23), the interaction model as

$$A * F : \log h = \beta_A x_A + \beta_F x_F + \beta_{AF} x_A x_F. \tag{6.9}$$

In this situation, a test for the presence of an interaction is equivalent to testing the null hypothesis that the regression coefficient $\beta_{AF} = 0$.

Again, it is useful to check that if this model is fitted using an 'automatic' selection procedure, then the method adopted by the computer package does not have the potential to exclude either β_A, β_F or both, yet still retain the coefficient β_{AF} in the final model. Thus, by analogy with the quadratic term for age, care should be taken to distinguish model $A*F$ from model $A + F + U$, where $U = A.F$ and $x_U = x_A x_F$. In this latter case, the automatic selection procedure may choose between $A + F$, $A + U$ and $F + U$ as alternatives to what appears to be a three-factor model, $A + F + U$; whereas the only sensible alternative to model $A*F$ of equation (6.9) is the model $A + F$. Here, model $A + F$ is nested within model $A*F$, but models $A + U$ and $F + U$ are not.

Example – interaction – influence of age in patients with and without diabetes

In the study described by Umen and Le (1986) there is some evidence of an interaction between age and presence or absence of diabetes. This led the authors to develop two separate models: one for those patients without diabetes and the other for those with diabetes. They did this in preference to developing a single model including a diagnosis by age interaction term. Their modelling approach was further complicated by the other four variables of Table 6.7 having a major influence on survival in non-diabetic patients, but having little influence on those with diabetes, as we indicated previously.

6.6   PRACTICAL CONSIDERATIONS

To illustrate the selection method options we have used an example which focuses on an ultimate goal of deriving a prognostic index, which is the topic for Chapter 8. However, as with all studies, thought should first be given to the actual main objective of the study in question and this may influence the final choice of selection method. As there is such a wide variety of possible situations it is difficult to be prescriptive in terms of the best selection method to use. So the advice we give below needs to be considered carefully.

MISSING VALUES

It is important that the proportion of data items that are missing or unknown in the data set is minimal. Experience suggests that as the number of variables requested by the researchers increases the proportion of 'missing' data also increases. Missing data may cause considerable 'biases' to arise in the modelling process and should be avoided if at all possible. Although there are no formal rules attached to an acceptable level of missing data, if more than 20% are missing for a particular variable then serious consideration should be given to excluding it from the modelling process. If the missing data comprise less than 5%, then the bias introduced may be regarded as small. These are only pragmatic suggestions, however, and may have to be varied with circumstance. No useful model can result if a vital piece of information cannot be easily collected.

Researchers should be aware of the problem of missing data in the consideration of variable selection. Variables that contain a lot of missing values are essentially not analysable, even if they are clinically important. One should also avoid considering too many candidate variables as they may collectively contain a very large amount of missing data. Furthermore, the LR test is not valid if the models being compared have a different number of observations. Users of the significance-tests strategy should carefully check that the models being compared do not have different numbers of observations because of missing values in different variables. If one is using an automated variable selection procedure from a statistical package, it is important to check the way the package deals with missing values before conducting any analysis.

One simple way to 'avoid' missing data at the analytical stage is to delete all patients from the analysis who have any missing data in the variables of interest. This makes all the analytical devices such as the LR test and the associated p-values comparable at every stage in the variable selection process. However, exclusion of patients on this basis may be very wasteful of information as this leads to, for example, excluding a patient with only a single missing value in a variable that turns out to be of little explanatory value. So in practice one may start by excluding all patients with missing values at the early stages of the selection process but bring them back into the process as it becomes clear which of the variables are likely to be in the final model. Some subjectivity will be required in making this judgement.

A useful approach, at least for categorical variables, is to create a distinct category for those variables for which data are missing. If the data are missing at random then this category should behave in a central manner since it will comprise a (random) mixture of the other category levels. This is similar to the 'Fluoride not classified' group given in Table 5.6 from the study of Samuelson and Kongerud (1994). Were the missing category to correspond to (say) the highest risk category, then this may indicate that 'missing' is a sign of poor prognosis. Perhaps it is then 'missing' as the patient was too ill for the measure to be recorded. For example, when a patient is an emergency admission time for less routine assessments may not be available and so they may go unrecorded. In which case the absence of these values may be indicative of a worse outcome and hence the fact that they are 'missing' is prognostic for outcome.

However, this strategy is no substitute for the 'real' data values and serious concern must be raised about a variable for which there is a large proportion of missing data.

WHICH SIGNIFICANCE LEVEL?

The significance-test method requires defining a level of 'statistical significance'. As for many statistical procedures, the choice of the level to decide between 'significant' and 'non-significant' is a subjective matter. Again, as for many procedures, the 0.05 level is often used to define statistical significance. However, another common level used in selecting variables for the purpose of exploratory analysis and prognostic studies is 0.1. The reason for this is that with such a level, we are less likely to reject a possibly important variable. The change-in-estimates method requires a level of 'practical (clinical) significance'. Again, there is no one-size-fits-all solution, but a significance level of 0.2 is often recommended. Often when building a Cox model, it may be better to err on the side of caution and to include a variable rather than exclude it.

BIVARIABLE SCREEN

As discussed by Sun, Shook and Kay (1996), it is common in the medical literature to screen potential explanatory variables by simple or univariate Cox regression analysis, relating them individually with the survival outcome variable, then only those explanatory variables reaching a certain statistical significance level are brought forward to a significance test-based stepwise (up or down) selection process. Indeed the study of Umen and Le (1986) on the survival of patients with end-stage renal disease summarised in Table 6.7 is one example. Despite its popularity, it is not to be recommended in practice.

The rationale for using such a bivariable screen appears to be as follows: if an explanatory variable is associated with an outcome variable in a univariate Cox regression model, this association may be the result of confounding. As such, this variable should be further examined in a multivariable regression framework. However, if an explanatory variable is *not* associated with an outcome variable in a univariate regression, there is no gain in further examining it in a multivariable regression model. This argument is flawed because it overlooks the possibility of 'negative confounding', that is, confounding which may suppress a genuine relation. In contrast, the more familiar type of confounding—a spurious relation being produced by a confounder—can be called 'positive confounding'.

For example, a higher level of education in women is associated with not giving birth (nulliparous), and higher education is also associated with lower cancer incidence. However, a nulliparous status is associated with higher breast cancer incidence. As a result, parity can 'suppress' (or reduce) a genuine social-economic gradient in breast cancer incidence. In the presence of 'negative confounding', the effects of variables may be 'neutralised'. Say, in this example, since more education relates to nulliparity, and since nulliparity relates to higher cancer incidence, in the bivariable analysis of associations between (a) education and time to-cancer, and (b) nulliparity and time-to-cancer, both can be non statistically significant. Therefore there is a chance that neither of them is selected in this screening procedure.

It may be argued that in epidemiological applications, 'positive confounding' is much more commonly seen than 'negative confounding', and therefore the use of a bivariable screening process is acceptable. However, it may be that the true situation is that while positive confounding is more commonly 'reported' in the medical literature, negative confounding is equally common but is 'under-reported' because of the lack of awareness of this issue.

AUTOMATED SEARCH

Many statistical packages include an automated algorithm to perform stepwise selection of variables based on the significance-test approach. This is so common that one may be misled into thinking that the significance-test strategy is equivalent to such automated search. This is not the case. In the examples in this chapter the selection was made 'manually' at each stage of the stepwise procedure.

In general, automated selection is not recommended. Firstly, it is easy to make the mistakes described in Section 6.5. The computer may not understand the nature of the variables. Secondly, statistical properties are not the only concerns in variable selection. In the development of a prognostic index, for instance, we care not only about the statistical findings from the training data set but also the cost of collecting future data for the application of the index. Thus if there are two strongly correlated predictors, the automated algorithm may select the more predictive variable which is more expensive to measure and leave out the less expensive one. However, the users of the derived prognostic index may prefer to use the less expensive predictor instead, even if it is slightly inferior. Such considerations—which will vary from study to study—require judicious use of selection methods. It is difficult to expect readily available software to perform such judgements.

7 Extensions of the Cox Model

Summary

This chapter introduces 'time-dependent' explanatory variables or covariates, which are those whose value, for any given individual, may change over time. These are also referred to as time-varying or updated covariates. These contrast with covariates that remain fixed for all time for that individual. The Cox proportional hazards model can be extended to incorporate such variables. We present this extension and discuss the practical implementation of this methodology and subsequent interpretation of the results from such analyses.

We also discuss aspects of stratified analysis which allows one to handle non-proportional hazards and clustered survival data, delayed entry, and truncation of follow-uptime.

7.1 INTRODUCTION

In the Cox models introduced in Chapter 5, we included only those covariates measured at a specific point in time, for example those recorded at the time of entry into a study, to help predict the future course of patients. In Chapter 6 we considered whether a history of fits, patient age and tumour grade determined at the time of entry to the trial predicted the future course of patients with brain cancer. Thus at entry to the study—the single-time point—a particular patient aged 40 may have a Grade 3 tumour but no prior history of fits. Such variables are known as 'fixed covariates' because they are observed or measured at a single point in time.

During the follow-up of patients, however, we will often obtain further information on some covariates which may, in fact, help us to better predict the subsequent course of the patient. For example, at a regular three-month check-up of patients with brain cancer, the grade of the tumour may be reassessed. The now updated grade of the tumour at this three-month check-up may then be a better indicator of future prognosis, as compared to the tumour grade recorded at entry into the trial. Biologically, one would anticipate that this may in fact be the case, since those patients with more aggressive disease at entry are likely to have a worsening tumour grade, indicating a progression of their disease. In contrast, those with less aggressive disease are more likely to have a static or even improving grade of disease at subsequent assessments following a period of treatment.

A further example of such a covariate is recurrent disease which may happen, at some later stage, in patients with brain cancer following surgical removal of their tumour. Those experiencing a recurrence are likely to have a poorer subsequent prognosis than those remaining free of recurrence.

For some situations, not all the subjects eventually recruited to an epidemiological study are recruited at the same time, and some may even leave for segments of the study. For example, a particular worker exposed to a specific hazard within the work place may be

Survival Analysis Second Edition David Machin, Yin Bun Cheung, Mahesh K.B. Parmar
© 2006 John Wiley & Sons, Ltd ISBN: 0-470-87040-0

transferred to another department for a period, then back again whilst new workers may join and some may retire at any time during the course of the study.

These situations of covariates being updated over time, 'truncation' and 'delayed entry', can all be accounted for when estimating the corresponding Cox *PH* model if a careful track of these changes is recorded by the investigation team.

7.2   TIME-DEPENDENT EXTENSION OF THE COX MODEL

CONSTRUCTING THE MODEL

Binary variable

In Chapter 1 we introduced the Stanford Heart Transplantation Program described by Turnbull, Brown and Hu (1974) and one may want to ask of these data whether transplant reduced mortality. One (incorrect) way of approaching this question is to define an independent variable with value equal to one for those who received a heart transplant and 0 for those who did not, and then use the Cox model we have introduced to compare the survival times of these two groups. Applying this approach to the data of Table 1.1 would give a $HR = 0.314$ (*p*-value < 0.0001), which shows that patients who received heart transplant had better survival. However, this analysis is not very meaningful as patients had to wait for a donor and hence 'survive' the period until one became available. So the receipt of a transplant was at least partly the result, instead of the cause, of sustained survival. Thus it is wrong to interpret the quoted *HR* as evidence of transplant reducing mortality. Such a research problem is not uncommon. For instance, medical researchers are sometimes tempted to study the impact of response to treatment on survival time. But patients who died quickly had no chance to develop a response to the treatment they were given, leading to the same problem of cause and consequence.

In the Stanford Heart Transplantation Program, transplant status may be considered a time-varying covariate. The survival and transplant experience of the second and tenth patients who did not, and the first two patients (patients 31 and 32) who did, receive a transplant are shown in Figure 7.1 for illustration. Patients 2 and 10 did not receive a transplant and they died on day $X = 5$ and day $X = 36$ respectively. In contrast, Patient 31 received a transplant on day 0, which (to avoid zeros) is considered to occur at 0.25 day after registration, and died on day 15, hence $X = 0.25$, $Y = 14.75$. Similarly Patient 32 received a transplant on day 35 and died three days later, hence $X = 35$, $Y = 3$.

Patients 2 and 10 had no change in transplant status. However, that of Patients 31 and 32 varied over time. The variable Transplant(t), with (t) denoting that it is time-varying, had a value 'No' before day 0.25 and day 35 for the two patients respectively. After that point the variable is updated to have a value 'Yes'. As shown in Chapter 5, the partial likelihood (*PL*) of the Cox model consists of calculations at the time-points when the outcome events take place. At the evaluation at $t = 5$ when Patient 2 died, Patients 10 and 32 had Transplant(t) equal to 'No' while Patient 31 had status 'Yes' because the value had been updated at day 0.25. At $t = 15$ when Patient 31 died, both Patients 10 and 32 remained to have Transplant(t) equal to 'No'. At $t = 36$, when Patient 10 died, however, the status of Patient 32 was 'Yes' as the value was updated on day 35. The *PL* of the Cox model makes it possible to let a subject's exposure status vary over time. Section 7.5 illustrates this technical point in more detail. Defining transplant status as a time-varying covariate, the *HR*

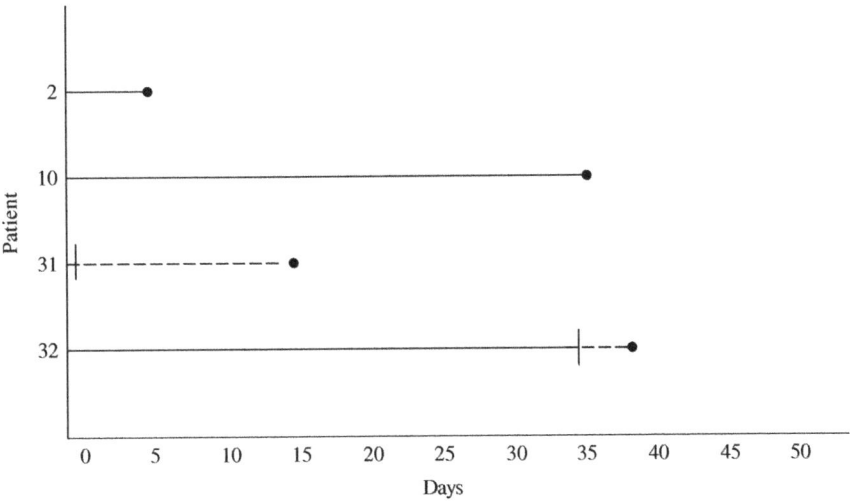

Figure 7.1 Time or censored time to transplant and subsequent death in four patients recruited to the Stanford Heart Transplantation Program

is estimated to be 0.992 ($p = 0.981$), showing that there was no evidence that transplantation had any effect on mortality in these patients.

Fixed and time-varying covariates

In the above example the time-varying covariate transplant status was updated at most once in each subject. The updating did not occur at regular intervals; it occurred whenever someone received a transplant. But the idea of time-varying covariates is general. There is no limit to the number of times updating takes place and there is no limit on the timing or regularity of the updating. Furthermore, a Cox regression model may contain both time-varying and fixed covariates.

> **Example** – *time-varying covariate* – *influence of marital status on mortality*
>
> Korenman, Goldman and Fu (1997) examined the effect of widowhood on mortality. Obviously marital status can vary over time so, in this study, the participants were interviewed every two years, when their marital status was enumerated. One analysis was based on marital status updated using information from these regular interviews. The researchers concluded that widowhood was associated with a higher mortality.
>
> A major problem in the studies of the health impact of marital status is that health status may affect marital status instead of the other way round. To remove this possible reverse causation, the analyses reported by Korenman, Goldman and Fu (1997) included various fixed covariates that represented health status at baseline interview in the models.

Continuous time-varying covariates

Although this need not be the case, the examples we have used so far concerned time-varying covariates whose values changed between 0 and 1 at different periods.

Example *– time-dependent covariates – graft versus host disease and changing granulocyte level*

Farewell (1979) investigated the relation between the time to appearance of an infection, using a time-dependent analysis of data arising from a randomised trial of laminar airflow (LAF), in patients with aplastic anaemia and acute leukaemia, receiving bone marrow transplants (BMT). In this trial, 89 patients were randomised following BMT, either to a LAF isolation room or to usual patient care.

The aim was to assess whether the protective environment of the LAF room (the 'treatment' variable) decreases the infection rate once an allowance for any other factors influencing risk of infection had been made. In addition to treatment (LAF or no LAF), the four fixed covariates recorded at entry to the trial were age, marrow cell dose, sex match of the donor, and whether or not recipient infections prior to transplantation were recorded. The two time-dependent covariates were the occurrence of graft versus host disease (GVHD) and granulocyte level post BMT, as these were also thought to influence a patient's risk of infection. GVHD is a binary variable and granulocyte count a continuous variable.

The analysis summarised in Table 7.1 includes only four of these variables. These were the 'treatment' allocated, the fixed covariate of evidence of prior infection and the two time-dependent covariates, GVHD and granulocyte count.

Table 7.1 Prediction of time to infection in 89 patients with aplastic anaemia and acute leukaemia using Cox's time-dependent covariate model (From Farewell, 1979, Reproduced by permission of Blackwell Publishing Ltd)

Covariate		Value	Regression coefficient	SE	HR	p-value
Fixed						
T: LAF room	x_T	No	0	–	1	–
		Yes	−0.909	0.346	0.403	0.008
I: Prior infection	x_I	No	0	–	1	–
		Yes	−0.183	0.627	0.833	0.780
Time-dependent						
G(t): GVHD	$z_G(t)$	No	0	–	1	–
		Yes	−0.225	0.773	0.799	0.780
LGr(t): log (granulocyte count)	$z_C(t)$		−0.151	0.086	0.860	0.080

The fixed covariate—prior infection—is clearly a binary variable taking the value 1 when a prior infection had been observed and 0 otherwise. Thus the values of the fixed covariates are $x_T = 1$ if the patient is allocated to the LAF room and $x_T = 0$ if not, together with $x_I = 1$ if prior infection is recorded and $x_I = 0$ if not. The time-dependent covariate GVHD occurs as an immunological reaction of the new marrow graft against the patient. This was defined as a binary variable with a value of 0 if no GVHD exists and the value one after GVHD occurs. It is also well established that the granulocyte count is of major importance in determining a patient's susceptibility to infection. Following transplantation, a patient's granulocyte level is expected to fall rapidly and then gradually to return to a normal level. This variable was recorded on a daily basis for all patients in the study and the log (granulocyte count) rather than the count itself was used as a time-dependent variable in the proportional hazards model. The values of the time-dependent covariates are therefore $z_G(t) = 1$ if GVHD occurs and $z_G(t) = 0$ if it does not, and $z_C(t) = $ log (granulocyte count) as at day t.

In this situation, the time-dependent Cox model can be specified as

$$T + I + G(t) + LGr(t) : \log h(t) = \beta_T x_T + \beta_I x_I + \gamma_G z_G(t) + \gamma_C \log[z_C(t)]. \qquad (7.1)$$

Here β_T and β_I are the regression coefficients for the fixed covariates of treatment and infection, and γ_G and γ_C are the regression coefficients for the time-dependent covariates.

The only two important factors resulting from this analysis appear to be treatment, with use of the LAF room having an associated $HR_T = 0.4$, (p-value $= 0.008$) and granulocyte count. The latter indicates that for every log (granulocyte count) increased by one unit, for example from 368 to 1000 since log $368 = 5.9$ and log $1000 = 6.9$, there is a reduced $HR_{Gran(t)} = 0.86$ (p-value $= 0.080$). Although granulocyte count appears of only marginal conventional significance, since the p-value $= 0.08$ is greater than 0.05, it should be retained in the model because earlier studies have established its relationship to infection.

NON-PROPORTIONAL HAZARDS

Discrete time intervals

Time-varying covariates can be used to detect non-proportional hazards. In a study of neonatal mortality in relation to size at birth described by Cheung, Yip and Karlberg (2001a), it was suspected that body thinness at birth might relate to mortality in different ways during different windows in the neonatal period (first four weeks of life). The variable *Pond*(Ponderal Index, a measure of body thinness) was measured in standard deviation scores. The timing of birth and death were recorded to the nearest minute in the database. The researchers partitioned the neonatal period into six sub-periods and created five binary, time-varying covariates to represent them, as shown in Table 7.2.

Again, the suffix (t) is used to highlight that the variables are time-varying. The variable *Time2*(t) took on the value 0 in the first 24 hours of life. Then it was updated to have value one at the start of the second day of life, which was updated again to have value 0 at the start of the fourth day. Variables *Time3*(t) to *Time6*(t) were created similarly to represent the subsequent periods of time. The time period $0 - 24$ hours has all five time-varying covariates set equal to 0. Two models representing *PH* and non-*PH* were fitted. Both models were

Table 7.2 Time-varying covariates representing different time periods

Variable	Day			Week		
	1 (0–24hrs)	2–3	4–7	2	3	4
$Time2(t)$	0	1	0	0	0	0
$Time3(t)$	0	0	1	0	0	0
$Time4(t)$	0	0	0	1	0	0
$Time5(t)$	0	0	0	0	1	0
$Time6(t)$	0	0	0	0	0	1

adjusted for other (fixed and time-varying) covariates such as gestational age but for brevity these covariates are not shown or discussed here:

$$PH : \log h(Pond) = \beta_1 \times Pond \tag{7.2}$$

$$Non\text{-}PH : \log h[Pond(t)] = \beta_1 \times Pond + \beta_2 \times [Pond \times Time2(t)] + \cdots + \beta_6$$
$$\times [Pond \times Time6(t)]. \tag{7.3}$$

The *PH* model in equation (7.2) estimates a single log *HR*, β_1, for the impact of *Pond* for the whole neonatal period. In contrast, the non-*PH* model allows the impact of *Pond* to interact with time periods. The coefficients β_2 to β_6 denote the interaction effects. The effect of *Pond* in the first 24 hours of life is given by the $HR \times \exp(\beta_1)$. That in Days two and three is given by $\exp[(\beta_1 + \beta_2) \times Pond]$ because $Time2(t)$ takes on the value one and the other time-varying covariates take on the value 0 at this time period. Similarly, the effect of *Pond* is allowed to be different in the subsequent periods and can be estimated by summing β_1 and the appropriate β_i, for $i = 3, 4, 5$ or 6 as shown in equation (7.3). The log-likelihood of the *PH* model among full-term neonates was found to be -15696.11, while that of the non-*PH* model was -15663.12. The likelihood ratio test statistic is therefore $-2 \times [-15696.11 - (-15663.12)] = -2 \times (-33.01) = 66.02$. Since the non-*PH* model has five more parameters, the test is on five degrees of freedom. Referring to Table T3 shows that the non-*PH* model fitted significantly better than the *PH* model (*p*-value < 0.0005). The time-varying impact of *Pond* in the six periods can be calculated using the estimated β_i of Table 7.3. The results showed that a higher *Pond* value at birth is related to a substantial reduction of mortality in the first day of life ($HR = 0.689$). From the second day to the end of the third week the *HR* fluctuates around 0.85. *Pond* has little association with mortality in the fourth week of life ($HR = 0.932$).

Though the *HR* in different time periods in the non-*PH* model can be obtained easily as described, the *p*-value and CIs require a bit more calculation to obtain as they involved the covariance terms between the regression coefficients β_i. For instance, the $SE(\log HR)$ in the second period is

$$SE(\beta_1 + \beta_2) = \sqrt{SE(\beta_1)^2 + SE(\beta_2)^2 + 2 \times Cov(\beta_1, \beta_2)}, \tag{7.4}$$

where $Cov(\beta_1, \beta_2)$ is the covariance between β_1 and β_2. Major statistical packages provide the *SE*s and covariances concerned in the outputs. Once the *SE* of the time-specific *HR* is

Table 7.3   Times-varying impact of Ponderal Index

Period	β_i	HR	p-value
0–24 hours	−0.373	$\exp(-0.373) = 0.689$	< 0.001
Day 2–3	0.169	$\exp(-0.373 + 0.169) = 0.815$	< 0.001
Day 4–7	0.221	$\exp(-0.373 + 0.221) = 0.859$	< 0.001
Week 2	0.175	$\exp(-0.373 + 0.175) = 0.820$	< 0.001
Week 3	0.225	$\exp(-0.373 + 0.225) = 0.862$	< 0.001
Week 4	0.303	$\exp(-0.373 + 0.303) = 0.932$	0.141

know, a z-test can be calculated and examined for significance using the hypothesis testing method described in Section 1.5.

Smooth time-varying hazard ratios

The previous neonatal mortality example of non-*PH* has it that the *HR* of Ponderal Index at birth changed at discrete time intervals. This need not be the case. For instance, one may define $z(t) = Pond \times t$, and formulate a model

$$\mathbf{Linear}: h[Pond(t)] = h[Pond, z(t)] = \exp[\beta_1 Pond + \beta_2 z(t)]. \qquad (7.5)$$

This model states that the effect of *Pond* on the log *HR* is described by $(\beta_1 + \beta_2 t) \times Pond$. In other words, the effect of *Pond* is assumed to increase (or decrease) linearly in relation to time. If one thinks that the effect of *Pond* changes non-linearly over time, one may define $z(t)$ as some non-linear function of time, say, $z(t) = Pond \times t^2$ or $z(t) = Pond \times (1/t)$ and substitute the new $z(t)$ into equation (7.5) to form a non-linear *HR* model.

7.3   STRATIFIED ANALYSIS

As in the use of the Logrank test, stratified analysis within the Cox model can remove confounding by (preferably major) explanatory variables. This is especially useful if one is not able to assume *PH* on the part of the confounding factor. Furthermore, a standard Cox model assumes independent random sampling so if the data are correlated, for example arising from clustered samples, stratification can be used to handle the clustering effect.

NON-PROPORTIONAL HAZARDS

A standard Cox model assumes *PH* for each explanatory variable. Stratification enables us to control for the effect of such a variable in a Cox model without making this assumption. Suppose that gender is a confounder of the effect of marital status on mortality and the associated complementary log plots are not parallel. We further assume that there are more widows than widowers. Instead of including gender as a covariate in the model to estimate the effects of widowhood, one may perform an analysis stratified by gender.

A stratified version of the Cox model works by setting up the partial likelihood (*PL*) functions for the strata separately. Thus, in an obvious notation, the *PL* in our example is

$$PL = PL_{Females} \times PL_{Males}. \qquad (7.6)$$

The components of this equation, that is $PL_{Females}$ and PL_{Males}, are the usual PLs for the Cox model, it is just that they are now restricted to the observations in the females and males respectively. This PL is then maximised in relation to the HR for widowhood, subject to the constraint that the effect of widowhood in the two strata is identical. This removes the gender effect without making the assumption of PHs and, indeed, without attempting to quantify the gender effect by a HR.

Stratified analysis is best used when the stratifying variables are potential confounders but their effects on the outcome are not of direct scientific interest. Note that one may not stratify by a variable and at the same time estimate its regression coefficient.

CLUSTERED DATA

Like most other statistical methods, the standard Cox model assumes independent observations. This assumption is not met if clustering is involved in the study design. Such examples abound, for instance, in studies of workers within different factories and children within schools or families. Observations within a cluster will probably be more similar to each other than to observations from other clusters, thereby violating the independence assumption of the standard Cox model. Stratification offers one way out of this problem. By defining each cluster as one stratum, the stratified Cox model now only assumes conditional independence, that is, the observations only need to be independent within clusters.

$$PL = PL_1 \times PL_2 \times \cdots \times PL_C, \tag{7.7}$$

where C is the total number of clusters in the study. The HRs are estimated subject to the constraint that they are identical in the strata.

The use of stratification to handle clustered data has a limitation that should be noted. Thus, as Hayes, Alexander, Bennett *et al.* (2000) discussed, in cluster randomised trials in which everyone in the same cluster receives the same intervention the within cluster HR for the intervention cannot be estimated. This implies that the stratified Cox regression model is therefore not able to estimate this HR.

7.4   TIME-SCALE AND DELAYED ENTRY

CHOICE OF TIME-SCALE

We have been discussing the use of time since an initial event as a time-scale. When we talked about age at death, it was equivalent to time since birth. Now consider a woman diagnosed with breast cancer on 01 January 1991, at the exact age of 35, who died on 31 December 2000. The length of the time-to-event is unambiguously 10 years, but there are (at least) two ways to 'label' the time-scale. These are, as indicated by Figure 7.2, by age, giving an interval from 35 to 45, or by the time since diagnosis of cancer, giving a survival time interval from $t = 0$ to $t = 10$. Both time-scales are correct if used and interpreted correctly.

Imagine that there are two cohorts of female breast cancer patients; one diagnosed at age 35 and one at age 40 and there are two choices of time-scale as we illustrated in Figure 7.2.

A common clinical question is whether an earlier diagnosis indicates a more aggressive disease and therefore is associated with poorer prognosis. Figure 7.2(a) illustrates this feature by showing a *higher* mortality curve for those aged 35 at diagnosis. The upward trend of

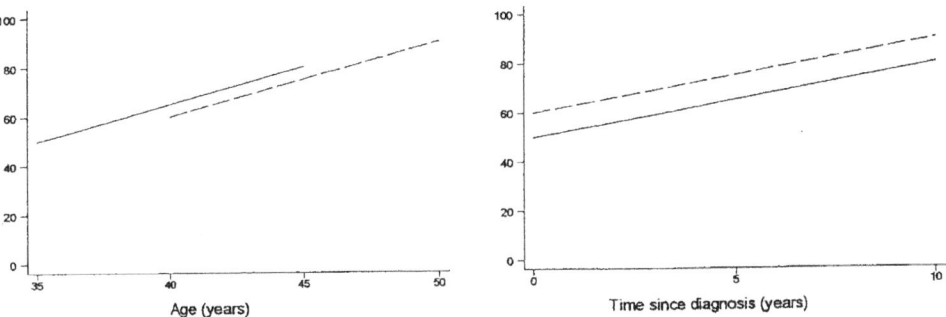

Figure 7.2 **(a)** Mortality rates in relation to age. Solid line for patients diagnosed at age 35; broken line for patients diagnosed at age 40. **(b)** Mortality rates in relation to time since diagnosis. Solid line for patients diagnosed at age 35; broken line for patients diagnosed at age 40

the curves corresponds to an increase in mortality as all the women get older. A Cox model essentially estimates the vertical distance between these curves. Figure 7.2(b) rearranges the same mortality curves using time since diagnosis as the time-scale. The stunning effect now is that those diagnosed at 35 have a *lower* mortality.

When age is used as the time-scale in Figure 7.2(a), the effect of attained age during follow-up (as opposed to age at diagnosis) is absorbed into the unspecified baseline hazard, $\lambda_0(t)$ of Section 5.2, of the Cox model. Hence this effect is removed when comparing the two cohorts.

When time since diagnosis is used as the time-scale the vertical distance between the two curves is affected by both age at diagnosis and attained age—the latter being positively correlated with mortality. Cheung, Gao and Khoo (2003) point out that if one simply wishes to predict which group of patients are more likely to die, say in the next 10 years, time since diagnosis may be preferred. Thus the cohort diagnosed at age 40 in Figure 7.2(b) has higher mortality not because their disease is more aggressive, but just because they are older.

In general time since randomisation is usually appropriate for clinical trials, as mortality is strongly associated with this, at least in patients with poor prognosis for survival as they will not be so much older when they die. However, age for the time-scale may be of more value in epidemiological studies as mortality will be strongly linked to attained age in many cases.

DELAYED ENTRY

Delayed entry, or late entry to the risk set, refers to the situation where a subject becomes under observation at a point after time zero. As in the example of using age as time-scale, patients enter into the study at age at diagnosis of cancer rather than at birth. Had they died before a cancer was diagnosed they would never have become under observation to begin with. Therefore their survival time from birth to the age at diagnosis is irrelevant. Delayed entry is sometimes called left truncation, referring to the fact that the period before entry is truncated from observation. It is also called staggered entry since usually the subjects enter into the study at different ages or time-points.

Furthermore, a subject may temporarily leave the 'at risk' population, or risk set, and then return later. This is called interval truncation. Suppose in a study of occupational accidents, a worker is initially employed in the industry concerned, then becomes unemployed, and then finds a job in the industry again. During the unemployment period, he is not at risk of occupational accidents. Should this fact be ignored in the analysis, the hazard will be under-estimated.

Example – *delayed entry – diagnosis of breast cancer*

Cheung, Gao and Khoo (2003) were interested in whether a younger age at diagnosis of breast cancer indicates a more aggressive tumour and therefore predicts a higher mortality. Since older people tend to have higher mortality no matter whether they have any cancers or not, they used age instead of time since diagnosis as the time-scale. This controlled for the age effect by absorbing the age pattern of mortality into the unspecified baseline hazard of the Cox model. The subjects became at risk at the age of diagnosis of cancer. Nobody had breast cancer at birth (age $= 0$)! Hence every subject had a delayed entry. The Cox model with delayed entry found that the hazard ratio of age in five-year bands was 0.78, indicating a negative association between age at diagnosis and mortality.

7.5   TECHNICAL DETAILS

PARTIAL LIKELIHOOD (*PL*)

Updated covariates

The partial likelihood for the Cox model is a product of components evaluated at the time of each observed event, that is,

$$PL = \prod_{i=1}^{n} \left[\frac{e^{\beta x_i}}{y_{(1)} \times e^{\beta x_1} + y_{(2)} \times e^{\beta x_2} + \cdots + y_{(n)} \times e^{\beta x_n}} \right]^{\delta_{(i)}}. \tag{7.8}$$

Censored cases, indicated by δ_i equal 0, have no real influence in the likelihood as anything raised to the power 0 is simply one. When the covariate is time-varying, the value of x has to be indexed by time and for clarity we have labelled such variables $z(t)$ and replaced the regression coefficients β by γ. Thus the expression (7.8) becomes

$$PL = \prod_{i=1}^{n} \left[\frac{e^{\gamma z_i(t)}}{y_{(1)} \times e^{\gamma z_1(t)} + y_{(2)} \times e^{\gamma z_2(t)} + \cdots + y_{(n)} \times e^{\gamma z_n(t)}} \right]^{\delta_{(i)}} \tag{7.9}$$

if only updated covariates are included. In most examples both types of covariates are possible.

For the four patients from the Stanford Heart Transplantation Program shown in Figure 7.1 their failure times were 5, 36, 15 and 38 days respectively. We will re-index them according to their rank of failure time as $i = 1, 2, 3$ and 4. The first event occurred $t = 5$ while the patient was still waiting for transplant, or $z_1(t) = 0$. This component of the PL is:

$$PL_1 = \left[\frac{e^{\gamma z_1(5)}}{y_{(1)} \times e^{\gamma z_1(5)} + y_{(2)} \times e^{\gamma z_2(5)} + y_{(3)} \times e^{\gamma z_3(5)} + y_{(4)} \times e^{\gamma z_4(5)}} \right]$$

$$= \left[\frac{e^{\gamma \times 0}}{1 \times e^{\gamma \times 0} + 1 \times e^{\gamma \times 1} + 1 \times e^{\gamma \times 0} + 1 \times e^{\gamma \times 0}} \right].$$

All four patients were at risk at this time and therefore all $y_i = 1$; whereas all but one had received a transplant by this time and therefore $z_2(5) = 1$.

The second event occurred at $t = 15$, leading to another component of the PL:

$$PL_2 = \left[\frac{e^{\gamma z_2(15)}}{y_{(1)} \times e^{\gamma z_1(15)} + y_{(2)} \times e^{\gamma z_2(15)} + y_{(3)} \times e^{\gamma z_3(15)} + y_{(4)} \times e^{\gamma z_4(15)}} \right]$$

$$= \left[\frac{e^{\gamma \times 1}}{0 \times e^{\gamma \times 0} + 1 \times e^{\gamma \times 1} + 1 \times e^{\gamma \times 0} + 1 \times e^{\gamma \times 0}} \right].$$

One of the four patients had died and was no longer at risk on day 15, so $y_1 = 0$. Only the patient who died on this day had received a transplant, $z_2(15) = 1$.

Another patient died at $t = 36$ so:

$$PL_3 = \left[\frac{e^{\gamma z_3(36)}}{y_{(1)} \times e^{\gamma z_1(36)} + y_{(2)} \times e^{\gamma z_2(36)} + y_{(3)} \times e^{\gamma z_3(36)} + y_{(4)} \times e^{\gamma z_4(36)}} \right]$$

$$= \left[\frac{e^{\gamma \times 0}}{0 \times e^{\gamma \times 0} + 0 \times e^{\gamma \times 1} + 1 \times e^{\gamma \times 0} + 1 \times e^{\gamma \times 1}} \right].$$

Two of the four patients had died and were no longer at risk on day 36 ($y_1 = y_2 = 0$). Note that one patient received a transplant on day 35 and therefore $z_4(36)$ is updated from 0 to one, in contrast to $z_4(15) = 0$ in PL_2.

The updating of time-varying covariates can be tedious but it is readily handled by the built-in functions of available statistical packages.

Delayed entry and truncation

The PL of equation (7.9) can accommodate delayed entry, that is the situation where a subject is not at risk of failure until he or she enters the risk group. Such a subject, say subject Q, would not be included in any PL_i if the events up to and including i all occur before Q is in the risk set. However, we can incorporate this subject Q into equation (7.9) by setting $y_q = 0$ for this subject when $i < q$ and thereafter setting $y_q = 1$.

Interval truncation is handled the same way. So, if a subject enters into a study late, temporarily leaves the at risk population and then rejoins it, and finally is censored, the y_q will be 0, 1, 0, 1, 0 for the five periods of time marked by his movements, that is, before joining, before temporary departure, before rejoining, before censoring, and after censoring.

The easiest way to analyse data with delayed entry and interval truncation is, of course, to use a statistical program that is designed for this purpose. If this is not available, one may use the time-varying covariate functions of some statistical programs to achieve the same purpose. That is, a covariate is defined as missing at times when the subject is not at risk. When the program formulates the component of the *PL* at these times, it is forced to exclude subjects with a missing value from the denominator of the components. This will trick the program into working as if the y_i indicator is set to 0.

8   Prognostic Indices

Summary

This chapter describes how to use a Cox model to determine a prognostic index to help classify patients into different risk groups. Discussion of which patient variables to include and how the risk groups are formed and used is presented. We stress the roles of training and confirmatory data sets, respectively, to establish and verify the prognostic index. Finally, we include a description of how a well established prognostic index may be updated.

8.1   INTRODUCTION

As we have seen, one important application of the Cox's proportional hazards (*PH*) model is to help identify variables which may be of prognostic importance. Often, there may be many potential characteristics of the patient, such as age, gender, weight, and features of the disease present, such as its severity, which may or may not influence outcome. Thus the requirement is that those variables that are strongly prognostic are to be identified, those clearly not prognostic set aside, whilst others may need to be more fully investigated in further studies.

Once identified, knowledge from the retained variables may be combined and used to define a prognostic index (*PI*), which in turn defines groups of individuals at differing risk. To use the prognostic index, key patient characteristics are recorded at diagnosis and from these a score is derived. This score gives an indication of whether, for example, the particular patient has a good, intermediate or poor prognosis for the disease. For example, it is well known that those patients with Ewing's sarcoma presenting with metastatic disease have a poorer prognosis than those who do not. Despite this the same treatment may be appropriate for both metastatic and non-metastatic groups. So if one treatment under investigation in a clinical trial turns out to be better than the standard, the relative prognostic effect of the presence of metastatic disease may or may not be modified.

It is common to find, although by no means always the case, that several variables contribute to the ultimate prognosis. For example, if in Ewing's sarcoma a pelvic site is involved this too is an adverse prognostic feature for subsequent survival. Thus note has to be taken of the four metastases (absent: present) by site (pelvic: non-pelvic) combinations in judging prognosis for these patients.

Factors prognostic for outcome are often determined by using multivariable regression techniques relating, for example, the time to resolution of the condition to the potential explanatory variables. Thus for Ewing's sarcoma the Cox regression model for the ultimate survival time will include (covariate) information on both the presence or absence of metastatic disease and pelvic involvement at diagnosis. Once established, this regression

Survival Analysis Second Edition   David Machin, Yin Bun Cheung, Mahesh K.B. Parmar
© 2006 John Wiley & Sons, Ltd   ISBN: 0-470-87040-0

model can help to quantify the risk, with respect to survival time, associated with these factors.

As for all studies, good design features are an essential ingredient for prognostic studies. Of critical importance are clear eligibility criteria for the patients involved, the identification of a distinct training data set, from which the *PI* is developed, a validation data set upon which the developed *PI* is evaluated, and careful choice of candidate variables.

8.2   CANDIDATE SUBJECTS

TRAINING DATA

Before establishing which individual patients are to be included in the prognostic factor investigation the basic patient population of interest has to be defined. So, just as one would do for any clinical study, clear eligibility criteria have to be established. Such eligibility requirements will usually include the particular diagnoses of interest as well as precise details of how these diagnoses are established. Further, it may be necessary to restrict the patients so selected to those that will receive a particular form of therapy. In some situations, this restriction may be made to ensure a relatively homogeneous set of patients so that the potential prognostic indicators are not obscured by varying degrees of efficacy of the (possibly) uncontrolled choice of therapies that may have been given to such patients. Clearly if the patients used for a prognostic study are those recruited to a randomised trial, then differences between patients (due to treatment received) can be accommodated in the prognostic modelling process in a systematic way. Once the eligible patients are identified, then these provide the 'training' data with which the *PI* is developed.

The choice of subjects may also (and should) be influenced by the quality of data that can be collected for the purposes of the study. Once again if these data come from a randomised trial then one may be reassured more easily that the data are well documented than for a study that involves extracting data from patient (retrospective) case notes which are designed principally for other purposes. Without good quality data, the conclusions drawn from studies of prognosis must be uncertain.

VALIDATION DATA

Once the *PI* is developed then a further key feature of the design is for the research group to identify a potential validation group, perhaps patients satisfying the same eligibility criteria as the training set but from a different institution. However, an important aspect of the process is to ensure the model to be validated is derived *before* detailed knowledge of the validation group data is available to the modelling team. Thus Altman and Royston (2000) state: "…considerations argue strongly for the need to evaluate performance of a model on a new series of patients, ideally in a different location". Thus if a research group is developing a *PI*, then to satisfy this requirement a validation group of patients is required.

This implies that the whole exercise is a two-stage process, involving the index or training group of patients as we have described above and a second validation group of patients. The device of splitting the data at random into two and using one half to develop the model and the other to test it is a common approach. However, this does not satisfy the requirement for: "…a new series of patients, ideally in a different location". What is more this may seriously reduce the ability of the training set (since the number of subjects is now halved) to select an appropriate *PI*.

8.3   CANDIDATE VARIABLES

STUDY ENDPOINT

Just as for any other study, the key endpoint (here survival time) has to be established. For example, in many circumstances this will be the time either to the resolution of the disease (cure) or, as would be the case in prognostic studies in patients with advanced cancer, the survival time of the patient. In either case the magnitude of the influence of any explanatory variable, x, on the survival time can be assessed using the univariate Cox *PH* regression model

$$\log h = \beta x. \tag{8.1}$$

For v potential prognostic variables, x_1, x_2, $x_3 \ldots x_v$ the Cox model takes the multivariable form, of equation (5.22) which we repeat here for convenience but express in terms of log h rather than h,

$$\log h = \beta_1 x_1 + \beta_2 x_2 + \beta_3 x_3 + \cdots + \beta_v x_v, \tag{8.2}$$

where β_1, β_2, $\beta_3, \ldots \beta_v$ are the corresponding regression coefficients to be estimated in the modelling process.

The structure of a prognostic factor study is to record for each of the N patients recruited, their basic characteristics at the time of diagnosis of their disease and their ultimate survival, t. In simple terms, once the regression model is fitted to these data, those $\xi (\leq v)$ variables for which a null hypothesis that the corresponding regression coefficient $\beta_i = 0$ is rejected, are retained in the model and are termed prognostic. The remaining $v - \xi$ variables that are 'not statistically different' from zero are removed from the model and are considered as not prognostic for outcome.

One should also give some thought as to how the prognostic factors once established are to be used. If the purpose is purely scientific, then the variables considered may be very esoteric in nature (perhaps determined by very complex assays). On the other hand, if the index is to be used to guide advice that will be given to patients in the clinic then it is probably best to focus on variables which can be measured easily with minimal time-consuming or sophisticated (laboratory-type) measures involved.

POTENTIAL PROGNOSTIC VARIABLES

Apart from the endpoint measure itself, it is also important to determine which variables are to be the candidate variables for the prognostic factor investigation.

Help with the choice of variables to study (or not) should be obtained by reviewing the literature for variables that have been investigated in previous studies. It is clear that those that have been shown to have major prognostic influence should also be included in the planned study. We will call these 'Level–In' variables and these correspond to those of type K in equation (6.1). A decision then has to be made as to which of the other variables so examined may be still unproven, 'Level–Query'—Q of equation (6.1), and which have already been found conclusively not to be useful, 'Level–Out'. The latter will clearly not feature in the subsequent modelling process.

Of course, the purpose of the current study may be to investigate entirely new variables, 'Level–New'. For this latter category it will be advisable to consider aspects in relation to their possibly ultimate causality. At this stage one also has to determine whether the objective of investigating 'Level–New' variables is to replace the 'Level–In' variables or rather to ask if their added inclusion 'enhances' the ability to distinguish more clearly prognostic groups. The approach to modelling is different in these two situations.

Considerable thought at the planning stage needs to be focussed on the selection of the variables and their associated Levels. There is a tendency for investigators to assign very few to 'Level–Out' for fear of 'missing something important'.

Example – *choice of candidate variables – node-positive breast cancer*

Although not using our categorisation, Sauerbrei, Royston, Bojar *et al.* (1999) imply for non-metastatic breast cancer that nodal status is the only Level–In variable associated with prognosis. In contrast Level–Query is attached to tumour size, tumour grade, histologic type, oestrogen (ER) and progesterone receptor (PR), menopausal status and age despite many investigations of their respective roles. They also point out that more then 100 Level–New factors have been proposed at various times for this disease.

8.4   SELECTING A MODEL

UNIVARIATE

As there are usually several, and sometimes many, variables as potential candidates for inclusion even after a careful preliminary screening as described above, the next step is often to reduce the options by fitting a univariate model for each in turn. Once fitted, then one only takes forward those of the candidate variables (all of which must be either Level-In, Level-Query or Level-New) for which the corresponding null hypothesis of $\beta = 0$ had been rejected. These retained variables are then studied using multivariable Cox regression models.

Example – *choice of variables – brain cancer*

From the data of a randomised trial of misonidazole plus radiotherapy versus radiotherapy alone for patients with cancer of the brain, conducted by the Medical Research Council Working Party on Misonidazole in Gliomas (1983), discussed in Chapter 6, a Cox's *PH* model was used to identify a set of variables influencing the duration of survival of these patients. In particular, two variables, age and length of history of fits, were useful in helping to predict survival time.

MULTIVARIABLE

Although individually the candidate variables in the univariate stage of the modelling may all be statistically significant, when included together in a multivariable model this need no longer be the case. Essentially this is because similar (or the same) information for one may be held in one or more of the other variables under consideration. The next stage of the modelling process is then to select those from within a multivariable model which together still appear to influence outcome and to discard those which do not.

Example – *step-up and step-down selection – patients with brain cancer*

In a complete analysis conducted by the Medical Research Council Brain Tumour Working Party (1990), four variables were identified that collectively were useful in predicting the length of survival of patients with brain tumours. These were age (A), categorised as <45, 45–59, ≥ 60 years; clinical performance status (C), categorised as 0–1, 2, 3–4; extent of neurosurgery (N), categorised as complete, partial, biopsy only; and length of history of fits (F), categorised as ≥ 3 months, <3 months, none.

The authors used both step-up and step-down variable selection procedures, as described in Chapter 6, with both procedures identifying these same four factors as the important variables. All other recorded variables were taken as not adding further prognostic information.

In the above example, the categorisation for history of fits contrasts with the analysis in Chapter 6, which categorised patients into a binary form as either having or not having a history of fits. It is useful to note here that all the categories are first ordered from good to bad with respect to prognosis. Clinical knowledge concerning this disease suggests the order. This choice helps the interpretation as, if we are correct in this knowledge, then the corresponding regression coefficients should all be positive and the HRs will be greater than one. Also, the three category levels of each factor were coded 0, one and two and treated as a numerical continuous variable measured on this three-point scale. By assigning these values, this implicitly means that one is assuming a linear trend in survival time across each factor. We do not know whether the corresponding regression coefficients are statistically significant until we fit and test the models.

The final form of the Cox model calculated from data for the 417 patients with brain tumours was

$$A + C + N + F: \log h = \beta_A A + \beta_C C + \beta_N N + \beta_F F. \tag{8.3}$$

The estimates of the regression coefficients of equation (8.3) are $b_A = 0.3366$, $b_C = 0.2084$, $b_N = 0.2279$ and $b_F = 0.2434$. These, together with the associated SEs and HRs for each level of these prognostic factors, are given in Table 8.1. For example, for patients who are 45–59 years of age, $HR = \exp(0.3366 \times 1) = \exp(0.3366) = 1.40$, whilst for those aged ≥ 60 the $HR = \exp(0.3366 \times 2) = \exp(0.6732) = 1.96$. Both these HRs are expressed relative to those patients of <45 years.

Table 8.1 Prognostic factors and prognostic index scores derived from 417 patients with brain cancer (data from Medical Research Council Brain Tumour Working Party, 1990, with kind permission from Springer Science and Business Media)

Prognostic factor	Category	Category score	Estimated coefficient $(b) \times$ Category score	$SE(b)$	HR	Index score
Age (A)	<45	0	0	–	1	0
	45–59	1	0.3366	0.0719	1.40	7
	≥60	2	0.6732		1.96	14
Clinical	0–1	0	0	–	1	0
performance	2	1	0.2084	0.0594	1.23	4
status (C)	3–4	2	0.4168		1.52	8
Extent of	Complete	0	0	–	1	0
neurosurgery	Partial	1	0.2279	0.0693	1.26	5
(N)	Biopsy only	2	0.4558		1.58	10
Length of history	≥3 months	0	0	–	1	0
of fits (F)	<3 months	1	0.2434	0.0714	1.28	5
	None	2	0.4868		1.63	10

PRACTICALITIES

Once the variables to be examined in the prognostic modelling have been determined the model can be fitted and the 'important' variables identified in a number of (statistically speaking) mechanistic ways. However, there is no 'best' method and so there is some subjective choice involved in which to use. However, with sufficient data, strongly influential candidate variables are likely to emerge whatever the method adopted.

Some care is needed in the use of any 'mechanistic' approach. Thus a statistically significant regression coefficient for a variable may be established, perhaps in a prognostic factor study of many patients, but its actual effect on patient outcome is very small. Conversely in a more modest study, a variable exerting a major prognostic influence but not statistically significant, could be eliminated.

Thus any judgement must be based on the magnitude of the regression coefficient and not just the associated p-value.

8.5   DEVISING A NEW INDEX

FITTING THE MODEL

Once the eligibility of each member of the training set has been established, the variables to consider have to be selected and the relevant data collected. The same type of process is used when developing a new PI as that in deriving the example of equation (8.3).

SCORING THE PATIENTS

Once the model has been established, to develop a PI for use with future patients with brain cancer it is first necessary to calculate the value of equation (8.3) for each of the 417 patients in the trial, using patient characteristics determined at entry to the study and at a post-resection review. This is done using the corresponding values for their individual categories, as set out in Table 8.1.

Thus, for example, a patient at presentation, aged 63 (Category score 2), with clinical performance status 2 (Category score 1), having complete neurosurgery (Category score 0) and no experience of fits (Category score 2) will have from equation (8.3) a relative hazard of

$$\log h = (0.3366 \times 2) + (0.2084 \times 1) + (0.2279 \times 0) + (0.2434 \times 2) = 1.3684. \qquad (8.4)$$

For the this patient the score, S, is simply

$$S = \log h = 1.3684. \qquad (8.5)$$

In a similar way, a patient less than 45 years old, with a clinical performance status of 2, having a partial resection and no history of fits, has the following score:

$$S = (0.3366 \times 0) + (0.2084 \times 1) + (0.2279 \times 1) + (0.2434 \times 2) = 0.9231$$

This calculation is then repeated for the remaining 415 patients in the trial. Since there are four factors for each of three possible values, or levels, there are theoretically $3^4 = 81$ different scores possible. These range in value from $S = 0$, for patients less than 45 years, clinical performance 0 or one, complete neurosurgery and a history of fits of duration in excess of three months, to $S = 2.0326$ for patients aged 60 years or more with clinical performance status 3 or 4, biopsy only and no history of fits.

The frequency distribution of the 417 resulting scores is given in Figure 8.1 and shows that the majority of patients have scores between 0.7 and 1.7. There are relatively few patients

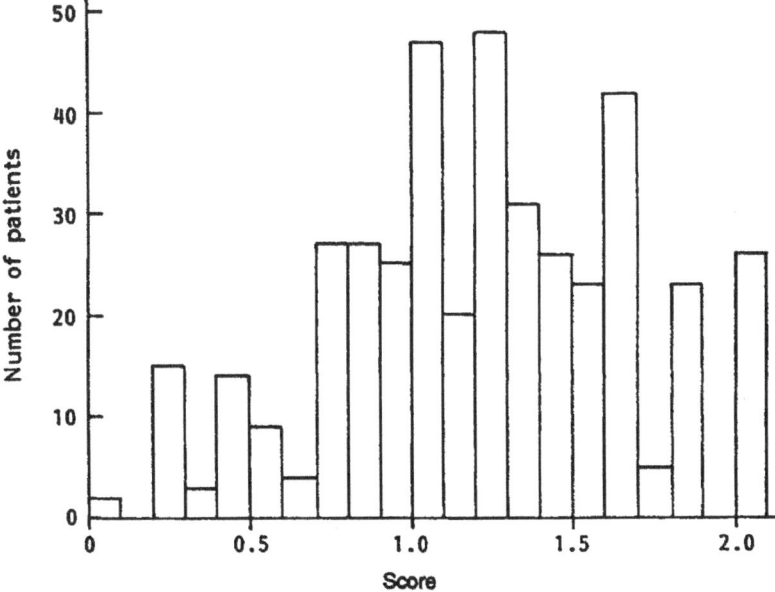

Figure 8.1 Grouped frequency distribution of scores derived from a Cox model fitted to the survival information of 417 patients with brain cancer (data from Medical Research Council Brain Tumour Working Party, 1990, with kind permission from Springer Science and Business Media)

with very low scores: only two patients with $S < 0.1$; but quite a few with very high scores: 26 patients with $S \geq 2.0$.

The next step, at least in theory, is to calculate the separate $K\text{-}M$ survival curves for the resulting 81 score groups. However, in this example, there are clearly too few patients per group for this purpose, since there will be an average of only five ($417/81 = 5.15$) patients per group. In point of fact, there are fewer than $3^4 = 81$ distinct groups as some of the combinations result in the same score. Nor would it be sensible to calculate the survival curves of patients in the 19 groups of Figure 8.1 as again there are too few patients in some of these groups. Instead, we first partition the scores into convenient, often arithmetically convenient, groups with sufficient patients per group. For example, we might identify patients with low scores ($S < 1$), medium scores ($1.0 \leq S < 1.5$) and high scores ($S \geq 1.5$). In this case, the low, medium and high score groups have 126, 172 and 119 patients, respectively.

We then calculate the corresponding survival curves estimated from the individual patients falling into these three groups. The survival curves are shown in Figure 8.2. These show the rather better outcome for the low score (better risk) patients, who have a median survival time of approximately one year. This contrasts with, for example, the poor risk group, who have a median survival of approximately four months. As one might expect, the survival curves also indicate a gradient of survival differences between the three score groups.

SIMPLIFYING THE MODEL

To derive a *PI*, which can be used more easily than calculating the rather difficult score, S, it is usual to simplify the regression coefficients in the fitted Cox model of equation (8.3). One

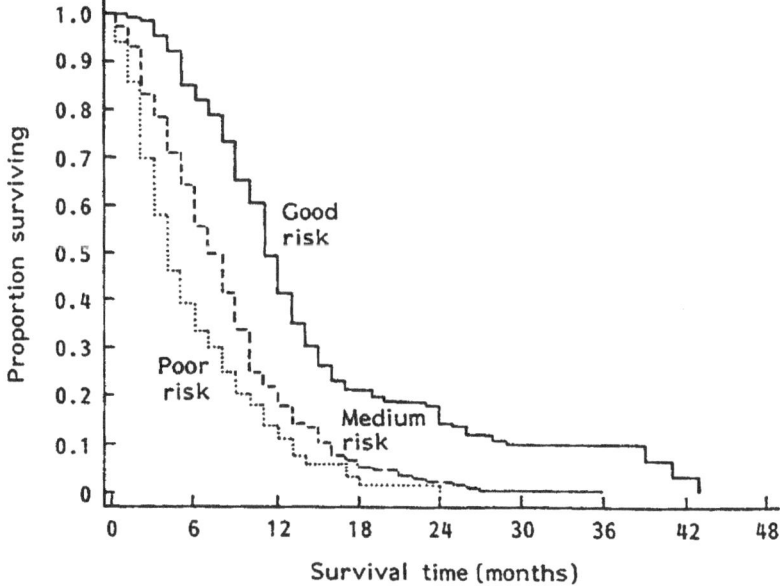

Figure 8.2   Kaplan-Meier survival curves for low, medium and high score groups derived from 417 patients with brain cancer (data from Medical Research Council Brain Tumour Working Party, 1990, with kind permission from Springer Science and Business Media)

method of doing this is as follows. We begin with the fitted Cox model of equation (8.3), that is

$$S = 0.3366A + 0.2084C + 0.2279N + 0.2434F. \qquad (8.6)$$

We first note the regression coefficients are in the ratio 3366 : 2084 : 2279 : 2434. The decimal place in equation (8.6) is of no consequence here since the same multiplicative change in all the regression coefficients affects all patients and hence preserves their rank order with respect to their values of S. This ratio is, after multiplying the coefficients by two and dividing by 100, approximately 67 : 42 : 46 : 49, which, in turn, is very similar to 70 : 40 : 50 : 50 or finally 7 : 4 : 5 : 5!

There is a balance here between strictly preserving the ratios of the regression coefficients as they appear in equation (8.6), while at the same time arriving at modified coefficients that are easy to work with. That is, they are both arithmetically simple to manipulate and easy to remember. Once derived, these modified coefficients are used to replace the score S of equation (8.6) by the PI. This is given by the equation

$$PI = 7A + 4C + 5N + 5F. \qquad (8.7)$$

As a consequence, we replace, for the patient who is aged 63, clinical performance status 2, having complete neurosurgery and no history of fits, the score $S = 1.3684$ by $PI = (7 \times 2) + (4 \times 1) + (5 \times 0) + (5 \times 2) = 28$. Similarly for the patient with $S = 0.9231$ we have $PI = (7 \times 0) + (4 \times 1) + (5 \times 1) + (5 \times 2) = 19$, and so on for the remaining 415 patients.

The PI can be calculated for each of the 417 patients in the study, and the values range from 0 to 42, corresponding to S equal to 0 and 2.0326, respectively. A high score of the PI indicates a worse prognosis than a low one. Not surprisingly the shape of the resulting frequency distribution of the individual PIs will be similar to that for the score S shown in Figure 8.1.

Finally, the distribution of the PI is examined and convenient subgroups of differing prognosis are identified. We choose three convenient groups as 0−19, 20−29 and 30−42 for this purpose. The boundaries of the risk groups, that is, 20 and 30, are chosen here for convenience of memory. Table 8.2 shows the number of patients in each of the groups, together with the corresponding median survival times and the K-M two-year survival rates. The corresponding survival curves of the patients divided into these three groups, classified as Good, Medium and Poor risk patients, are shown in Figure 8.3.

There are minor differences in the patients selected to each PI group from those of Figure 8.2, but these are most likely in patients with scores close to the boundaries of the

Table 8.2 Number of patients, median and two-year survival according to prognostic group for 417 patients with brain cancer (data from Medical Research Council Brain Tumour Working Party, 1990, with kind permission from Springer Science and Business Media)

Prognostic index	Risk group	Number of patients	Median survival (months)	2-year survival rate
0−19	Good	111 (27%)	12	16%
20−29	Medium	161 (39%)	8	3%
30−42	Poor	145 (35%)	4	0%

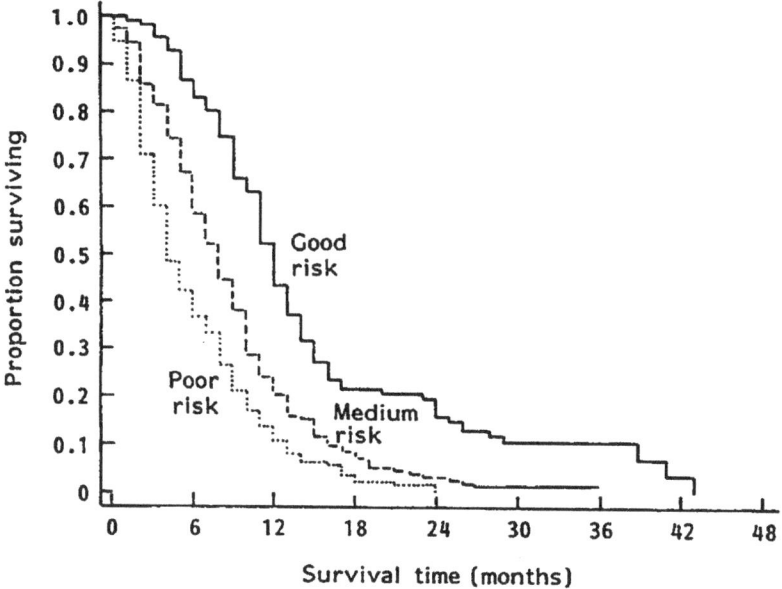

Figure 8.3 Survival curves for the three patient groups identified on the basis of a prognostic index (data from Medical Research Council Brain Tumour Working Party, 1990, with kind permission from Springer Science and Business Media)

respective risk groups. Thus, there are 111 patients in the good risk group of Table 8.2 (*PI* of 0–19), in contrast to 126 with good risk as classified by $S < 1$. This is due to both the modified regression coefficients used in the calculations and to changes in the relative positions of the convenient boundaries chosen to define the Good, Intermediate and Poor risk patients.

Example – *prognostic index* – *low-grade non-Hodgkin's lymphoma*

Leonard, Hayward, Prescott and Wang (1991) present a *PI* for low-grade non-Hodgkin's lymphoma (NHL), derived from survival information on 506 patients. Their *PI* requires information on ECOG performance status, age, stage of disease, sex and haemoglobin levels at presentation as summarised in Table 8.3.

This *PI* includes the continuous variable haemoglobin which is treated as such in the Cox model. Thus, although very simple scores are attached to performance status, age, stage of disease and sex, and these are easily summed, it is also necessary to subtract the score for haemoglobin. This makes the calculation of the final *PI* somewhat less straightforward.

The authors give three examples of patients with NHL and the characteristics of these are summarised in the final columns of Table 8.3 against the corresponding variable category and associated component score contributing to the *PI*. The score for patient *A* is, therefore, $1 + 0 + 1 + 0 + (-0.27 \times 13) = 2 - 3.51 = -1.51$.

Table **8.3** Relevant presentation features and scores for three patients with non-Hodgkin's lymphoma (From Leonard, Hayward, Prescott *et al.*, 1991. Reprinted by permission of Kluwer Academic Publishers)

Presentation feature	Category	Score	Patient *A*	Patient *B*	Patient *C*
ECOG performance status	0	0			
	1 or 2	1	ECOG 2	ECOG 2	ECOG 1
	3	2			
	4	4			
Age (years)	≤ 49	0	49 years		
	50 - 65	2		65 years	
	66+	4			66 years
Stage	1	0			
	2, 3 or 4	1	Stage 4	Stage 3	Stage 2
Sex	Female	0	Female	Female	
	Male	1			Male
Haemoglobin	g/dl	−0.27	13 g/dl	12 g/dl	10 g/dl
		Score	−1.51	+0.76	+4.30

In this example, those with a negative score (Patient *A*) are regarded as having the best prognosis, those with a score between 0 and 3 (Patient *B*) intermediate prognosis and those with a score ≥3 (Patient *C*) as the worst prognosis group. It is then easy to remember that a negative *PI* suggests the best prognosis and a *PI* of three or more the worst. Use of haemoglobin as a continuous variable, in this way, has the advantage of not introducing rather artificial break points for this variable, above which a patient is of good prognosis, below which, bad. However, it does have the drawback of being more cumbersome and less easy to remember.

It is worth noting that the groups derived by Leonard Hayward, Prescott *et al.* (1991) were established on the basis of those 25% (lower quartile) with the worst prognosis, the intermediate 50% and finally 25% (upper quartile) with good prognosis. This approach guarantees sufficient patient numbers in the risk groups, but does not necessarily give convenient boundaries.

Example – *deriving a PI* – *inoperable hepatocellular carcinoma*

Tan, Law, Ng and Machin (2003) use a Cox regression analysis on variables potentially prognostic for survival in patients with inoperable hepatocellular carcinoma (HCC). In their context, they established from their training set of 397 patients, three variables as prognostic and derived a score, *S*, based on these. They give

$$S = 0.683A + 0.327P + 0.290F,$$

where *A* denotes ascites, *P* physical performance by Zubrod performance score (ZPS) and *F* serum AFP level. Dividing the terms on the right-hand side of this equation by the smallest regression coefficient, namely 0.290, and rounding to the nearest integer gives a simplified survival score, S, of

$$S = 2A + P + F.$$

Here the scores for A can take the values 0 or 1; P: 0, 1 or 2 and F: 0, 1, 2 or 3.

On this basis the minimum possible for $S = 0$ and the maximum is $S = 7$. Plots of the corresponding eight survival curves suggested that there were three groups (Low, Medium, High Risk) of sufficiently different prognosis. The K-M survival curves for these three groups are given in Figure 8.4(a). At six months the estimated proportions alive for Low, Medium and High Risk groups are approximately 60%, 20% and 5% respectively.

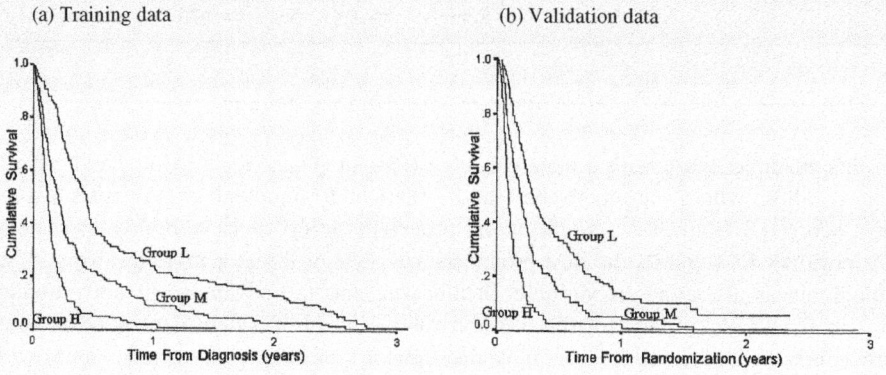

Figure 8.4   Training and validation Kaplan-Meier estimates of Low, Medium and High-risk prognostic groups for patients with inoperable hepatocellular carcinoma (from Tan, Law, Ng and Machin, 2003, reproduced by courtesy of the American Society of Clinical Oncology)

PREDICTED PROGNOSTIC INFORMATION

If the K-M plots of the different risks groups are sufficiently separated then this suggests that these groups may be used for prognosis. Altman and Royston (2000) provide a measure of the prognostic information contained in these groups as that summarised by the *P*redicted *SEP*aration (*PSEP*)

$$PSEP = p_{High} - p_{Low}. \tag{8.8}$$

Here p_{High} is the predicted probability of dying for the patients in the worst prognosis group (High Risk) at a fixed time t, and p_{Low} is the predicted probability of dying for the patients in the best prognosis group (Low Risk) at the same time-point.

***Example** – PSEP – inoperable hepatocellular carcinoma*

The six-month death rates for the training set of 397 patients with inoperable HCC are given in Table 8.4. Thus the proportions of deaths at $t = 6$ months in the High and Low Risk groups are $p_{High} = 0.947$ and $p_{Low} = 0.571$ respectively, so $PSEP = 0.947 - 0.571 = 0.376$.

Table 8.4 Estimated six-month death rates, *PSEP* for training and *OSEP* for validation groups according to survival score (*S*) in patients with inoperable hepatocellular carcinoma (from Tan, Law, Ng and Machin, 2003, reproduced by courtesy of the American Society of Clinical Oncology)

		Patient Group			
		Training Data Set		*Validation Data Set*	
Risk Group	*S*	*n (%)*	6-month death rate (*p*)	*n (%)*	6-month death rate (*p*)
Low	0–2	105 (26.4)	0.571	142 (43.8)	0.666
Medium	3–4	160 (40.3)	0.787	111 (34.3)	0.855
High	5–7	132 (33.3)	0.947	71 (21.9)	0.972
		PSEP	0.376	*OSEP*	0.306

8.6 TESTING THE PROGNOSTIC INDEX (*PI*)

PROCESS

As with all exploratory procedures, it is almost inevitable that a *PI* derived from one data set will not perform as well on a second. There are many reasons for this but an important one is because of random differences (perhaps exaggerating the effects of a particular variable on prognosis) that will be picked up by the modelling process. In contrast, where random differences happen to reduce the effects of the particular variable it will then tend to be excluded from the model chosen. In the former case, the 'exaggeration' may be revealed on later investigation whereas there is a real danger in the second case that the one omitted may go unnoticed. It is clear also from the procedures we have described above that 'subjective' judgement comes into the modelling process.

VALIDATION SET

The *PI* developed for the brain tumour patients appeared to provide good discrimination between poor, medium and good risk groups. However, as the same data has been used to develop the *PI*, it is hardly surprising that we observe such good discrimination between the risk groups. In short, we cannot use a single set of training data both to develop and test a *PI*. As we have indicated, to test the *PI* appropriately we need an independent or confirmatory data set.

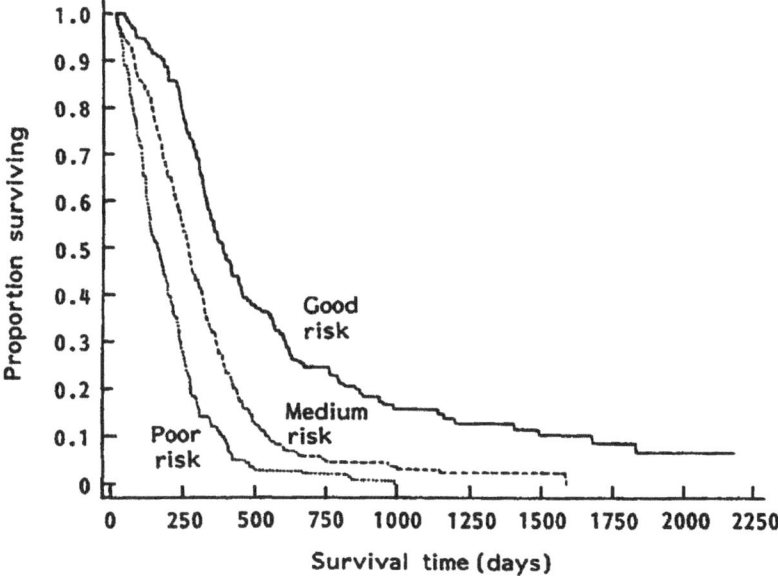

Figure 8.5   Survival curves of good, medium and poor prognosis groups of patients with astrocytoma
(data from Bleehen and Stenning, 1991)

For our example, a confirmatory data set is provided by a subsequent Medical Research Council multi-centre trial of two doses of radiotherapy in patients with cancer of the brain (Bleehen and Stenning, 1991) in which stage, age, performance status and duration of history of fits were also recorded. In this (second) trial, patients with brain tumours of either Grade 3 or 4 astrocytoma were randomised to receive either 45 or 60 Gy of radiotherapy treatment.

Using the information from these patients, the earlier derived *PI* of equation (8.7) was used to score each patient. The patients were then placed in the appropriate risk groups, defined with boundaries at 20 and 30, respectively, as previously specified. The *K-M* survival curves for the three prognostic groups for these 'confirmatory' patients are shown in Figure 8.5.

OBSERVED SEPARATION

It can be seen from Figure 8.5 that, although there is still a clear distinction between 'Good', 'Medium' and 'Poor' risk groups, the separation between the three confirmatory data groups is not quite as marked as that of Figure 8.2. In particular, the Medium and Poor risk groups have 'shrunk' closer to each other, although the Good risk group appears to have a relatively, but small, improved prognosis. These differences are no more than we might expect because the *PI* is unlikely to provide such a good separation between groups in an independent data set, as was observed in the data set used to derive it. The 'shrinkage' is, in fact, a well-known phenomenon that is often observed in confirmatory data sets.

This shrinkage can be quantified by calculating from the corresponding validation *K-M* survival curves, the equivalent of *PSEP* of equation (8.8) but now termed the *O*bserved *SEP*aration (*OSEP*).

Example – *validation group* – *OSEP* – *inoperable hepatocellular carcinoma*

Tan, Law, Ng and Machin (2003) used patients from the Asia-Pacific wide multi-centre trial for treatment of inoperable HCC and recruited over the period 4 April 1997 to 8 June 2000 to validate their *PI*. These were 329 patients randomised in a double-blind fashion to either tamoxifen treatment or placebo. Survival information was available on all but five of these patients. All patients had their baseline characteristics recorded at the time of diagnosis of their HCC, following which they were randomised to the trial and routinely followed up until death.

Survival was calculated from the date of randomisation. The *S* derived from the training group was used to calculate, for each new patient, the corresponding value for him or her. On the basis of this score the patient was then assigned to one of the proposed Low, Medium and High-risk groups as previously defined and the survival experience summarized using the *K-M* technique. From these curves, shown in Figure 8.4(b), the proportion alive at six months was estimated giving $OSEP = p_{High} - p_{Low} = 0.306$. This is close to the corresponding $PSEP = 0.376$ obtained from Figure 8.4(a), hence demonstrating validity of the *PI*.

In addition, the use of the validation group, obtained from a prospective multi-national multi-ethnic randomised controlled clinical trial with high quality data, provides additional reassurance. The training model was established three years before the prospective validation data became available.

PRACTICALITIES

We have indicated some necessary steps required when constructing a *PI*. The aim of such an index is to identify patients with differing risk. It must be remembered that the divisions established for the risk groups are arbitrary, so that even within a *PI* group there may be substantial variation in prognosis.

Prior to easy access to powerful and inexpensive personal computers, emphasis was placed on deriving a *PI* that was very easy to compute and the boundaries of the 'at risk' groups easy to define. Thus, arithmetically simple and memory-jogging numbers were often used in the *PI*. However, it is relatively easy to write a menu-driven computer program that can calculate a *PI* directly from, for example, the regression coefficients of Table 8.1. The examining clinician merely records the patient details and feeds them into the program, which then returns the *PI* group and associated risk for that patient.

THE ROLE OF TREATMENT

In developing the *PI* with the brain tumour patients, a regression coefficient to account for the treatment received by the patient was not included in the model of equation (8.3). This was because no survival difference between patients allocated to the two treatments was observed. However, for the patients of the confirmatory data set, a survival difference between the two treatments allocated was observed. The results reported by Bleehen and Stenning (1991) gave an $HR = 0.81$ for survival, with 95% CI of 0.66 to 0.99, in favour of the

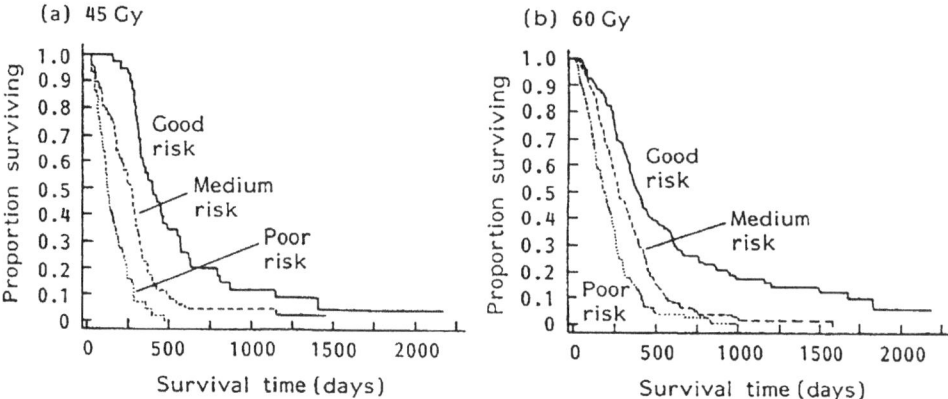

Figure 8.6 Survival curves for each prognostic risk group by treatment allocated in patients with astrocytoma (data from Bleehen and Stenning, 1991, reproduced by permission of The Macmillan Press Ltd)

high dose regimen. This difference obviously accounts for some of the variability observed, in that those patients who received the 'better' treatment had on average a better survival time. In this context, it is of interest to assess whether the *PI* appears relevant to patients in both treatment groups. Figure 8.6(a) shows the survival curves by prognostic group for those patients allocated to receive a low-dose radiotherapy of 45 Gy and Figure 8.6(b) shows the same for those allocated to receive a high-dose radiotherapy of 60 Gy.

It can be seen that the separation between the three prognostic groups is maintained in both treatment groups. It is a common experience that, in many cases, prognostic factors are often independent of the treatment given. However, we should note that although the separation between the groups remains, the actual curves for the individual groups receiving the two treatments may differ. For example, the survival for the good risk group who receive 60 Gy is likely to be higher than for the same good risk group but who receive 45 Gy and this is confirmed by Figure 8.6.

When the data to develop a *PI* come from a randomised trial, the differing treatments are well defined and can be included in the model with ease. In contrast, if the data arise from, say, a retrospectively inspected series of case records, there may be many different treatments employed. To take account of these, we would need either to add many terms to the model by use of dummy variables or attempt to summarise the numerous possibilities into treatment groupings. In the latter case, we may, for example, classify the treatments into broad categories of chemotherapy, radiotherapy or surgery. Once summarised in this way, 'type of treatment' could then be added to the models for developing the *PI*.

8.7   UPDATING THE INDEX

Once the *PI* has been tested on a confirmatory data set, it may be appropriate to refine and update the index by pooling the data from both sets. In such cases, it is not sensible to begin the model selection process all over again, since we have, at least in our example, firmly established the four important prognostic factors. What we do instead is to fit these factors to the combined data set and thereby obtain modified estimates of the corresponding regression coefficients. A new and updated *PI* will be derived from these for use with prospective patients.

However, there are two further aspects that have to be considered. First, there may be a significant survival difference observed between the training and validation data sets, perhaps as a consequence of a change in therapy over time. Second, if we are combining data from two or more trials conducted in parallel, then the type of treatments used in each may differ and it is possible that the magnitude of the effect of a prognostic factor may also differ, depending on the therapies utilised.

Consider again the example of patients with brain tumours. To allow for the treatment effect both over time and within each trial, we incorporate a term for treatment, *T*, into the Cox model of equation (8.3) as follows:

$$T + A + C + N + F : \log h = \beta_T T + \beta_A A + \beta_C C + \beta_N N + \beta_F F. \qquad (8.9)$$

For brevity, we have indicated in equation (8.9) that only one regression coefficient, β_T, is needed in order to include the effect of treatment in the model. In fact, how the treatment effect is included in the model will depend on the treatment-specific features of the training and confirmatory data sets. For example, with the data from the two trials in patients with brain tumours, the patients of the training data received either placebo or misonidazole in addition to radiotherapy of a minimum dose of 45 Gy, while those of the confirmatory data received radiotherapy at doses of either 45 or 60 Gy. In this situation, we can describe the effect of treatment in different ways in the model of equation (8.9) as summarised in Table 8.5.

In one method, the four different treatments are regarded as such and, therefore, are classified as four levels of a non-ordered categorical variable. This can then be incorporated into equation (8.9) using the three dummy variables g_1, g_2, g_3. This is referred to as Model I in Table 8.5. Each of the three dummy variables will have the associated regression coefficients γ_1, γ_2 and γ_3. The estimates of these are given as c_1, c_2 and c_3 in the second (updated) column of Table 8.6.

Comparing these results with those of Table 8.1, which are reproduced in the 'original' column in Table 8.6, we see that the regression coefficient for age has increased somewhat, from 0.3366 to 0.4678. In contrast, the coefficient for extent of neurosurgery has become smaller, from 0.2279 to 0.1571. The regression coefficients for clinical performance status and length of history of fits have stayed largely unchanged. This suggests that, by including the patients from the confirmatory data set into the model, age has become a more important prognostic factor, while the extent of neurosurgery has become less important. Following

Table 8.5 Models for including treatment in the development of a prognostic index for patients with brain tumours

Data set	Treatment	Model I			Treatment	Model II	
		g_1	g_2	g_3		g_4	g_5
Training	45 Gy + Placebo	0	0	0	Control	0	0
	45 Gy + Misonidazole	1	0	0	Test	0	1
Confirmatory	45 Gy	0	1	0	Control	1	0
	60 Gy	0	0	1	Test	1	1

Table 8.6 Fitting Model I of Table 8.5, together with the confirmed prognostic variables from an earlier analysis, to the combined data of two randomised trials in patients with brain tumours (data from Bleehen and Stenning, 1991, reproduced by permission of The Macmillan Press Ltd)

| Factor | | Estimated regression coefficients | | |
		Original (from Table 8.1)	Updated	SE
Treatment				
Placebo		–	0	–
Misonidazole	c_1	–	−0.1959	0.0954
45 Gy	c_2	–	−0.0919	0.1079
60 Gy	c_3	–	−0.3558	0.0898
Prognostic variables				
A	b_A	0.3366	0.4678	0.0500
C	b_C	0.2084	0.2403	0.0436
N	b_N	0.2279	0.1571	0.0471
F	b_F	0.2434	0.2411	0.0487

these changes in the estimates of the regression coefficients through, by the process described in Section 8.5, results in an updated *PI* of the form

$$PI_{Updated} = 9A + 5C + 3N + 5F. \tag{8.10}$$

We note that $PI_{Updated}$ does not contain terms associated with the effect of treatment, despite treatment being included in the model. This is because treatment was included in the model only to obtain adjusted estimates of the coefficients of the *PI*. When the *PI* is used for future patients, the treatment employed is chosen, and may in fact be different from those used in the patients in our examples. The four other variables, however, are intrinsic characteristics of the patient at the time of their diagnosis.

This updated *PI* implies, in broad terms, that age is now approximately twice as important as clinical performance status and length of history of fits, and three times as important as the extent of neurosurgery. Previously in the *PI* of equation (8.7) there was less variation in the weights attached to the prognostic factors.

Two further aspects should be noted in Table 8.6. First, the *SE*s for the estimates are smaller than in Table 8.1. This is because the number of deaths available for this analysis is approximately twice that of the earlier analysis. Second, the estimate for the treatment effect has no straightforward interpretation. Note, however, that fitting treatment-specific coefficients will, in general, also contribute to smaller *SE*s for the regression coefficients of each prognostic factor.

Model II of Table 8.5 recognises explicitly that there are two data sets and models this with $g_4 = 0$ and 1, respectively, with associated regression coefficient γ_4. Control and test therapies within these data sets are then modelled with $g_5 = 0$ and one respectively, with associated regression coefficient γ_5. Fitting this model to the data gives estimates of these regression coefficients as −0.1317 and −0.2268 respectively. More importantly, for our example, the corresponding estimates for the regression coefficients for age, clinical performance status, extent of neurosurgery and length of history of fits of 0.4670, 0.2411, 0.1571 and 0.2421 differ very little from those of Model I, summarised in Table 8.6. As a result, the updated *PI* with this form of the model remains as equation (8.10).

A third possible model, to include the effect of treatment in the process of updating the *PI*, adds a treatment by data set interaction term to Model II. This Model III replaces the term $\gamma_4 g_4 + \gamma_5 g_5$ in Model II by $\gamma_4 g_4 + \gamma_5 g_5 + \gamma_{45} g_4 g_5$, the latter representing the interaction term. Fitting this model to the data gives estimates of these regression coefficients as -0.1599, -0.2638 and 0.0679 respectively. The first two of these are very close to the values of -0.1317 and -0.2268 for the corresponding Model II values and the coefficient for the interaction term is close to zero. More importantly for our application, however, the regression coefficients for age, clinical performance status, extent of neuro-surgery and length of history of fits of 0.4678, 0.2408, 0.1571 and 0.2411, respectively, are very close to those of Model II. As a result, the updated *PI* with this model again remains as equation (8.10).

8.8   CONFIRMING AN ESTABLISHED INDEX

VERIFICATION

If a prognostic model for a situation has been developed by others and perhaps reported in the literature, then one may reasonably wish to verify if the *PI* so derived is applicable to another set of patients. This published *PI* is equivalent to the 'training' set in circumstances where an entirely new *PI* is being developed. However, before proceeding it is useful to check the exact details of how the *PI* was produced and to be sure that the methodology (both clinical and statistical) is acceptable. For example, if the methodology appears flawed then this may affect judgement with respect to the level of verification that one might expect. Of course if 'pure' verification is required then care has to be taken in defining the patient eligibility in precisely the same way as for those for whom the model was constructed. On the other hand, if one is interested to see if the model is applicable to a wider range of patients then as wide a range as considered relevant is appropriate. However, the expectations for the original *PI* must be duly adjusted, depending on the extent of the overlap between the patient groups concerned. The criteria for judging the model must be defined in advance of the verification process.

For pure verification purposes, a measure such as *PSEP* should first be obtained for the data constructing the original model, perhaps from the relevant publication itself. Then the score for each patient in the new data group is obtained using the exact model formulation as published and, on the basis of their individual scores, they are assigned to the recommended prognostic groups. The corresponding *K-M* curves are then estimated and the *OSEP* calculated and compared to the original *PSEP*. Close agreement in these values would verify the utility of the *PI*.

A common mistake, rather than to check the exact model published on the new data, is to build one's own model and see if the process of model building chooses the same variables. However, it is often quite difficult to replicate some of the more 'subjective' criteria involved in a modelling process so differences may result as a consequence of this. This distinguishes the verification of a *PI* published by others from that of developing an entirely new *PI* in which the investigator has full control of the design and analytical processes. Nevertheless, if this process selects the same variables, then a check is made of whether or not the corresponding regression coefficients are similar in value. This may or may not verify the prognostic value of the published *PI*.

MODIFICATION

In certain circumstances, a *PI* is so well established that to change it on the basis of new information may not be very practicable. Clearly, if the new information suggests that the very basis of the *PI* needs to be questioned, then that is a different matter. Suppose that the *PI* is indeed well established, implying that the model from which it derives is also well established, both in terms of the variables it contains and also the value of the corresponding regression coefficients. To establish if any new information is going to influence the estimates of the regression coefficients, one can use the procedure described in the following example.

We assume our model includes only age and history of fits and is of the form $A + F$ of equation (6.3). Thus $\log h = S = 0.6528 x_A - 0.4647 x_F$. We now wish to determine if we need to modify the estimates of the regression coefficients of this model with our new data. The procedure is first to calculate the score, S, for all the new patients. We then fit the model

$$\log h = S + \beta_{SA} x_A + \beta_{SF} x_F \tag{8.11}$$

to the data. Here, β_{SA} and β_{SF}, represent any extra information in the new data on the influence of age and history of fits on prognosis.

We now test the two null hypotheses for the respective regression coefficients, that is, $\beta_{SF} = 0$ and $\beta_{SA} = 0$. If both these hypotheses are not rejected, the model remains that of equation (6.3). This implies that the regression coefficients for calculating S remain unchanged. On the other hand, if either of the null hypotheses is rejected, then the corresponding regression coefficients in S are modified by adding the estimates of b_{SA}, b_{SF} of β_{SA}, β_{SF} or both, to b_A and b_F as appropriate. Such a change or changes are then carried through to the *PI*, which may or may not be affected depending on the magnitude of these changes in the regression coefficients.

If the possibility of adding a single (entirely new) variable, V, is under consideration, then equation (8.11) is modified to include that variable as

$$\log h = S + \beta_V V. \tag{8.12}$$

In this case, the null hypothesis of $\beta_V = 0$ is tested. Once more, if the null hypothesis is not rejected, then the model S is not modified. On the other hand, if the hypothesis is rejected, then S is updated by addition of the new variable, V. In which case, the process of simplifying the regression model may have to be repeated. The new variable will clearly affect the *PI*, perhaps in a substantial way and should provide extra discrimination between the risk groups.

If both modifications to existing regression coefficients and the possibility of new variables are being considered then equations like (8.11) and (8.12) can be combined in an obvious way.

Special computational procedures have to be used to fit these models. These procedures essentially force the model both to give S a regression coefficient of one, as S can be written $1 \times S$ in equations (8.11) and (8.12) to emphasise this, and also to lock the variable S into the model if a selection procedure for the other variables is used.

9 Sample Sizes

Summary

This chapter describes how sample sizes can be determined for survival studies comparing the survival curves of two treatment groups. To obtain such sample sizes, it is necessary to specify at the planning stage of the study the size of the effect that is anticipated together with the size and power of the Logrank test to be used for the comparison. We stress that the sample size is chosen in such a way as to ensure that sufficient endpoint events are observed, as their numbers are more crucial than the number of subjects recruited. A method of estimating the total duration of a study accounting for both recruitment and follow-up stages is given. We highlight the approximate nature of sample size calculations and indicate that proposed studies with inadequate power should be considered carefully before their implementation. Extensions to sample size problems associated with Cox models in general are indicated.

9.1 INTRODUCTION

One important problem to address once the design of a particular investigation has been decided is an appropriate sample size. A study that is too small may not be able to answer the question posed; one that is too large will be wasteful of resources. As we have indicated earlier, the majority of studies are comparative in nature. Thus a randomised controlled trial will compare two or more possible interventions given to patients to determine if there are real differences in therapeutic benefit. More generally, many studies, whether in the laboratory, clinic or elsewhere, will also compare two or more predefined groups, such as patients with different types of genetic markers or histological subtypes. The analysis of such examples can be conducted through the Logrank test or by use of the Cox model and focus on the type D (design) variables defined in Chapter 6.

On the other hand, in a more epidemiological context, one may wish to investigate factors influencing survival time, such as the influence of birth weight on neonatal survival, taking account of other characteristics of the babies concerned. These lead more naturally to consider sample sizes for regression problems involving type D and K variables. However, the main focus remains the influence of birth weight so the study design, and sample size, should focus on the estimate of the $HR(s)$ for that.

The same effectively applies to a clinical trial, but here practice usually dictates that only factors known to have major influence on outcome should be recorded and hence accounted for in the analysis. Randomisation to the different intervention groups tends to obviate the need to record (and hence adjust for) variables of less prognostic influence. The main focus remains, for example, the estimate of relative efficacy for a therapeutic trial as expressed through the corresponding HR. So sample size too focuses on reliably estimating this HR.

Survival Analysis Second Edition   David Machin, Yin Bun Cheung, Mahesh K.B. Parmar
© 2006 John Wiley & Sons, Ltd   ISBN: 0-470-87040-0

In contrast, although prognostic factor studies also depend on the Cox *PH* regression models, interest is now in identifying all the variables that are important for prognosis. So in this case, we are concerned that all the regression coefficients of the variables contributing to the final prognostic index (*PI*), discussed in Chapter 8, are well established. So adequate sample size is required to satisfy this.

The number of subjects, more strictly the number of events to be observed, necessary for a particular clinical or epidemiological study to achieve its design goals depends on several factors. These include: the anticipated difference between groups as expressed by the *HR*, often termed the effect size; the level of statistical significance required, and the power or size of the chance of detecting the effect size postulated.

9.2   GENERAL CONSIDERATIONS

EFFECT SIZE

The effect size is the true difference between the groups under consideration in a comparative study. In the context of a survival time study this may be expressed as a *HR*, the different medians or a difference between two survival rates at a fixed point in time.

To assist in the description of sample size calculations, we use the notation indicated in Figure 9.1, which shows two Exponential survival curves representing two treatment groups in a randomised trial and each of the form of Figure 4.1 although differing in the hazard rates. There is one curve corresponding to the survival of patients receiving control treatment, *C*, and one for those receiving the test treatment, *T*. However, these could equally represent the survival in any two groups arising from many different types of study.

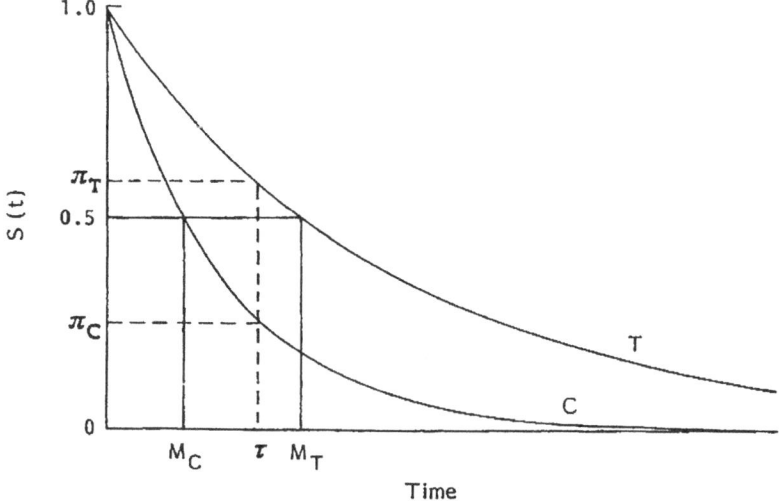

Figure 9.1   Anticipated Exponential survival curves of patients receiving control, *C*, and test, *T*, therapies for a particular disease

The difference between groups of Figure 9.1 can be summarised by the *HR*, which is

$$\Delta = \frac{\lambda_T}{\lambda_C}. \tag{9.1}$$

where λ_T and λ_C are the constant hazards for groups T and C respectively.

In the circumstance of an Exponential survival distribution the proportion, π, alive at a fixed time τ is related to the hazard rate by means of equation (4.3), so that for example,

$$\pi_T = S_T(\tau) = \exp(-\lambda_T \tau). \tag{9.2}$$

From which

$$\lambda_T = -\log \pi_T / \tau, \tag{9.3}$$

with a similar expressions for group C.

As a consequence, the hazard ratio Δ can be expressed as

$$\Delta = \frac{\lambda_T}{\lambda_C} = \frac{\log \pi_T}{\log \pi_C} \tag{9.4}$$

since τ divides out.

In some situations it is more natural to think of anticipated differences in terms of a difference in median survival times. However, for Exponentially distributed survival times, there is a direct relationship between the median survival time and the survival rate observed at a fixed time.

Suppose the anticipated median survival time for one of the treatment groups is M. By definition, the proportion surviving to the median time is 0.5 and so $\exp(-\lambda M) = 0.5$. This in turn gives, using equation (9.3) with $\tau = M$, the hazard

$$\lambda = -\log 0.5 / M. \tag{9.5}$$

We can then substitute the anticipated median survival times for groups C and T into equation (9.5) in turn to obtain the corresponding values for λ_C and λ_T. These lead to the anticipated *HR* of equation (9.4) as

$$\Delta = \frac{\lambda_T}{\lambda_C} = \frac{M_C}{M_T}. \tag{9.6}$$

Thus Δ is merely the inverse of the ratio of the corresponding median survival times for treatments T and C. If necessary therefore, at the planning stage of a study, we can provide planning values for the corresponding medians, and hence obtain Δ_{Plan} through equation (9.6).

It is clear from equations (9.4) and (9.6) that if any two of Δ, π_T, π_C or of Δ, M_T, M_C are provided, then the third can be derived.

Since we are currently planning the study we use, for example, Δ in the above rather than *HR* as this is the quantity or parameter we wish to estimate with the study data once collected.

Example – *colonisation-free rates* – *patients with cystic fibrosis*

Valerius, Koch and Hoiby (1991) described a small trial of 26 patients with cystic fibrosis who were randomised to receive either no treatment (*C*) or anti-pseudomonas treatment (*T*) for *Ps. aeruginosa* in their sputum. In this trial 12 patients were randomised to *C* and the remaining 14 to *T*. The survival time recorded in this case is the time that the patients' sputum is free of colonisation by *Ps. aeruginosa* as measured from the date of randomisation to the date of the first positive test of their sputum.

The results are shown in Figure 9.2, which gives the approximate colonisation-free rates at 12 months for groups *C* and *T* as $p_C = 0.50$ (50%) for the untreated patients and $p_T = 0.85$ (85%) respectively. This difference can be expressed as an observed advantage to the treated group of $p_T - p_C = 0.35$ (35%) at one year. From which equation (9.4) gives the estimated $HR = \log 0.85 / \log 0.50 = 0.23$.

Also from the figure one can estimate the median survival time for *C* as between 12 and 16 months but that for *T* cannot be estimated.

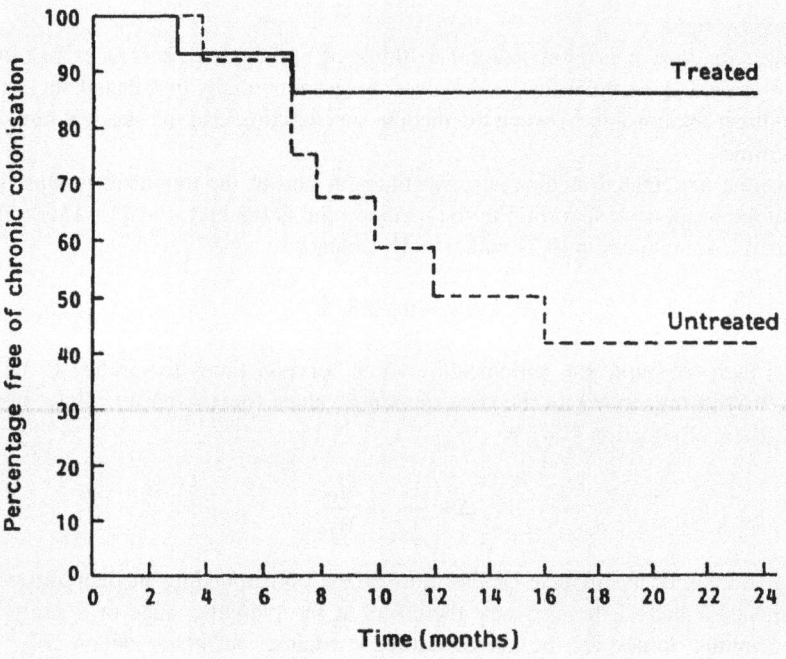

Figure 9.2   Probability of *Ps. aeruginosa*-free sputum in untreated and treated patients with cystic fibrosis (Reprinted from *The Lancet*, **338**, Valerius, Koch and Hoiby, 1991, Prevention of chronic Pseudomonas aeruginosa colonisation in cystic fibrosis by early treatment, 725–726, © 1991, with permission from Elsevier)

CLINICALLY IMPORTANT DIFFERENCE

A key element in the design is the 'effect size' that it is reasonable to plan to observe—should it exist. Sometimes there is prior knowledge, which then enables an investigator to anticipate what effect size between groups is likely to be observed, and the role of the study or trial is to confirm that expectation. In some situations, it may be possible to state that, for example, only a doubling of median survival would be worthwhile to demonstrate in a planned trial. This might be because the new treatment, as compared to standard, is expected to be so toxic or expensive that only if substantial benefit could be shown would it ever be utilised. In such cases the investigator may have definite opinions about the difference that it is pertinent to detect.

Example *– planning a confirmatory trial – patients with cystic fibrosis*

Suppose a group of investigators were sceptical of the results given by Valerius, Koch and Hoiby (1991) and so wished to conduct a confirmatory trial. It would seem reasonable to consider the estimated values obtained from that trial as a basis for this planning. Thus they may consider the estimated $HR = 0.23$ as the planning value for Δ. However, they are aware that this estimate was based on a trial including only 26 patients and consider this may overestimate the true benefit of T. As a consequence, they may postulate an effect somewhat smaller than this, but which if demonstrated would still be clinically important (see Section 1.5). For example, they may think that $\Delta = 0.5$ or 1/2 is more realistic than 0.23. In this case, they may prefer to design their trial with this effect size in mind.

Although the anticipated effect size has been described specifically for the case of two Exponential survival distributions, the same process applies if only PHs can be assumed. This enables the same quantities to be used for planning purposes in this wider context.

TEST SIZE

As we are making a comparison, the null hypothesis, H_0, states that the true value of the HR is one or alternatively expressed as the absolute difference in survival rates is 0. On these two scales the null hypothesis of no group differences are equivalently $\Delta_0 = 1$ and $\delta_0 = 0$. The subscript 0 reminds us that these are the effect sizes anticipated by the null hypothesis.

Now, even if this null hypothesis is actually true, that is, there is truly no difference between treatment and control, we may observe at the conclusion of our new trial a value of the HR which is not exactly equal to 1. Under the assumption of no difference this will only be a random departure from the underlying $\Delta_0 = 1$. In this instance the difference between the observed HR and the value 1 will be due to chance alone and the associated p-value will not be small. On the other hand, if the p-value is small we are led to question whether the null hypothesis is indeed true. In fact, if the p-value is small enough we may reject the null hypothesis and conclude that the two treatments actually differ in their efficacy. This is equivalent to concluding that $\Delta \neq 1$ and hence Δ_{Plan}, the anticipated value of the HR under the alternative hypothesis, H_a, is perhaps more likely.

When designing a trial or any other comparative study, we have to decide at what level this p-value (probability) should be set, such that if a smaller p-value is observed we would reject the null hypothesis. The value we set at the design stage for this probability is often termed the test size and is denoted by α. It is also called the significance level or type I error. It is important to distinguish α from the p-value. The former denotes, at the planning stage, our pre-specified design significance level, while the latter is calculated at the analysis stage once our study is completed. At this latter stage, if we observe a p-value $\leq \alpha$ then we reject the null hypothesis of, for example, equal treatment efficacy and conclude that the treatments do indeed differ in their relative efficacy.

Another way of viewing α is that it is the probability of falsely rejecting the null hypothesis. That is, if there is in truth no difference between the two groups, it is our design probability, which is set reasonably small, that we will actually claim a difference between the two. Although the choice of α is arbitrary, it has become common to set it at either 0.05 (5%) or 0.01 (1%). In general, the *smaller* the test size specified by the design team the *larger* the study will be.

ONE- OR TWO-SIDED COMPARISONS?

When designing a study to compare groups, with the aim of showing that one is superior to another, it is necessary to state whether a one-sided or two-sided test is going to be performed at the analysis stage. The decision depends upon the alternatives considered possible at the design stage. If we consider that there is a chance that, for example, a new treatment may be worse than the standard although we anticipate it will be better, then we allow the possibility that the observed difference between treatment survival rates can be less than 0 (new treatment worse) as well as more than 0 (new treatment better). This situation would lead to a two-sided test being performed. In this case at the analysis stage if, from a significance test, the value of $z = -2.581$, indicating indeed that the new treatment has done *worse* than the control, the p-value is nevertheless obtained by summing the areas to the left of $z = -2.581$ and that to the right of $z = +2.581$ in Table T1. This totals $2 \times 0.0099 = 0.0198$.

In rare circumstances it may be decided *a priori* that there is no possibility that, for example, the new treatment is worse than the control. In this one-sided situation the only alternative to the null hypothesis $\delta_0 - 0$ is that $\delta > 0$ (equivalently expressed as $\Delta_0 = 1$, and $\Delta < 1$) then a one-sided statistical test would be performed. In this case, if at the analysis stage a value of $z > 0$ is obtained, as one would expect, then it is referred to Table T1 but the area in the upper tail of the distribution alone gives the p-value. Thus with $z = +2.581$, Table T1 gives p-value $= 0.0099$. On the other hand if, and totally unexpectedly, $z = -2.581$ then we cannot claim any difference between the groups.

In fact, in most instances we are performing a study because we do not know whether there is a difference or not between two groups. Thus two-sided tests are most often used. Since one-sided tests are so unusual, the discussion presented here assumes two-sided tests will be performed.

POWER

Once we have specified the anticipated effect size, Δ_{Plan}, we need to ensure that the study we have designed has a high probability of detecting this should it, in fact, be the true underlying effect size. This probability is called the power of the study. Consequently, we require a small probability that the planned study will not detect this benefit should it, in truth, exist. This small probability, β, is often called the false negative probability or the type II error. The power of a study is $(1 - \beta)$ and is usually expressed as a percentage. In randomised trials the power is typically demanded to be high, for example at least 80% and quite commonly 90%. In general, the *larger* the power specified by the design team the *larger* the study will be.

9.3   TWO-GROUP COMPARATIVE STUDIES

DESIGN

To illustrate the sample size calculations for comparative studies, we will assume that we are planning a clinical trial of two alternative therapies with survival from randomisation until death as the outcome variable. Further, the design team are aware of the results of a preliminary trial and will use this information for planning purposes. In this case the design team need to specify the anticipated effect size, Δ_{Plan}. The hope is that the observed HR, which estimates the true Δ, will be close to this value. They will also need to provide an anticipated proportion alive at some fixed time in one group, π_{Plan-C}, or equivalently the corresponding median survival time, M_{Plan-C}.

They must further consider the proportion of patients to be allocated to the groups C and T (Test), which we assume are in the ratio 1 to φ. For example, if $\varphi = 1$ then patients are assigned equally, whereas if $\varphi = 2$ then twice as many receive treatment T as C. The reverse is the case if $\varphi = \frac{1}{2}$.

For randomised trials, equal allocation is most often used but it should be emphasised that the randomised trial is only one of many possible illustrations of a two-group comparison. Indeed, in many comparative studies members of one of the two groups of concern may not be so easy to find so that it is easiest for the investigators concerned if φ is not restricted to unity.

Finally the test size α and power $1 - \beta$ have to be specified.

NUMBER OF EVENTS

The primary concern in any survival type study is the presence of censored observations whose presence implies that the reliability of a study does not depend on the total study size, N, but rather on the total number of events observed, E. This implies that a study should recruit the N subjects and then wait until the required E events are observed before conducting the analysis and reporting the results. In a study without censored survival times N and E will be equal but this is unusual.

It can be shown that if patients are allocated to each group in the ratio $1 : \varphi$, the number of events for the C group, e_C, that need to be observed in a clinical study comparing two groups, with an anticipated benefit of Δ_{Plan}, test size α and power $1 - \beta$, is given by

$$e_C = \frac{(z_{1-\alpha/2} + z_{1-\beta})^2}{\varphi} \left[\frac{1 + \varphi \Delta_{Plan}}{1 - \Delta_{Plan}} \right]^2. \tag{9.7}$$

The terms $z_{1-\alpha/2}$ and $z_{1-\beta}$ are defined in Section 1.3, and specific values corresponding to α and β are obtained from either Table T1 or Table T2 of the Normal distribution.

The corresponding number of events for the second group, T, are $e_T = \varphi e_C$, giving the total number of events required as $E = e_C + e_T = e_C(1 + \varphi)$.

NUMBER OF SUBJECTS

It should be noted that equation (9.7) contains the benefit as expressed by the single summary Δ_{Plan} and leads to the total number of events required, E. However, in order to calculate the number of subjects required for this number of events to be observed, it is necessary to specify the anticipated values for π_T and π_C as we have indicated previously. The total number of subjects required is then given by

$$N_{Total} = \frac{(1 + \varphi)E}{[(1 - \pi_{Plan-C}) + \varphi(1 - \pi_{Plan-T})]}. \tag{9.8}$$

The subjects would then be recruited from the two groups on a $1 : \varphi$ proportionate basis.

Example – study size – patients with cystic fibrosis

Suppose in the confirmatory trial using the anti-pseudomonas therapy in patients with cystic fibrosis the investigators had decided that, since the proposed therapy is new, they would like to gain some experience with the therapy itself whereas they are very familiar with the (no treatment) control option. In such a situation it may be appropriate to randomise patients in blocks of five in a ratio of 2:3 in favour of the test treatment, that is, $\varphi = 3/2 = 1.5$. This implies two patients receive C for every three receiving T. In such circumstances it is usual to randomise patients in blocks of size, $b = 5$ (or size $2b$), each block containing two (or four) C and three (or six) T patients receiving the respective allocation.

Use of the two-sided column of Table T2 with $\alpha = 0.05$ gives $z_{0.975} = 1.9600$ and the one-sided column with $\beta = 0.2$ gives $z_{0.8} = 0.8416$. Substituting these together with $\varphi = 1.5$ and $\Delta_{Plan} = 0.23$ in equation (9.7) gives $e_C = \dfrac{(1.9600 + 0.8416)^2}{1.5}\left[\dfrac{1 + 1.5 \times 0.23}{1 - 0.23}\right]^2 = 16.0$ events.

From which $E = 16.0 \times (1 + 1.5) = 40$ events. Substituting this into equation (9.8) with $\pi_{Plan-C} = 0.50$ and $\pi_{Plan-T} = 0.85$ gives a total of $N = 78.4$. Rounding this to the nearest but larger integer divisible by the block size of five gives $N = 80$. Then, dividing these in a ratio of 2:3, gives 32 to receive C and 48 T.

In general, unless the allocation ratio is more extreme than 2:1, that is, the value of φ is greater than two, then unequal allocation does not make a substantial difference to the total numbers of events and subjects required.

SAMPLE SIZE TABLES

For the case of equal group sizes, that is $\varphi = 1$, equation (9.8) is tabulated in Table T4. Tabulations are for a two-sided $\alpha = 0.05$, $1 - \beta$ of 0.8 and 0.9, values of π_C ranging from

0.05 to 0.9 and the anticipated difference $\delta = \pi_T - \pi_C$ ranging from 0.05 to 0.5 (The subscript *Plan* is omitted). Differences in the number of patients provided by direct use of equation (9.8) and Table T4 arise from rounding both in the calculations themselves and the final tabular entry, which is always rounded up to the nearest even number in order to be divisible by two since the groups are to be of equal size.

From this table we can see that small changes in δ can have an enormous impact on the number of subjects required. For example, if we set $\pi_C = 0.45$, $\alpha = 0.05$, $1 - \beta = 90\%$ then for $\delta = 0.10$, 1020 patients are required. However, for $\delta = 0.05$, 4014 patients are required. This is nearly four times as many—for a halving of the absolute effect to be estimated! We can also see from this table that a change in $1 - \beta$ from 80% to 90% can also influence N, although not in as marked a manner as changes in δ. Finally, large changes in our estimate of an appropriate π_C can also have a considerable influence on N.

To adapt expression (9.7) and hence (9.8) to allow for a one-sided comparison merely involves replacing $z_{1-\alpha/2}$ by $z_{1-\alpha}$. For example, if we set our test size, α, to be 0.05 then a two-sided test would give $z_{1-\alpha/2} = 1.9600$, while $z_{1-\alpha} = 1.6445$, leading to a smaller value of E for the one-sided design. This will mean that a one-sided test design will always require fewer events to be observed than the corresponding two-sided design.

LOSS TO FOLLOW-UP

One aspect of a study which will affect the number of subjects recruited, is the anticipated proportion who are subsequently lost to follow-up. Since these subjects are lost, we will never observe and record the date of the critical event, even though it may have occurred. Such subjects have censored observations, in the same way as those for whom the event of interest has still not occurred by the time of analysis of the study. Such lost subjects, however, do not, and will never, contribute events for the analysis and, therefore, we need to compensate for their loss.

If the anticipated loss or withdrawal proportion is w or $100w\%$, then the required number of patients, N, given by equation (9.8) should be increased to

$$N_{Adjusted} = N/(1 - w). \tag{9.9}$$

The estimated size of w can often be obtained from reports of studies conducted by others. If there is no such experience to hand, then a pragmatic value may be to take $w = 0.1$. We are assuming that the loss to follow-up is occurring at random and is not related to the current (perhaps health) status of the subject. If this cannot be assumed then the basis of the Logrank analysis is brought into question.

Example – adjusting for patient losses – patients with resectable colon cancer

An adjuvant study of the drug levamisole is proposed for patients with resectable cancer of the colon (Dukes' C), in which the primary objective of the study is to compare the efficacy of levamisole against a placebo control, with respect to relapse-free survival. How many patients need to be recruited in the trial if a decrease from 50% to 40% in relapse rates at one year is anticipated, and a power of 80% is required? A patient loss rate of 10% is anticipated.

Here we wish to increase the success rate, that is, failure to relapse, from 50% to 60%, so $\pi_{Plan-C} = 0.5$ and $\pi_{Plan-T} = 0.6$. These give $\delta = 0.6 - 0.5 = 0.1$

and $\Delta = \log 0.6 / \log 0.5 = 0.74$. Assuming a two-sided test with $\alpha = 0.05$, $1 - \beta = 0.8$, and equal randomisation $\varphi = 1$, then Table T4, with $\pi_{Plan-C} = 0.5$ and $\delta = 0.1$, gives $N = 764$ patients required.

Allowing for a loss to follow-up rate $w = 10\%$ and using equation (9.9) we obtain $N_{Adjusted} = 764/(1 - 0.1) = 849$. Thus, a total of approximately 850 subjects should be recruited to the trial, half of which will receive placebo and half levamisole.

STUDY DURATION

We have noted earlier that it is the total number of events that determines the power of the study or equivalently the power of the subsequent Logrank test. For any study with a survival time endpoint there is clearly a period of accrual during which subjects are recruited to a study and a further period of follow-up beyond the end of accrual during which time more events are observed. To observe a pre-specified number of events we can either (i) keep the accrual period as short as possible and extend follow-up; or (ii) have the accrual period as long as practicable and have a short post-recruitment follow-up; or (iii) achieve a balance between accrual and follow-up. The approach taken depends on the scarcity of subjects available for study, the event rate in the control arm, and practical considerations, such as the costs of accrual and follow-up. For example, in rare diseases it may be considered that it is best to minimise the number of patients required while maximising the follow-up period.

Alternatively, in a more common disease it may be more appropriate to minimise the total study time, which comprises the sum of the accrual and follow-up periods.

The duration of a two-group comparative study can be estimated, at least in the circumstances where we can assume an Exponential distribution of survival times in each group. This is a *PH* assumption which leads to estimates that can be used as approximations to other *PH* situations, such as comparisons using the Logrank test which does not require constant hazards within each group.

If we define D as the duration of patient entry, after which patient recruitment is stopped and follow-up is closed, then this is determined by the solution of the following rather complex equation.

$$\left(D - \frac{E}{R}\right)\left(\frac{1}{\lambda_C} + \frac{1}{\lambda_T}\right) - \frac{[1 - \exp(-\lambda_C D)]}{\lambda_C^2} - \frac{[1 - \exp(-\lambda_T D)]}{\lambda_T^2} = 0, \qquad (9.10)$$

where R is the anticipated subject entry rate during a period equivalent to the median survival time of group C, that is M_C. The median survival time, M_C, is used as the unit of time in calculating D. Since for the Exponential distribution, $M = \log 2/\lambda$, then M_{Plan-C} and M_{Plan-T} can be used in this expression to provide values for λ_C and λ_T for equation (9.10).

Unfortunately, there is no explicit solution to this equation and the value for D has to be found using an iterative method. Nevertheless, a lower limit for D is provided by

$$D_{Lower} = E/R, \qquad (9.11)$$

which is very easy to calculate.

Example – *trial duration – patients with resectable colon cancer*

We previously calculated that the number of patients required, allowing for a 10% loss to follow-up, for the adjuvant study of levamisole in resectable cancer of the colon (Dukes' C) was 850 subjects. This was to ensure, although we did not give this explicitly, a total of approximately $E = 700$ events would be observed.

Under the assumption of Exponential survival in the control group which has a median survival of approximately $M_{Plan-C} = 2$ years and an assumption by the investigators that $R = 250$ patients will be recruited in the equivalent period, then equation (9.11) gives $D_{Lower} = 700/250 = 2.8$ units or duration of patient entry being $M_{Plan-C} \times D_{Lower} = 2 \times 2.8 = 5.6$ years.

This then provides the investigators with an estimate of the planned duration of the trial of about six years

---

Machin, Campbell, Fayers *et al.* (1997) and Elashoff (2000) provide numerical solutions for D and tabulations for some situations.

9.4 REGRESSION PROBLEMS

TWO GROUPS

As we have indicated, a two-group comparative study can be analysed either by means of the Logrank test or using Cox's univariate *PH* regression. Thus sample sizes, for this simplest of regression models can be determined by use of equations (9.7) and (9.8) above. If there are covariates present, then these will tend to account for some of the variability in survival times so that the study size as determined by considering the design variable D may be somewhat more than needed. However, it is difficult to be certain of this, so this possibility is often ignored in the sample size determination process.

LINEAR RELATIONSHIPS

If the relationship between the survival time and the covariate, x, is thought to be linear, then the object of the study is to estimate the slope of this relationship that is expressed by a single parameter, β_{Linear}. A minimal sample size can be determined by first choosing the minimum and maximum values of the covariate x that will be included in the study. If x corresponds to a dose of a drug, for example, then this choice may be under the direct control of the investigating team, whereas if it is birth weight then only a possible range of values can be postulated. The values $x_{Minimum}$ and $x_{Maximum}$ essentially define two extreme groups to compare and again the calculations of sample size as for a two-group comparison can be made to give (say) N_1. A second estimate may be obtained by contrasting $x_{Minimum}$ (or equivalently $x_{Maximum}$) with the value midway between the two extreme values to give (say) N_2. The final sample size chosen may be taken as a value somewhere between these two, a final choice perhaps depending on resources available.

This somewhat *ad hoc* procedure can be extended to more complex situations but it is difficult to give specific guidance.

Example – *Three-dose comparison* – *inoperable hepatocellular carcinoma*

In a randomised trial of the use of tamoxifen in patients with inoperable hepato-cellular carcinoma, Chow, Tai, Tan *et al.* (2002) summarised the justification for the sample size chosen as follows: "The trial was designed to compare placebo (P) with tamoxifen 120 mg/d (TMX120). To assess a possible dose response, an intermediate group of tamoxifen 60 mg/d (TMX60) was included and patients were randomized into one of 3 groups (P, TMX60, and TMX120) in a ratio of 2:1:2. It was assumed that the 6-month survival rate with P would be 40% and that the minimum clinically important difference to detect was 20% greater than this value. For a 2-sided test size of 5% and a power of 80%, this gave approximately 200 patients. The 3-arm trial comparing P, TMX60, and TMX120 in the ratio 2:1:2 would test the possibility of a dose response with survival and require 250 patients. This was increased to 300 (120, 60, and 120 patients respectively) to account for a possible 10% attrition rate".

NUMBER OF VARIABLES

For k potentially prognostic variables, $x_1, x_2, x_3 \ldots x_v$ the Cox model takes the multivariable form, of equation (5.20) which we repeat here for convenience,

$$\log h = \beta_1 x_1 + \beta_2 x_2 + \beta_3 x_3 + \cdots + \beta_v x_v, \qquad (9.12)$$

where $\beta_1, \beta_2, \beta_3, \ldots \beta_v$ are the corresponding regression coefficients to be estimated in the modelling process.

In equation (9.12) the number of variables, v, that can be included is clearly without end but for every variable added there is a least one further regression coefficient to be estimated. It is easy to imagine that there can be more candidate variables than patients. So a simple rule is to never allow into the model more variables than subjects. If there are more variables than subjects, then the screening process to determine Level-In, Level Query, and Level-Out as defined in Chapter 8 must ensure the number is reduced accordingly. It has to be realised that if a g-group categorical variable is included, then this adds $g - 1$ regression coefficients to the model. Thus it is really the number of regression coefficients, $k(\geq v)$, to be estimated that should, at the very least, be less then N. In fact, for survival type studies, it is the number of events observed, O, that is critical rather than N itself. Thus a very large study with few events may have the same limit to k as a small study with a proportionately larger number of events.

There is no easy way to calculate study size for prognostic modelling to cover all exigencies including their unknown number, and strength, of any truly prognostic variable of those candidates being considered.

Although dealing with univariate logistic regression rather than Cox regression, Peduzzi, Concato, Kemper *et al.* (1996), recommend that about 10 events per regression coefficient to be estimated are necessary in order to get reasonably stable estimates of the regression coef-ficients. This suggests that the number of *Events Per Regression Coefficient (EPRC)* ≥ 10 which implies a total of $O \geq 10 \times k$ events are required.

For actual survival time studies using Cox *PH* models, we suggest that k should be a maximum of $O/10$ and preferably closer to $O/20$.

Example – *number of variables* – *inoperable hepatocellular carcinoma*

For the Index group of Tan, Law, Ng and Machin (2003) there were $N = 397$ patients all but seven of whom had died and none were lost to follow-up. Thus the number of events is $O = 397 - 7 = 390$. This gives the suggested number of regression coefficients that might be estimated as between $390/10 = 39$ and $390/20 = 18$. In the actual study, there were a total of $k = 30$ regression coefficients arising from the $v = 11$ candidate variables under consideration and so this study is within that suggested range.

Example – *study size* – *non-small cell lung cancer*

Piffarré, Rosell, Monzó *et al.* (1997) investigated the prognostic value on survival of replication errors (RER) on chromosomes 2p and 3p amongst 64 patients with non-small-cell lung cancer using Cox's proportional hazards model.

Amongst these patients only $O = 19$ (30%) had died, which suggests that the number of regression coefficients appropriate to estimate in a multivariable Cox model is between 19/20 and 19/10 which indicate at the most $k = 2$. In fact the authors appear to have investigated at least $v = 8$ candidate variables (involving $k \geq 10$ regression coefficients) including age; gender; histological type (squamous cell carcinoma, adenocarcinoma, large-cell carcinoma); tumour stage (I, II, IIIA); K-ras (mutated, non-mutated); p53 (mutated, non-mutated); LOH (complete loss of one or both alleles of the repeat locus), and RER (positive, negative). As a result of a non-specified selection procedure they derived a prognostic model including RER and Stage. The numbers of events was clearly too few for such an investigation.

TRAINING AND VALIDATION GROUPS

The above considerations may help one to determine an appropriate size for the training data set for a *PI* study. It is difficult to be prescriptive about the required size of the validation group. Clearly the number of candidate variables to include is now stipulated by the *PI* derived from the Index group. Thus one might argue that the number of regression coefficients relevant to validation group, $k_{Validation}$ is likely to be much smaller than the number considered when deriving the *PI*, $k_{Training}$, so a pragmatic way is to suggest $O_{Validation}$ is somewhere in the order of $10 \times k_{Validation}$ to $20 \times k_{Validation}$.

Example – *size of validation group – inoperable hepatocellular carcinoma*

The final *PI* derived in this study included $v = 3$ variables (involving $k_{Validation} = 3$ regression coefficients). Thus the above suggestion indicates that $O_{Validation}$ should be between $10 \times k_{Validation} = 30$ and $20 \times k_{Validation} = 60$. The data set actually used comprised 296 patients of whom 276 (93%) had died. This would appear to more than sufficient for the validation process.

PARAMETRIC MODELLING

If the regression model utilises a parametric model, then the associated parameters as well as the regression coefficients will need to be estimated. This suggests that sample sizes required are likely to be larger than those indicated by the methods above. Our suggestion is that a further 10 to 20 events are required for each parameter of the survival distribution concerned. Thus for the Weibull distribution with parameters γ and κ to be estimated, this implies observing an extra 20 to 40 events in addition to those required to estimate the corresponding β's.

9.5   PRACTICALITIES

USE OF SAMPLE SIZE CALCULATIONS

Sample size calculations play an essential part in the design of any study. However, it must be recognised that there are a number of assumptions and 'guesstimates' which go into the calculation of the required sample size.

In particular in equation (9.7), although there are commonly accepted values for the test size, α, and the power $1 - \beta$, there is often considerable uncertainty over the values of Δ_{Plan} or π_{Plan-C} and π_{Plan-T}. Equivalently, we can say there may be considerable uncertainty over the values of π_{Plan-C}, and δ_{Plan}. The uncertainty in the specification of these components and their subsequent influence on the calculations, taken together with the necessary assumption of *PH* used for the calculations, serves to emphasise that sample size calculations provide no more than a guide to the number of patients that may be required.

In practice a range of plausible effect size options are considered before the final planning effect size is agreed. For example, an investigator might specify a scientific or clinically useful difference that it is hoped could be detected, and would then estimate the required sample size on this basis. The calculations might then indicate that an extremely large number of subjects are required. As a consequence, the investigator may next define a revised aim of detecting a rather larger difference than that originally specified. The calculations are repeated, and perhaps the sample size now becomes realistic in that new context. This being said the overriding consideration in this feasibility process is to ensure that, if the trial is to be conducted with the chosen sample size, it really is scientifically and clinically worthwhile.

However, one additional problem when planning comparative clinical trials is that investigators are often optimistic about the magnitude of the improvement of new treatments over the standard. This optimism is understandable, since it can take considerable effort to initiate a trial and, in many cases, the trial would only be launched if the investigator were enthusiastic about the new treatment and sufficiently convinced about its potential efficacy. However, experience suggests that as trial succeeds trial there is often a growing realism that, even at best, the earlier expectations were optimistic. There is ample historical evidence to suggest that trials that set out to detect large treatment differences nearly always result in 'no significant difference was detected'. In such cases there may have been a true and worthwhile treatment benefit that was missed, since the level of detectable differences set by the design was unrealistically high, and hence the sample size too small to establish the true (but less optimistic) size of benefit.

Finally, whatever the context, if we have underestimated Δ by Δ_{Plan} then our study will be more than sufficient in size. If Δ_{Plan} is an overestimate then the study may fail to detect this and possibly a smaller but scientifically important difference may be missed.

LIMITED RESOURCESS

A common situation is one where the number of subjects—who may be patients—that can be included in a study is governed by non-scientific forces such as time, money or human resources. Thus with a predetermined (maximal) sample size, the researcher may then wish to know what probability he or she has of detecting a certain effect size with a study confined to this size. If the resulting power is small, say $<50\%$, then the investigator may decide that the study should not go ahead. A similar situation arises if the type of subject under consideration is uncommon, as would be the case with a clinical trial in rare disease groups. In either case the sample size is constrained, and the researcher is interested in finding the size of effects which could be established for a reasonable power, say, 80%.

MULTIPLE ENDPOINTS

We have based the above discussion on the assumption that there is a single identifiable endpoint or outcome, upon which comparisons are based. Often there is more than one endpoint of interest, such as in patients undergoing hip replacement surgery, the time to become mobile post surgery, time to hospital discharge, or time to final healing in the two groups. If one of these endpoints is regarded as more important than the others, it can be named as the primary endpoint and sample-size estimates based on that alone. A problem arises when there are several outcome measures that are all regarded as equally important. A commonly adopted approach is to repeat the sample-size estimates for each outcome measure in turn, and then select the largest of these as the sample size required to answer all the questions of interest.

However, it is well recognised that if many endpoints are included in one study and the groups are tested for statistical significance for all of these, then the p-values so obtained are distorted. To compensate for this, smaller observed p-values may be required to declare 'true' statistical significance at level α. In such cases, the sample-size calculations will be similarly affected so that to retain the level at α for all the tests conducted a value depending on the number of endpoints, k, is sometimes substituted in, for example, equation (3.15). A common value chosen is simply α/k. Even when $k = 2$, this substantially increases the size of the planned study.

Theory, formulae and tables for the calculation of sample sizes for the Logrank test and other aspects of survival studies are given by Machin, Campbell, Fayers et al. (1997) and they, as well as, Elashoff (2000) also provide computer programs for this purpose.

10 Further Topics

Summary

This chapter describes modifications of the standard form of the Logrank test for circumstances where specific sections of the survival curve are thought to be more important for comparison purposes than others that essentially arise if the hazards are non-proportional. The use of survival techniques in systematic reviews of medical evidence, for cure models in which a fraction of the subjects remain as long-term survivors and may be regarded as cured, and their application in the situation where the subject is at risk from several competing events, are discussed. In some circumstances, paired survival times may be recorded and the analysis of crossover trials with such data is described. This is extended to a discussion of correlated data in general, including recurrent events.

10.1 INTRODUCTION

As with many methodologies once the ideas have been developed to a certain stage there is then often a period of rapid development, both in terms of the methodology and the fields where it has been applied. This is no less true for the survival techniques following the groundbreaking work of DR Cox in the 1970s. In the medical context, survival techniques are now commonplace in all areas of research activity from the laboratory bench and clinic to large-scale clinical trials and epidemiological studies. It is not the purpose of this chapter to review the considerable statistical and medical progress that has ensued but rather to highlight some of the developments. These include modifications of the standard form of the Logrank test to allow for non-*PH*, applications to the important field of overviews in which evidence from pertinent studies is combined through a meta-analysis, together with developments for competing risks, cure models, paired comparisons and correlated data.

10.2 TESTS WITH NON-PROPORTIONAL HAZARDS

We have described in Section 3.2 the Logrank test and in Section 3.3 the Mantel-Haenszel test for comparing two survival curves. These two tests are statistically the most powerful in assessing differences between two survival curves when the ratio of the hazard rates (hazards) for the two groups remain approximately constant as time progresses. In this case, the hazards are termed proportional. In circumstances when the hazards are not proportional, the tests can still be used, but they may not be the most powerful tests available. Thus, in instances in which non-*PH* are anticipated, it may be better to use alternative methods of analysis.

In Chapter 4 a method of assessing whether the hazard within a particular group remains constant with time is given and an illustration, using data from patients with colorectal

Survival Analysis Second Edition   David Machin, Yin Bun Cheung, Mahesh K.B. Parmar
© 2006 John Wiley & Sons, Ltd   ISBN: 0-470-87040-0

cancer, is given in Figure 4.4. This method can be extended to assessing constancy of the ratio of the relative hazards in two patient groups by calculating such a plot for each as in Figure 4.5. This involves plotting the complementary log, $\log\{-\log[S(t)]\}$, against $\log t$ for each group.

Example – complementary log plots – patients with brain cancer with and without a history of fits at diagnosis

Figure 10.1 shows the $\log\{-\log[S(t)]\}$ against $\log t$ plots for two groups of patients with brain cancer. One group of patients had a history of fits prior to diagnosis and the other group did not. From Figure 10.1 we can see that the hazard is approximately constant within each group, as each plot is approximately linear. The two lines are approximately parallel, which indicates a constant ratio of relative hazards between the two groups as time progresses. This in turn suggests that an overall summary by use of the *HR* is likely to be appropriate.

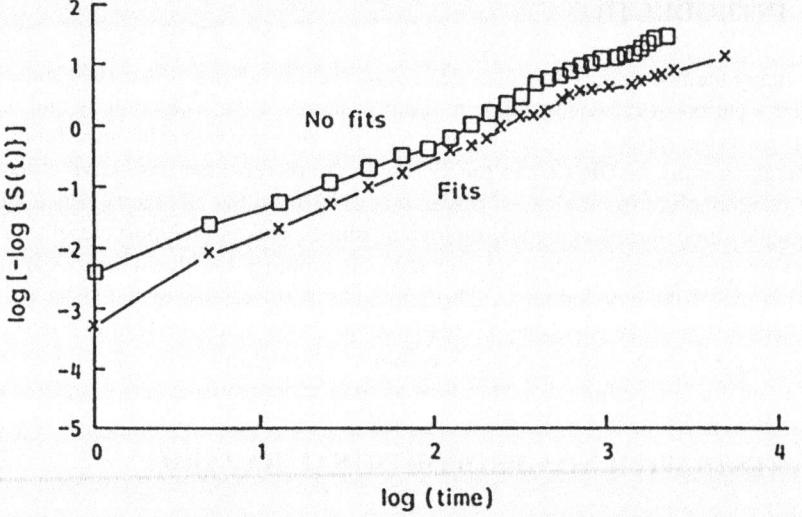

Figure 10.1 Graph of $\log\{-\log[S(t)]\}$ against $\log t$ in two groups of patients with brain tumours (From Medical Research Council Working Party on Misonidazole in Gliomas, 1983, with permission from the British Institute of Radiology)

However, and in contrast, Figure 10.2 shows the same type of plot for the patients contributing to Figure 10.1 but now divided into three groups on the basis of their age. From this plot we see that although the hazards for the 45–59 and 60+ years groups are approximately constant over time, they are not proportional, as the two lines converge as time increases. There is also a suggestion that the hazard for the younger patients does not appear to be constant, since there is some flattening of the plot for values of $\log t$ greater than 2.5. Thus, comparing the three groups, it would appear that the assumption of *PH* may not be appropriate, particularly for the comparison of the 45–59 and 60+ age groups.

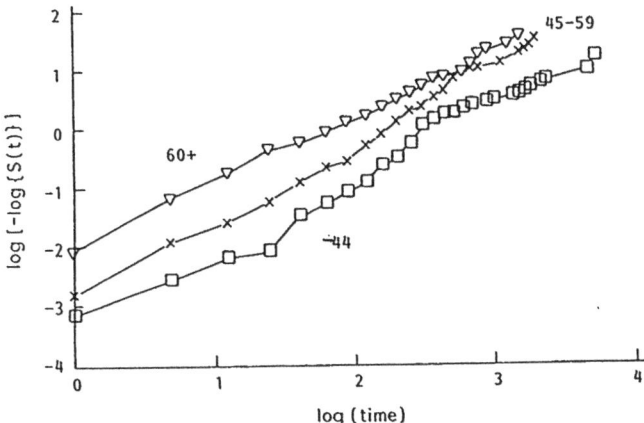

Figure 10.2 Graph of $\log\{-\log[S(t)]\}$ against $\log t$ in three age groups of patients with brain tumours (From Medical Research Council Working Party on Misonidazole in Gliomas, 1983, with permission from the British Institute of Radiology)

Example – non-PH – time to remission from incontinence

Nolan, Debelle, Oberklaid and Coffey (1991) give the time to resolution of incontinence in a randomised trial of two laxatives. They compare a multimodal therapy (*MM*) and behaviour modification only (*BM*), in 169 children: 86 receiving *BM* and 83 *MM*. The *K-M* estimates of the corresponding resolution of incontinence times of the two groups are shown in Figure 10.3. In this example, the lower survival curve indicates an advantage to that therapy, as patients receiving that therapy have a faster remission of their incontinence.

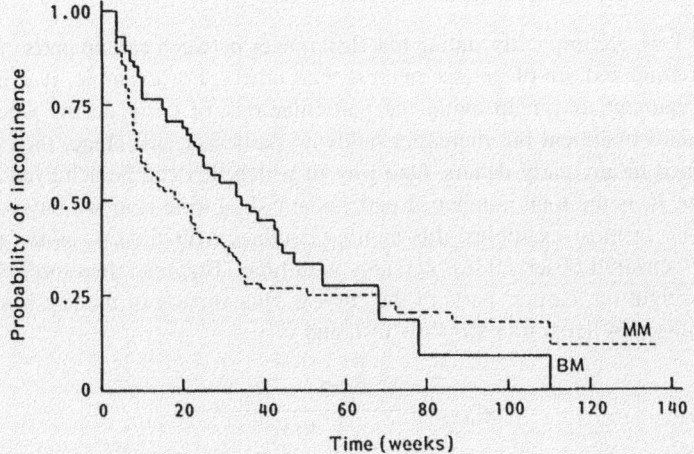

Figure 10.3 Kaplan-Meier curves for time to resolution from incontinence by treatment group (Reprinted from *The Lancet*, **338**, Oberklaid, and Coffey, 1991, Randomised trials of laxatives in treatment of childhood encores, 523–527, © 1991, with permission from Elsevier)

The two *K-M* curves cross at approximately 70 weeks, with an apparent advantage to the *MM* group prior to this time and thereafter a disadvantage. In this situation the complementary log plots would also cross, suggesting that the relative hazards do not remain proportional. However, it should be stressed here that the curves become less reliable with time so that the crossing at 70 weeks could merely be a consequence of small numbers of events observed in that region.

WEIGHTED MANTEL-HAENSZEL

A number of tests have been proposed which compare two survival curves for the non-*PH* situation. These tests can be generated from one basic formula and are known as weighted Mantel-Haenszel tests. For a two-group comparison of A and B, these are defined as

$$\chi^2_{MHw} = \frac{\sum w_t (O_{At} - E_{At})^2}{\sum w_t^2 V_t} \tag{10.1}$$

Here, E_{At} and V_t are calculated as described by equations (3.1) and (3.11) respectively. The weights are the w_t and can vary as time, t, changes. These tests all give a statistic which is distributed as χ^2 with $df = 1$ for the two group comparisons discussed here.

If we set $w_t = 1$, for all values of t, then this assigns equal weight to each death at whatever time, t, it occurs. In this situation, equation (10.1) becomes that of the (unweighted) Mantel-Haenszel test of equation (3.12). This is the most powerful test when the hazards are (at least approximately) proportional.

GEHAN

If we set $w_t \neq 1$ we are implicitly stating that differences between certain parts of the survival curves being compared are of greater interest than others. For example, if it is anticipated that a new treatment may help avoid the particular risk of early deaths when compared with the standard treatment but thereafter holds no particular advantage, then extra weight may be assigned to any early deaths. One way in which this can be achieved is by setting $w_t = R_t$, where R_t is the total number of patients at risk at time t, as we have described for equation (2.11). In most examples, this number declines over time, t, as the total number of deaths and censored observations increases with time. This test, therefore, places greater emphasis or weight on 'earlier' parts of the curves. This version of the test is known as the Gehan, generalised Wilcoxon or Breslow test, and is

$$\chi^2_{Gehan} = \frac{\sum R_t (O_{At} - E_{At})^2}{\sum R_t^2 V_t}. \tag{10.2}$$

To calculate χ^2_{Gehan} it is necessary to calculate the components of both the numerator and denominator at each death time, that is O_{At}, E_{At} and V_t, as was done in Table 3.3, and R_t.

> **_Example_** _– weighted Mantel-Haenszel and Gehan tests – time to remission from_ _incontinence_
>
> Nolan, Debelle, Oberklaid and Coffey (1991) quote both the Mantel-Haenszel version of the Logrank test with p-value $=0.12$, corresponding to $\chi^2_{MHw} = 0.82$, $df = 1$, and the Gehan test, with p-value $=0.012$, corresponding to $\chi^2_{Gehan} = 6.30$, $df = 1$. They also comment that: "The proportionality assumption was not satisfied for the full follow-up period".
>
> The difference in the p-values given by the two tests leads to quite different interpretations of the data and demonstrates how important it is to plot the survival curves for the two groups so that an appropriate interpretation of the significance tests can be made.

Care must be taken in applying the Gehan test as it can be very misleading when there are many censored observations or when the censoring is unequal in the two groups. These situations can arise in the early life of a prospective study, for example in a clinical trial which is still in the recruitment phase. In this case there may be many patients recently entered and therefore insufficient observation time for the critical events to occur. Unequal censoring can occur if, for whatever reason, information is systematically received on events occurring earlier in one group than in the other. For example, in a randomised trial to compare patients using a regular and predetermined appointments system against a system in which patients present only when they notice symptoms of recurrence, one could argue that those patients with fixed appointments will be examined more rigorously and early signs of recurrence thus detected and reported. In contrast, patients assigned to the other group will only report recurrence once the symptoms are clearly obvious to the patient.

TARONE-WARE

A similar but less extreme means of weighting the earlier part of the survival curve, than through the Gehan test, is given by using the Tarone-Ware version of the test. This is

$$\chi^2_{TW} = \frac{\sum R_t^{1/2}(O_{At} - E_{At})^2}{\sum R_t V_t} \tag{10.3}$$

where the w_t of equation (10.1) are set equal to $R_t^{1/2}$. This still gives more weight to the early deaths observed in the study but in a less extreme way than that of equation (10.2).

PETO-PRENTICE

Another definition for the weights has been suggested by both Peto and Prentice and their test is

$$\chi^2_{PP} = \frac{\sum w_{PPt}(O_{At} - E_{At})^2}{\sum w_{PPt} V_t} \tag{10.4}$$

where

$$w_{PPt} = \prod_{j=1}^{t} \frac{(R_j - d_j + 1)}{(R_j + 1)}.$$

Here d_j is the number of events at time j. The weighting for this χ^2_{PP} test is similar to the corresponding estimate of the K-M survival curve at each event given by equation (2.5) but with n_j replaced by $R_j + 1$. The aim of these weights is similar to both the Gehan and Tarone-Ware weights, in that the earlier parts of the curves are given greater weighting than the later sections. The Peto-Prentice test has the advantage that it is not susceptible to unequal censoring patterns in the different groups.

Example – *weighted Logrank tests – patients with cervical cancer*

Using the data from 30 patients with cervical cancer analysed in Table 3.3 the calculation of the various χ^2 statistics for the Mantel-Haenszel, Gehan, Tarone-Ware and Peto-Prentice tests are summarised in Table 10.1. For brevity of presentation, the censored survival times are omitted and the death times for treatment B are indicated in bold.

Table 10.1 Weights (w_t) and relative weights (W_t) for four weighted Mantel-Haenszel tests applied to survival data from 30 patients with cervical cancer

Death Time (t)	$O_{At} - E_{At}$	V_t	w_t (Mantel-Haenszel)	W_t (Mantel-Haenszel)	R_t (Gehan)	W_t (Gehan)	R_t (Tarone-Ware)	W_t (Tarone-Ware)	w_{PPt} (Peto-Prentice)	W_t (Peto-Prentice)
90	0.46667	0.24889	1	0.0625	30	0.1027	5.47723	0.0836	0.96774	0.0886
142	0.48276	0.25000	1	0.0625	29	0.0993	5.38517	0.0822	0.93548	0.0857
150	0.50000	0.25000	1	0.0625	28	0.0959	5.29150	0.0808	0.90323	0.0827
269	0.51852	0.24966	1	0.0625	27	0.0925	5.19615	0.0793	0.87097	0.0798
272	−0.46154	0.24852	1	0.0625	26	0.0890	5.09902	0.0778	0.83871	0.0768
291	0.52000	0.24960	1	0.0625	25	0.0856	5.00000	0.0763	0.80645	0.0739
362	−0.45833	0.24826	1	0.0625	24	0.0822	4.89898	0.0748	0.77419	0.0709
373	−0.47826	0.24953	1	0.0625	23	0.0788	4.79583	0.0732	0.74194	0.0679
680	0.41177	0.24222	1	0.0625	17	0.0582	4.12311	0.0629	0.70072	0.0642
827	−0.56250	0.24609	1	0.0625	16	0.0548	4.00000	0.0611	0.65950	0.0604
837	0.40000	0.24000	1	0.0625	15	0.0514	3.87298	0.0591	0.61828	0.0566
1037	0.36364	0.23141	1	0.0625	11	0.0377	3.31663	0.0516	0.56676	0.0519
1153	0.42857	0.24490	1	0.0625	7	0.0240	2.64575	0.0404	0.49591	0.0454
1297	0.50000	0.25000	1	0.0625	6	0.0206	2.44949	0.0374	0.42507	0.0389
1307	−0.40000	0.24000	1	0.0625	5	0.0171	2.23607	0.0341	0.35422	0.0324
1429	0.33333	0.22222	1	0.0625	3	0.0103	1.73205	0.0264	0.26567	0.0243
Total	2.564586	3.910995	16	1	292	1	65.62	1	10.92	1
χ^2				1.682		1.292		1.513		1.742
p-value				0.1947		0.238		0.2186		0.1869

For all the tests we only have to calculate the contribution to the test statistic at each death time. In Table 10.1 the actual weight w_t, with each method is presented, together with the relative weight W_t, which is the weight at time t divided by the sum of all the weights, for each death, that is $W_t = w_t / \Sigma w_t$. The latter is given because it allows more direct comparisons between the different statistical test weights, given to each death. Thus, for example, we see that the Mantel-Haenszel method gives the first death at time 90 days (at the earliest part of the curve) a weight of 6.25%, while the Gehan, Tarone-Ware and Peto-Prentice tests give weights of 10.27%, 8.36% and 8.86% respectively, to this first death. In contrast, if we consider the last death at 1429 days the relative weights for the four tests are 6.25%, 1.03%, 2.64% and 2.43%, respectively. Of all the tests, the Mantel-Haenszel statistic gives the most weight to the tail end of the curves. This is a weight equal to that for all other deaths, whenever they occur. The Gehan test gives the least weight amongst these four tests to the longest surviving patients. The corresponding χ^2 statistics and p-values for the four tests are also summarised in the last rows of Table 10.1. The corresponding value of $\chi^2_{Logrank} = 1.649$, $df = 1$, p-value $= 0.2005$. In this example, all five tests give rather similar results.

It is important to emphasise that, whatever test is used, its intended use should be specified at the design stage of the study, that is *before* the data are collected and analysed. Any test specified either after the data are collected or as a consequence of inspection of the resulting *K-M* survival curves must be regarded as secondary or exploratory. Such 'data-snooping' tests should be interpreted with great care for the presence of spurious statistical significance. In practice, it will often be very difficult to anticipate the shape of the survival curves with any degree of certainty. In such situations, and in general therefore, the Mantel-Haenszel version of the Logrank test is recommended for the primary analysis.

10.3   META-ANALYSIS

There are many situations in which medical studies done by different investigators have addressed the same or similar questions. In the context of clinical trials, which we will discuss in some detail, these studies may be a group of randomised trials. It is good practice to consider these groups of studies together to assess whether there is evidence of a difference between groups and also to estimate the likely size of this effect. Such a formal quantitative review of all relevant studies is called a meta-analysis or overview.

Meta-analysis can range from one extreme of the combination of a few summary statistics retrieved from published papers, to the other extreme in which every effort is made to identify and collect updated individual subject data from every relevant study (published or unpublished) that has been performed. The first approach can, in particular for survival data, provide misleading results as it may not include all relevant data.

We note that in a survival time context updated data imply that, for example, the current status of any patient alive at the time of reporting the individual trials is requested. In this way the overview will often include more events and longer follow-up than the combined number reported by the trials at their respective times of publication.

We emphasise that meta-analyses of individual patient data aim to include both trials that have been published in the literature and those that, for whatever reason, have not been published. Thus, such an overview aims to summarise all the available evidence relevant to the question.

Example – *meta-analysis – patients with advanced ovarian cancer*

The Advanced Ovarian Cancer Trialists' Group (1991) describe the results of all known, at the time, randomised trials investigating the role of chemotherapy in advanced ovarian cancer. The meta-analysis of these trials included updated survival information from more than 8000 patients. The largest trial amongst these was of 200 patients which, given the current expectations with respect to the magnitude of treatment benefits that are likely to arise in cancer treatment trials, is itself too small for the purpose intended. None of these trials individually had been able to establish the role of chemotherapy.

If there are k randomised trials, each comparing a test treatment, T, with a control or standard treatment, C, then each trial provides an observed number of events in each treatment arm together with the corresponding expected number of events obtained from the Logrank test calculations. From these

$$U_i = O_{Ci} - E_{Ci} \qquad (10.5)$$

for $i = 1, 2, \ldots, k$ can be calculated. This expression is of the form of the numerator in the exponential part of equation (3.13).

The corresponding variance, V_i, is equal to that given by summing equation (3.11). Thus

$$V_i = \sum_t \frac{m_t n_t r_t s_t}{N_t^2 (N_t - 1)} \qquad (10.6)$$

In this way, each trial in the overview provides an estimate of $HR_i = \exp(U_i/V_i)$. An overall estimate of the treatment effect obtained by combining information from all k trials, and which assumes that the true effect does not differ across trials, is given by

$$\log HR_{Average} = \frac{\sum[(\log HR_i)/V_i]}{\sum[1/V_i]} \qquad (10.7)$$

This averages the HRs obtained from each trial in such a way as also to take account of the relative information provided by each trial. In this way a trial with a large number of events will influence the average more than that which includes few events. This estimate has a SE given by

$$SE(\log HR_{Average}) = \sqrt{\frac{1}{\sum(1/V_i)}}. \qquad (10.8)$$

An approximate 95% CI for $HR_{Average}$ is therefore given by

$$\exp\left[\log HR_{Average} - 1.96\sqrt{\frac{1}{\sum(1/V_i)}}\right] \text{ to } \exp\left[\log HR_{Average} + 1.96\sqrt{\frac{1}{\sum(1/V_i)}}\right]. \qquad (10.9)$$

Example – meta-analysis – azathioprine for patients with multiple sclerosis

Yudkin, Ellison, Ghezzi *et al.* (1991) conducted a meta-analysis of randomised controlled trials of azathioprine treatment to avoid relapse in patients with multiple sclerosis. The analysis reports comparisons at fixed time-points only and that is why relative odds (*OR*) rather than *HRs* and var(log *OR*) rather than var(log *HR*) are used.

Figure 10.4 shows, for each of the seven trials in one part of their meta-analysis, the estimate of the *OR* for freedom from relapse at one year, together with the associated 95% *CI*. The analogous values of *U* of equation (10.5) and variance *V* of equation (10.6) are also given, together with the number of patients and relapses observed per treatment group.

We note that six of the seven trials have an estimate which indicates a more favourable outcome for the azathioprine-treated group. However, five of these seven have very wide 95% *CIs*, leaving considerable uncertainty surrounding the result of each trial. Only the largest trial (trial 16) showed an advantage to azathioprine treatment that is significant at the 5% level.

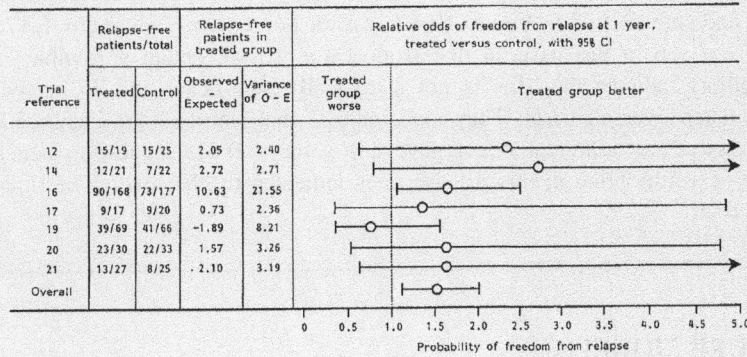

Trial reference	Relapse-free patients/total		Relapse-free patients in treated group		Relative odds of freedom from relapse at 1 year, treated versus control, with 95% CI	
	Treated	Control	Observed – Expected	Variance of O – E	Treated group worse	Treated group better
12	15/19	15/25	2.05	2.40		
14	12/21	7/22	2.72	2.71		
16	90/168	73/177	10.63	21.55		
17	9/17	9/20	0.73	2.36		
19	39/69	41/66	−1.89	8.21		
20	23/30	22/33	1.57	3.26		
21	13/27	8/25	.2.10	3.19		
Overall						

Figure 10.4 The overview analysis of trials of azathioprine for patients with multiple sclerosis (Reprinted from *The Lancet*, **338**, Yudkin, Ellison, Ghezzi *et al.*, 1991, Overview of azathioprine treatment in multiple sclerosis, 1051–1055, © 1991, with permission from Elsevier)

In general for each trial, the null hypothesis is that there is no difference between treatments with respect to survival: $\log HR = 0$ or $HR = 1$. Hence, for k trials addressing the same question in a meta-analysis, the combined null hypothesis that the treatment effect is zero in all trials is

$$\log HR_1 = \log HR_2 = \ldots = \log HR_k = 0.$$

If this combined null hypothesis is true, then it can be shown that

$$\chi^2 = \frac{\sum[(\log HR_i)/V_i]^2}{\sum[1/V_i]} \tag{10.10}$$

has a χ^2 distribution with $df = 1$.

If this combined null hypothesis is rejected this would indicate that at least one of the log *HR*s is different from zero and a real difference between treatments is indicated. However, this does not imply that this difference is the same in all trials. As a consequence, it is usual to test for the homogeneity of the treatment effect across all studies concerned by calculating

$$Q = \sum_{i=1}^{k} \left[\frac{(\log HR_i - \log HR_{Average})^2}{V_i} \right]. \tag{10.11}$$

Under the null hypothesis of the same, that is homogeneous, treatment differences across the k trials, Q follows a χ^2 distribution with $df = (k - 1)$. A large value of Q may indicate that the trials should not be averaged using equation (10.7).

***Example** – test for treatment effect homogeneity – azathioprine for patients with multiple sclerosis*

For the seven trials of azathioprine reported by Yudkin, Ellison, Ghezzi *et al.* (1991) and summarised in Figure 10.4 a test for homogeneity gave $Q = 5.17$. The $df = 7 - 1 = 6$ in this case so that from Table T3 we obtain a p-value > 0.2. The authors indicate that this is not statistically significant and so an average can be taken over all trials. They also indicate that a test of the combined null hypothesis of no treatment effect gave a p-value < 0.01, suggesting benefit to the use of azathioprine in this disease as is indicated by the 'overall' estimate in Figure 10.4.

10.4   CURE MODELS

In general, the proportion of patients who remain alive gradually declines with time until all are dead. Although this is true of us all, it is particularly so of patients with life-threatening disease who may die rather more rapidly than do the non-diseased of the same age. As we discussed in Chapter 4, one statistical description for survival time is the Weibull distribution model in which case the proportion alive, $W(t)$, at time t is given by

$$W(t) = \exp[-(\lambda t)^\gamma], \tag{10.12}$$

where λ and γ are the scale and shape constants which have to be estimated from the survival time data. The Weibull model is very flexible as, depending on the values of λ and γ, a wide range of shapes of hazard function are possible, as we illustrated in Figure 4.6. However, despite this flexibility, ultimately all patients die with this model as, when $t = \infty$, $W(\infty) = \exp[-(\lambda \times \infty)\gamma] = \exp(-\infty) = 0$.

In certain, happier circumstances, patients with a serious disease may be 'cured' in the sense that their life expectancy returns to that of their age-specific contemporaries. Thus in young patients, where death from other causes is unusual, the ultimate survival curve of a group of such patients, calculated as from the date of diagnosis of their disease, may plateau for a considerable period of time thereby indicating a fraction of them apparently cured.

To model this type of survival experience what are termed 'mixture' and 'non-mixture' models have been proposed. Sposto (2002) describes these models and also gives examples from studies of children with cancer.

MIXTURE MODELS

For a mixture model, patients are regarded (in the statistical sense) as those who are potentially curable and those who are not. If the fraction cured is π, then the survival curve will eventually plateau at this level and the cure model can be expressed as:

$$Cure(t) = \pi + (1 - \pi)W(t). \tag{10.13}$$

For this model, and for that of (10.12), when $t = 0$, $W(0) = \exp[-(\lambda \times 0)\gamma] = 1$, and so $Cure(0) = \pi + (1 - \pi) = 1$ also. That is, all are alive at $t = 0$. However, as we have shown for $t = \infty$, $W(\infty) = 0$ and so all patients die with the Weibull model while $Cure(\infty) = \pi + (1 - \pi) W(\infty) = \pi + (1 - \pi) \times 0 = \pi$ and there remain a proportion cured with the latter.

The 'cure' fraction π of equation (10.13) may depend on the particular treatment the patient receives, x_1, as well as patient specific characteristics, x_2, and this relationship can be expressed as

$$\pi = 1/[1 + \exp\{-(\beta_0 + \beta_1 x_1 + \beta_2 x_2)\}]. \tag{10.14}$$

Here β_0, β_1 and β_2 are the regression coefficients to be estimated from the data. Clearly this equation can be extended to include more explanatory variables.

The cure model is fitted by maximum likelihood, which provides estimates for λ, γ and those parameters associated with π. A program for this is available from Sposto (2000). We use the Weibull distribution for illustration but the other survival distributions of Chapter 4 may be employed.

Example – *mixture model for cure* – *children with Stage I Hodgkin's lymphoma*

Capra, Hewitt, Hayward *et al.* (Submitted) used the mixture model to estimate the proportion cured in children with Stage I Hodgkin's lymphoma. In this case, there was no covariate. The probability of 'cure' can be obtained by substituting β_0 into equation (10.14), ignoring the $\beta_1 x_1 + \beta_2 x_2$ part for a covariate. This gives $\pi = 0.9116$. Figure 10.5 plots the cure model survival curve, which shows a plateau beginning some 10 to 15 years post diagnosis.

It is of note that the shape parameter $\gamma = 2.4$ of the Weibull distribution is far from the value of unity which would correspond to the Exponential distribution of survival times.

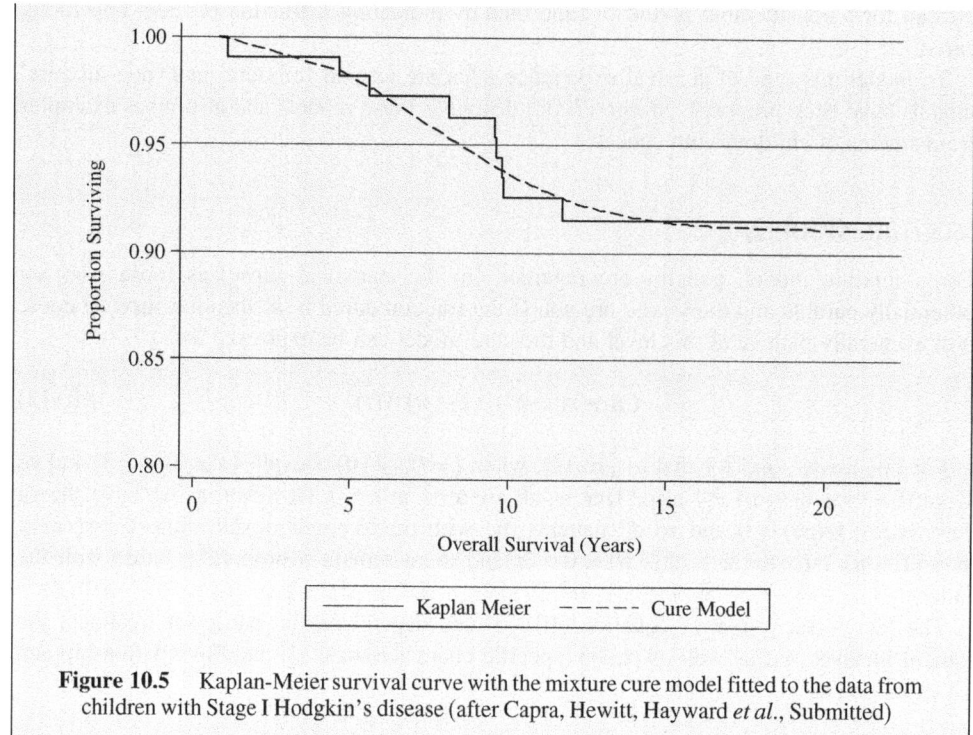

Figure 10.5 Kaplan-Meier survival curve with the mixture cure model fitted to the data from children with Stage I Hodgkin's disease (after Capra, Hewitt, Hayward *et al.*, Submitted)

Table 10.2 Estimated cure model for 111 children with Stage I Hodgkin's disease (from Capra, Hewitt, Hayward *et al.*, Submitted)

Parameter	Estimate	SE	z	p-value	π (%)
Intercept, β_0	2.3318	0.3596	6.48	< 0.0001	91.2
Scale, λ	0.1098				
Shape, γ	2.4354				

NON-MIXTURE MODELS

In contrast to the mixture model in which there are essentially two groups of patients having the diagnosis (those curable and those not), a non-mixture model allows all patients the potential of cure and is expressed by

$$Cure(t) = \pi^{[1-W(t)]}. \tag{10.15}$$

For this model, we have when $t = 0$, $W(0) = 1$ and so $Cure(0) = \pi^{[1-1]} = \pi^0 = 1$ as one would expect. Further when $t = \infty$, $W(\infty) = 0$ and so $Cure(\infty) = \pi^1 = \pi$ and there remain a proportion cured.

Just as for the mixture model, π itself may depend on the value of patient covariates.

Example – *non-mixture model for cure* – *children with Ewing's sarcoma*

Weston, Douglas, Craft *et al.* (2004) used the non-mixture cure model to estimate the proportion cured in children with metastatic and non-metastatic Ewing's sarcoma who were treated on two protocols (ET-1 and ET-2). The survival curves for the four metastatic status by treatment received groups are shown in Figure 10.6. This shows a plateau for each group beginning some five years post

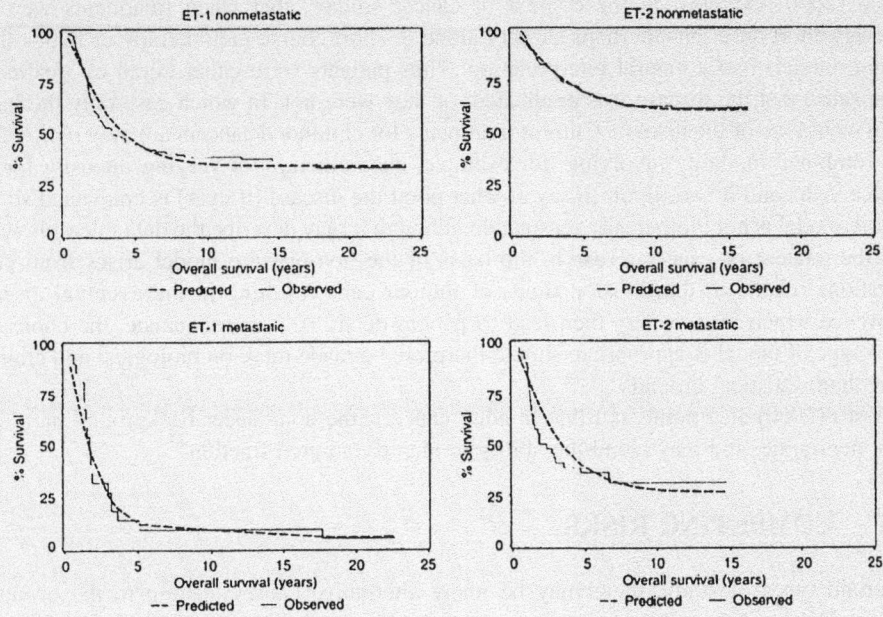

Figure 10.6   Kaplan-Meier estimates of the survival of patients in studies ET-1 and ET-2 by presence of metastases at diagnosis with the corresponding fitted cure models. (From Weston, Douglas, Craft *et al.* (2004). Reproduced by permission of the *British Journal of Cancer*).

Table 10.3   Estimated cure fractions (%) for patients with Ewing's sarcoma by treatment, metastatic status, age and pelvic involvement group (from Weston, Douglas, Craft *et al.*, 2004)

Pelvis involved	Age (years)	ET-1		ET-2	
		Metastatic disease			
		No	Yes	No	Yes
No	< 10	45	15	70	43
	≥ 10	34	7	61	31
Yes	< 10	25	3	53	22
	≥ 10	15	1	42	13

diagnosis with an estimated cure fraction greater in the non-metastatic patients and those treated by the ET-2 protocol.

The estimated fraction cured also appeared to depend on age at diagnosis and whether the pelvis was involved, as indicated in Table 10.3.

MIXTURE OR NON-MIXTURE MODEL?

Sposto (2000) explains, in the context of cancer studies, that when treatments were of relatively short duration—perhaps surgery alone or short course radiotherapy or both—then mixture models had a natural interpretation. Thus patients were either cured by treatment, in the sense that the disease was eradicated, or they were not. In which case only the latter group would die of the disease. Current treatments for childhood cancers are now more often of a combined modality involving, for example, chemotherapy of varying intensity for up to three years and it is difficult to say at what point the disease (if ever) is eradicated so the mixture model is not biologically reasonable although it may describe the data tolerably well.

In the context of cancer research, the basis of the non-mixture model arises from considerations related to the division times of tumour cells resulting in the eventual disease recurrence which in turn may then lead to patient death. As a consequence, the choice of which type of model is appropriate should therefore be made more on biological and clinical rather than statistical grounds.

Sposto (2000) also points out that in adult cancers, the non-cancer background mortality is not negligible, and may cloud the ability to identify a cured fraction.

10.5   COMPETING RISKS

In certain types of study, there may be many alternative causes leading to the event of concern. For example, suppose a study is conducted in workers at a nuclear installation who are exposed to the risk of dying from leukaemia, which is the *main* risk. However, they may also die from *competing risks* such as accident, cardiovascular disease, diabetes, and so on. These causes can be regarded as all competing within each individual to be responsible for their ultimate death. Thus, in a sense, we can think of these causes all racing to be the first and hence to be 'the' cause of the death and thereby preventing the 'other' causes from being responsible. This implies that if the death is caused by a cardiovascular accident (CVA), then t_{CVA} is observed while, for example, $t_{Accident}$, t_{Cancer} and $t_{Diabetes}$ will never be observed but have the corresponding censored survival times $t_{Accident}$, t_{Cancer} and $t_{Diabetes}$ censored at t_{CVA}. One field of application in which there are often many competing events is in the testing of alterative contraceptives in clinical trials.

CONTRACEPTIVE STUDIES

Clinical trials of contraceptive methods are a major area in which survival methods have been used and adapted. The primary objective of a contraceptive method is to permit intercourse but prevent conception, thereby allowing planned parenthood. A failure of a contraceptive method is an unplanned pregnancy whilst using the method. However, studies of contraceptive efficacy and use effectiveness often differ from other medical areas in that there is often no single primary endpoint. Typically, subjects in a contraceptive study are healthy women aged between 20 and 45 years and the incidence of pregnancy among such women is high in the absence of any contraceptive method. However, the efficacy of contraceptive drugs or devices under trial is also very high. Thus annual pregnancy rate among intrauterine device (IUD) users ranges from 2–10%, whereas the corresponding rate among women not using contraceptives, and who are exposed to the risk of pregnancy, is 80–90%.

In addition to pregnancy, there are other reasons, such as side effects, for discontinuing usage of contraceptive methods. As a result it is usual to define additional endpoints, usually termed discontinuation reasons, in these trials. However, once one of these is observed, then this prevents observation of the others and this leads to a competing risk situation.

DISCONTINUATION REASONS

Some of the types of event usually considered as endpoints for an IUD study are listed in Table 10.4. There are often two broad categories: one of 'use-related' discontinuations, essentially involuntary pregnancy, expulsion and medical removals, and the second of 'other' discontinuations, essentially non-medical removals, loss to follow-up and other. Each use-related discontinuation is regarded as pertaining to measures of the efficacy of the device and so is usually reported both separately and then as a combined group.

It should be noted that 'lost to follow-up' is also regarded as an event. This is because, in contraceptive trials, one method of expressing dissatisfaction with a method is not to return for the next follow-up visit, at which time it had been planned to supply the contraceptive for the next period of the study.

In many contraceptive studies, the only truly censored observations arise from subjects who complete the study without discontinuing method use. In these women no 'events' have

Table 10.4 Twelve-month post-insertion cumulative Kaplan-Meier Censor (also denoted *NR*) and Cumulative Incidence Method rates (also denoted *CR*) in women using two IUDs, either TCu380A or TCu220C, for each discontinuation reason (after Tai, Peregoudev and Machin, 2001)

Discontinuation reason	$K\text{-}M_{Censor}$ or Net rates (*NR*)		*CIM* or Crude rates (*CR*)	
	TCu380A	TCu220C	TCu380A	TCu220C
Involuntary pregnancy	2.20	5.79	1.29	3.51
Expulsion	12.49	12.79	8.09	8.74
Medical removals				
Pain	13.03	11.28	7.88	5.80
Bleeding	22.01	22.55	7.88	5.80
Pain and bleeding	4.92	4.31	2.44	2.08
Pelvic inflammatory disease	1.14	0.89	0.36	0.50
Other medical removals	6.12	6.54	2.94	2.58
Total	40.15	39.09	23.29	21.20
Non-medical removals				
Wish to become pregnant	26.96	24.29	15.69	13.68
No further need	24.40	29.05	9.38	10.89
Other non-medical removals	16.54	14.27	5.73	5.37
Total	53.92	53.95	30.80	29.94
Loss to follow-up	38.41	38.76	19.13	19.48
Other discontinuations	15.19	15.17	5.09	5.16

occurred in any of the categories of Table 10.4. It is common for contraceptive efficacy trials to have a fixed duration, often of one year and follow-up ceases at this anniversary. Thus on completion of the year, those women who had not discontinued the method earlier provide the only truly censored observations.

It is common practice to quote cumulative discontinuation rates, for each discontinuation reason, separately and for all reasons combined. Although these categories of discontinuation are mutually exclusive they do not necessarily represent independent risks.

KAPLAN-MEIER CENSOR ESTIMATE

In general terms, when considering competing risks instead of one type of failure there may be F such types and if all could be observed in an individual they would occur at times: $\Gamma_1, \Gamma_2, \ldots, \Gamma_F$. Now in fact, although there are several types of failure, we only observe the first to occur, say failure f, so that, the time to this (first and only observable) failure is Γ, where

$$\Gamma = \text{minimum}(\Gamma_1, \Gamma_2, \ldots, \Gamma_F) = \Gamma_f. \qquad (10.16)$$

If any event, of whatever type, is regarded as a failure then the corresponding K-M estimate provides an estimate of the *Event Free Survival* (*EFS*) time and is calculated by the methods described in Section 2.2. This is often used when a composite of events (whatever type of failure comes first is regarded as 'the' event) is of importance.

Equally, if failure type f alone is being considered, the K-M estimate of the associated survival time, $S_f(t)$, can be calculated. In this situation, if a different event occurs (necessarily before f) then the associated survival time is regarded as a censored observation for this calculation. Censored observations also arise from subjects who have not (yet) experienced (any) failure. The method, for one failure type and only one f, is termed the K-M censor method (K-M_{Censor}).

This process provides K-M estimates for each of the F failure types, as $S_1(t), S_2(t), \ldots, S_f(t), \ldots, S_F(t)$ and their product equals the *EFS*, that is $EFS(t) = S_1(t) \times S_2(t) \times \ldots \times S_f(t) \times \ldots \times S_F(t)$.

However, the estimate of K-M_{Censor} can only be meaningfully interpreted as cause-specific failure probabilities by relying on the unrealistic assumption of independence between all discontinuation reasons, and on the equally unrealistic assumption that the probability of failing prior to time t from reasons other than the one of interest is zero. This may result in an inflated estimate of the cumulative discontinuation rate for each reason leading to a possible total event rate in excess of 100% as has been pointed out by Tai, Peregoudov and Machin (2001).

Example *– cumulative discontinuation rates – randomised trial of two IUDs*

Table 10.4 shows the 12-month cumulative discontinuation rates calculated using $(1 - K$-$M_{Censor})$ estimates, for 12 distinct discontinuation reasons, in 2792 females randomised to be fitted with either the TCu380A or TCu220C IUD for a period of 1 year.

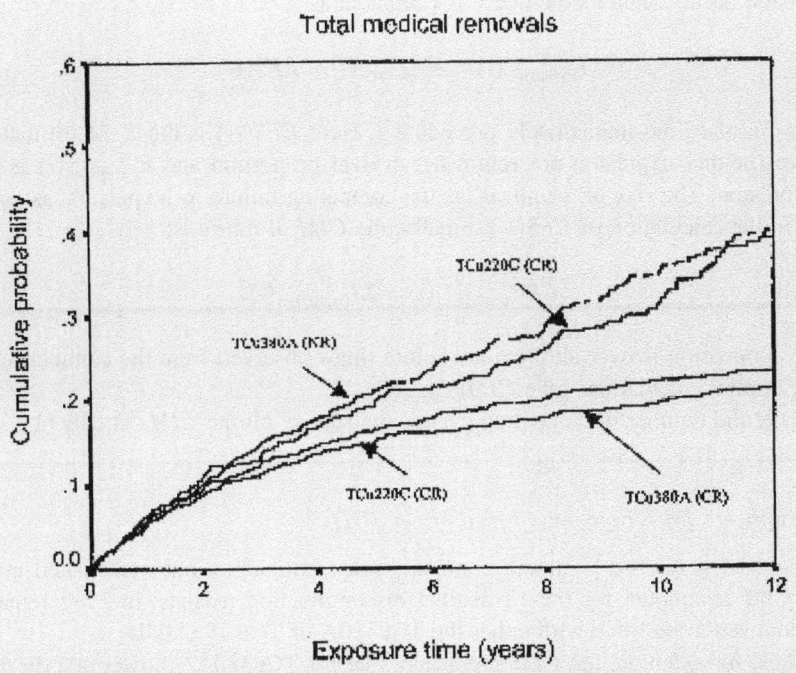

Figure 10.7 Comparative discontinuations for 'Total medical removals' in women using two types of IUD as calculated by the Kaplan-Meier Censor (denoted *NR**) method and by the Cumulative Incidence Method (denoted *CR**). (Tai, Peregoudev and Machin, 2001, with permission from John Wiley & Sons, Ltd)

Thus, for example, it is apparent from Table 10.4 that the cumulative involuntary cumulative pregnancy rate for TCu380A is lower at 2.20 than for TCu220C at 5.79%. In contrast, those for 'Total medical removals' are similar at 40.15% and 39.09% respectively as is shown in Figure 10.7.

However, summing the 12 distinct rates for each IUD give totals of 183.41% and 185.69% respectively, which are both far in excess of 100% that one might anticipate.

*The terms net rate (*NR*) and crude rate (*CR*) are common abbreviations for $(1-K-M_{Censor})$ and *CIM* respectively in contraceptive evaluation studies.

CUMULATIVE INCIDENCE

In the presence of competing risks, the *Cumulative Incidence Method* (*CIM*) estimates the cumulative probability for each cause of failure, in the presence of all risks acting on the index population.

Suppose the IUD is to be used for one year and there are just two causes of failure, expulsions and removals (for medical reasons). Thus in this period 'expulsion' and 'removal' are competing to be the first (failure) event to occur. Further suppose at time t in the trial an expulsion occurs, then its incidence is estimated as

$$I_{Expulsion}(t) = h_{Expulsion}(t) \times EFS(t\text{-}), \tag{10.17}$$

where $(t\text{-})$ is the time immediately preceding t. Here $EFS(t\text{-})$ is the $K\text{-}M$ estimate of the event-free (neither expulsion nor removal) survival proportion and $h_{Expulsion}(t)$ is the risk of an expulsion. The risk of 'removal' as the competing failure to 'expulsion' is taken into account in the calculation of $EFS(t\text{-})$. Finally, the CIM at time t is:

$$CIM_{Expulsion}(t) = \Sigma I_{Expulsion}(t), \tag{10.18}$$

Here the summation is over all previous failure times observed from the commencement of the trial. Similar calculations give $CIM_{Removal}(t)$.

Whatever the number of competing events, the sum of all the CIMs equals $(1 - EFS)$.

Example – CIM – randomised trial of two IUDs

Table 10.4 gives the 12-month cumulative discontinuation rates calculated using the CIM technique, for the 12 distinct discontinuation reasons, in 2792 females randomised to be fitted with either the TCu380A or TCu220C IUD.

Thus, for example, the CIM pregnancy rate for TCu380A is lower at 1.29 than for TCu220C at 3.51%, while those for 'Total medical removals' are similar at 23.29% and 21.20% respectively as is shown in Figure 10.7.

Summing the 12 distinct CIM rates for each IUD give totals of 87.69% and 88.03% respectively which, as one might expect, both do not exceed 100%. Thus the corresponding EFS are $(100 - 87.69) = 1.31\%$ and 11.97% respectively

Although $K\text{-}M_{Censor}$ and CIM suggest the same relative efficacy of the two IUDs, there is are major differences in the rates quoted.

The necessary calculations can be made using, for example, Stata as described by Coviello and Boggess (2004).

10.6   PAIRED OBSERVATIONS

CROSSOVER TRIAL

As we have indicated previously, survival methods have been developed principally from the study of mortality in human populations. Clinical trials to investigate the effect of interventions on such endpoints are generally designed as randomised parallel group studies, in which two or more groups are compared with regard to endpoints such as disease recurrence or death.

In these situations, because of the nature of the disease many and usually all patients, will not return to a condition similar to that observed at the time of randomisation. Clearly, in such circumstances, a two-period crossover trial in which patients, for example, receive both therapies under test, either in the order A followed by B, or B followed by A, is not usually appropriate. This is because it is assumed in such designs that, once the first treatment is completed, patients return to baseline values following an interval in which neither treatment is given (a washout period). Such a return to baseline is very unlikely in patients receiving therapy for a life-threatening disease such as cancer. However, in certain circumstances crossover trials including 'survival' time endpoints may be appropriate.

Example *– two period - two treatment - crossover trial – time to segment depression*

France, Lewis and Kay (1991) describe a crossover trial to compare the efficacy of atenolol (*A*) alone, with that of a combination of atenolol and nifedipine (*C*), in patients with angina pectoris. The trial design is summarised in Figure 10.8. Briefly, all patients underwent a run-in period on atenolol alone of four weeks. Patients then underwent an exercise test and were selected for entry into the randomised component of the study. Randomisation was to four weeks of *A* followed by four weeks of *C*, or four weeks of *C* followed by four weeks of *A*. At the end of each treatment period, there was no 'washout' period, the patients performed a treadmill exercise test, in which the patient's ECG (electrocardiogram) was monitored and the time to 1 mm ST segment depression was recorded. Patients stopped the test prematurely when they suffered excessive anginal pain, tiredness, breathlessness or other symptoms, and thus generated censored times.

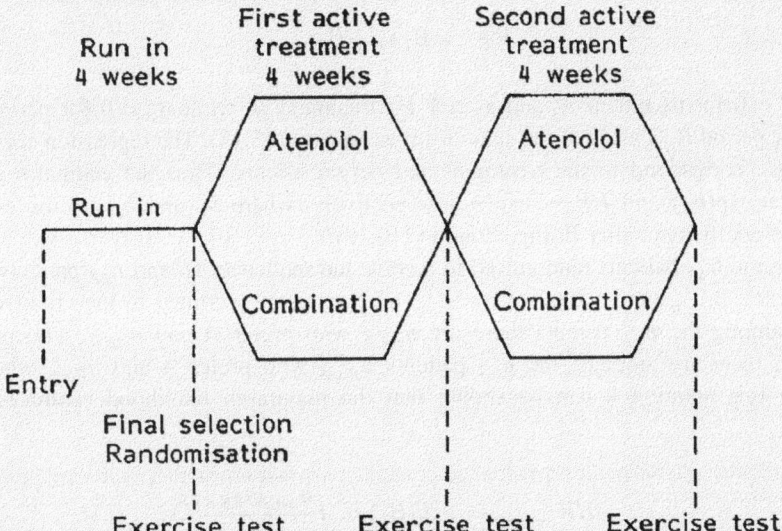

Figure 10.8   Design of a two-period crossover trial of atenolol and the combination atenolol plus nifedipine, for patients with angina pectoris (reproduced from France, Lewis and Kay, 1991, with permission from John Wiley & Sons, Ltd)

We note that the survival data is 'paired' because we have two survival times for each subject. One simple method of analysis is to count patient 'preferences'. Thus patients who experience an event on one treatment in a shorter time than they experience it on the other are said to 'prefer' that treatment.

However, there are three situations in which a patient preference cannot be determined. Two of these arise if censored observations are present. In the first situation the event of interest may not occur before the observation period is complete on either treatment. Perhaps one patient developed headaches that became so severe that emergency medication had to be instituted in both periods of the trial. In the second, the time to relief of the headache may occur on one treatment only, but this event time occurs *after* the time at which observation was prematurely stopped on the other treatment. These situations provide 'no information' on relative treatment effectiveness. The third situation is when there is a tie, in that the event occurs with the same survival time with each treatment and so consequently there is 'no preference'. For the headache study use of a stopwatch graded in seconds may avoid this problem entirely.

COX MODEL

A trial such as that described by France, Lewis and Kay (1991) is called a two-period, two-treatment, crossover trial and can be described by use of a Cox proportional hazards regression model. In this model, each patient has a separate underlying hazard which is influenced by both treatment T, (A or B) and period P, (I or II). Thus, we can specify the relative hazard as

$$\log h = \beta_T x_T + \beta_P x_P, \tag{10.19}$$

where $x_T = 0$ for treatment A, and $x_T = 1$ for treatment B, while $x_P = 0$ for period I and $x_P = 1$ for period II. This is of the same form as equation (5.18). The regression coefficients β_T and β_P correspond to the treatment and period effects. Thus the estimates of these are $HR_T = \exp(b_t)$ and $HR_P = \exp(b_P)$ respectively, where b_T and b_P are the estimated regression coefficients after fitting equation (10.19).

We assume n_{AB} patients randomised to receive the sequence AB and n_{BA} patients receive the sequence BA, giving a total of $n = n_{AB} + n_{BA}$ patients recruited to the crossover trial. Further, among the n_{AB} patents there are $n_{AB,A}$ who prefer A and $n_{AB,B}$, who prefer B. Similarly, there are amongst the n_{BA} patients $n_{BA,A}$ who prefer A and $n_{BA,B}$ who prefer B. Using this notation it can be shown that the maximum likelihood estimates of the HRs are:

$$HR_{Treatment} = \exp(\beta_T) = \sqrt{\frac{n_{AB,B} n_{BA,B}}{n_{AB,A} n_{BA,A}}} \tag{10.20}$$

and

$$HR_{Period} = \exp(\beta_P) = \log \sqrt{\frac{n_{AB,B} n_{BA,B}}{n_{AB,A} n_{BA,A}}}. \tag{10.21}$$

The details of the corresponding expressions are given by France, Lewis and Kay (1991).

Example – HRs for treatment and period – crossover trial

In the crossover trial described by France, Lewis and Kay (1991), $n_{AC} = 54$ patients completed the sequence AC. Of these $n_{AC,A} = 12$ preferred A, and $n_{AC,C} = 33$ preferred C, with nine patients providing ties or no information. Similarly $n_{CA} = 52$ patients completed the sequence CA, of which $n_{CA,A} = 14$ preferred A, and $n_{CA,C} = 29$ preferred C, again with nine providing ties or no information. Substituting theses values in equations (10.20) and (10.21) respectively gives $HR_{Treatment} = \sqrt{\dfrac{33 \times 29}{12 \times 14}} = 2.387$ suggesting an advantage to C, the combination treatment, in delaying the segment depression. Similarly $HR_{Period} = \sqrt{\dfrac{12 \times 29}{33 \times 14}} = 0.868$ which is relatively close to $HR = 1$ suggesting little evidence of a Period effect.

SURVIVAL CURVES

In a crossover trial, or in other circumstances that may provide paired survival data, the K-M estimates of the survival curves for each treatment group can be calculated in the standard way. However, in such a calculation every patient contributes to both curves but no account is taken of the paired nature of the data. These curves, therefore, do not make the best use of the information available.

To overcome this difficulty France, Lewis and Kay (1991) suggest that survival curves for all observations on each treatment A and B are first calculated separately and are then combined into an average survivor function, $S_{Average}(t)$. The average is:

$$S_{Average}(t) = \sqrt{S_A(t)S_B(t)}, \tag{10.22}$$

where $S_A(t)$ and $S_B(t)$ are the K-M estimates for all observations on treatments A and B, respectively. Using this average survival curve, the individual survival curves for each treatment group are then calculated as

$$S_A^*(t) = [S_{Average}(t)]^{\exp(+\beta_T/2)} \text{ and } S_B^*(t) = [S_{Average}(t)]^{\exp(-\beta_T/2)}, \tag{10.23}$$

where β_T is as defined in equation (10.19).

Example – survival curves from a crossover trial – time to segment depression

For the crossover trial of France, Lewis and Kay (1991) the K-M estimates of the survival curves calculated on the basis of the data from each separate treatment arm are shown in Figure 10.9(a). The apparent small difference in median exercise time does not reflect the magnitude of the treatment effect shown by the Cox analysis ($HR_T = 2.4$).

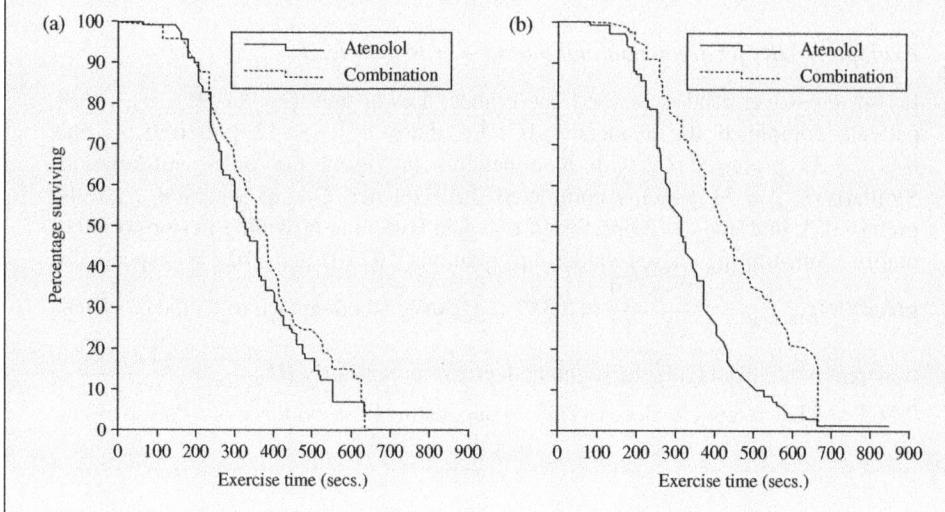

Figure 10.9 Estimated survival curves for 1 mm segment depression based (a) on the individual survival curves and (b) on the average survival function and Cox model regression coefficient (From France, Lewis and Kay, 1991, with permission from John Wiley & Sons, Ltd)

In contrast, Figure 10.9(b) shows the corresponding curves but now calculated from the average survivor function, which by the nature of their construction are consistent with the Cox analysis.

The median exercise time is approximately 300s with A and 420s with C. This indicates an increased exercise time by use of the combination therapy.

The crossover trial is one example which provides paired data and this type of design arises frequently in clinical studies. Paired, or more accurately matched-pairs, data are also common in epidemiological follow-up studies. However, pairs also arise naturally in some organs such as eyes, kidneys and ears and their survival either as expressed by loss of sight, kidney dysfunction or loss of hearing, in the respective organs, would generate paired survival times.

A general extension of survival methods from paired organs, such as the kidneys, to consider the time to development of, for example, rheumatoid arthritis in the digits of one hand, both hands or the whole body is clearly possible. Similarly we may be concerned with the time from birth to develop dental caries in each tooth of children.

10.7   ANALYSIS OF CORRELATED DATA

Most statistical analysis methods, including the standard Cox model and the parametric models of Chapter 4, assume that data are independent. This assumption is violated in some situations. One of them is when data are collected from clusters, such as children from the same families, patients of the same medical practitioner, and workers from the same factory. Observations within the same clusters: families, factories, or, in the case of a crossover trial, patients who receive both interventions, are likely to be more similar than observations from different clusters. Another situation is when the outcome event is recurrent. For instance, children may have multiple episodes of acute respiratory illness during a study period, and patients who have just been discharged from a hospital may subsequently have multiple episodes of readmission. Both clustered and recurrent data violate the independence assumption. They may be more generally termed correlated data, that is, the observations within clusters or multiple time-to-event data within patients are correlated. There are a variety of methods to handle such correlated data. We will discuss only a relatively simple one.

ROBUST STANDARD ERROR (*SE*)

The main problem when using the standard Cox model with correlated data is that the corresponding *SE*s are likely to be under-estimated, and consequently the *p*-value is also under-estimated. A popular approach to analysis in these circumstances is to ignore the correlation and estimate the regression parameters as usual. However, once calculated the standard *SE*s are replaced by estimates that are 'robust' to the correlation in the data when it comes to calculating *p*-values and *CI*s. One such robust estimator of variance (whose square root is a robust *SE*) is interchangeably called the 'sandwich', 'empirical', 'White', after the name of its originator, or simply the 'robust (variance) estimator'.

ANALYSIS OF CLUSTERED DATA

Clustered data occur if there are several observations (units) nested within the same (but higher-level) units. Examples are children within schools, workers within factories and residents within communities, and a pair of organs within patients.

Example – *cluster randomised trial – Access to Care*

The Zimbabwe Project on Access to Care and Treatment (ZIMPACT) provided two alternative types of intensified primary health care. A total of 22 factories, with a total of more than 7000 employees, were randomly allocated on a 1:1 basis to receive one of these. The unit of randomisation was the factory and as a consequence all employees in the same factory received the same form of primary health care. The primary object was to encourage workers to seek *V*oluntary *C*ounselling and HIV *T*esting (*VCT*). At the end of the study period of about two years approximately two-thirds of the participants did receive *VCT* and the 'time-to-*VCT*-uptake' was recorded.

Since staff members of the same factory are likely to influence each other in *VCT* uptake, the assumption of independence is unlikely to be valid.

It is important, for an appropriate analysis of correlated data that there is a variable in the data set that identifies the cluster of which the subject is a member. For instance, a small subset of the ZIMPACT data is shown in Table 10.5. The variable SiteID identifies participants from the same factories, and the calculations to obtain the robust *SE* require this information.

Table 10.5 Partial data from the ZIMPACT study (Data courtesy of Dr Liz Corbett, Biomedical Research and Training Institute, Zimbabwe)

SiteID	Age	Gender	Time (months)	VCT
1	35	1	23.92	0
1	44	1	8.38	1
1	30	1	23.92	0
...	...	...	...	...
2	50	1	23.88	0
2	35	0	11.11	1
2	42	1	23.88	0
...	...	...	...	

Example – *cluster randomised trial – Access to Care*

In the ZIMPACT study, one objective was to see whether the time to *VCT* uptake was related to age and gender. We will contrast the use of the standard Cox model and the Cox model with the robust *SE*. Using age as a continuous variable, and hence a linear effect on log(HR), in the *standard* Cox model gives the results summarised in Table 10.6. Older age was found related to a lower *VCT* uptake rate, with $b_{Age} = \log(HR_{Age}) = -0.0064$ and $SE = 0.0019$. From these $z = -0.0064/0.0019 = -3.37$ and, referring to more extensive tables than Table T1, we obtain the *p*-value $= 0.0006$. Hence age might be regarded as a significant predictor of *VCT* uptake were the independence assumption valid.

However, the corresponding *robust SE* $= 0.0090$, which is much larger than the standard estimate, reflecting the influence of within cluster correlation. Based on the robust *SE*, $z = -0.0064/0.0090 = -0.71$ and Table T1 gives $p = 0.478$. Hence there is now no evidence to conclude an age effect.

Similarly, the robust *SE* for the $b_{Gender} = \log(HR_{Gender})$ for male gender is larger than that estimated by the standard method and the *p*-value indicates a less significant finding increasing from 0.503 to 0.842.

We should emphasise that the analysis summarised here is only illustrative and should not be taken as the ultimate findings from this study.

Table 10.6 Results using two different estimators of *SE*. (Data courtesy of Dr Liz Corbett, Biomedical Research and Training Institute, Zimbabwe)

Type of Estimator		Standard			Robust	
Explanatory variables	$b = \log(HR)$	SE	*p*-value		SE	*p*-value
Age (years)	−0.0064	0.0019	0.001		0.0090	0.478
Gender (male)	0.0413	0.0643	0.503		0.2167	0.842

In Section 7.3 we discussed the use of stratification to remove the clustering effect. We noted that the stratification method could not be used to analyse cluster-randomised trials. The use of robust *SE* does not have this limitation and it is possible to use it to make inferences about the effect of the intervention in cluster-randomised trials. However, Donner and Klar (2000) suggest that for the robust *SE* to work properly in such a situation, there should be at least 20 clusters per intervention group. Thus this approach would not be recommended, when analysing the effect of the two types of primary health care in the ZIMPACT study because there are only 11 factories (clusters) per group.

ANALYSIS OF RECURRENT EVENTS

One fairly common approach to the analysis of recurrent events is to analyse only the time to the first event, ignoring data on the subsequent events. While this has the advantage of simplicity, it does not fully utilise the data. There are a variety of perspectives on how to conceptualise multiple failure times arising from recurrent events in the context of the Cox model. We describe one approach using the model for analysis of time from the previous event proposed by Prentice, Williams and Peterson (*PWP*), sometimes called a conditional risk set model, which is recommended by Kelly and Lim (2000) who give a useful review of this topic.

The *PWP* formulation of the Cox model has the following features. First, it analyses time from the previous event instead of time from the start of observation. Second, it only includes subjects who have experienced the previous $(k-1)$ events in the risk set of the kth event. For example, only subjects who have experienced the first event are counted in the risk set for the second event. Third, the baseline hazard function for each event is allowed to be different from that of the other events. This is achieved by stratifying on the order of the events. Therefore, the first event has one baseline hazard, the second event has another, and so on. Finally, from a data management point of view, the subjects have a variable number of observations. Suppose the maximum number of events observed is M, then subjects with k ($<M$) events contribute k uncensored observation(s) and one censored observation to the data set. Those subjects experiencing M events contribute M uncensored observations and no censored observations.

To apply the *PWP* model, it is *very important* that the data are set up in the correct form. This often requires a lot of careful data management and programming.

Since multiple events from the same subjects may be correlated, it is common to use the robust estimator of *SE* in association with the *PWP* model.

Example – recurrent events – anti-malarial cluster randomised clinical trial

A randomised anti-malarial combination trial (ACT) among children with uncomplicated malaria was started in September 2003 in The Gambia. The first dose of the medication was given at the clinic and the parents and children went home with the remaining doses for unsupervised administration. The parents were encouraged to bring the children back to the study clinics for care if they remained sick.

Table 10.7 Partial data from a randomised anti-malarial combination trial (ACT03) in The Gambia (Data courtesy of Dr Paul Milligan, London School of Hygiene and Tropical Medicine)

ID (1)	DateEnter (2)	Visit (3)	VisitDate (4)	Treat (5)	Centre (6)	Time (7)	Sick (8)
6732	10 Sep 03	1	.	A	1	143	0
0013	10 Sep 03	1	15 Sep 03	A	2	5	1
0013	10 Sep 03	2	.	A	2	138	0
6763	10 Sep 03	1	31 Oct 03	B	2	51	1
6763	10 Sep 03	2	07 Nov 03	B	2	7	1
6763	10 Sep 03	3	.	B	2	92	0
6744	10 Sep 03	1	13 Oct 03	B	2	33	1
6744	10 Sep 03	2	30 Oct 03	B	2	17	1
6744	10 Sep 03	3	05 Jan 04	B	2	67	1

Although the trial randomly allocated the children to receive one of three combinations of anti-malarial drugs, for illustration we use only two of the treatments and simply call them A and B. The data set consists of observations from 1096 children, who had up to three return visits. The numbers of first, second and third return visits were 299, 66 and 20, respectively. Table 10.7 shows selected observations from four children with 0, 1, 2 and 3 return visits, all of whom were recruited on 10 September 2003. The maximum number of events, M, is equal to three.

Just as in the analysis of clustered data, a subject identifier is essential for subsequent analysis using the robust SE. Thus column (1), of Table 10.7, is the variable that uniquely identifies each child. The study involved three centres and randomisation was stratified by centre (6).

The first row of data shows the values for subject (ID 6732) who did not have any event, that is, did not return to the clinic; hence the VisitDate for Visit 1 is absent. As the child did not experience the first event, he was not at risk of the second and third events and having only one row in the data set reflects this. The analysis was censored at 31 January 2004 and so Time $= T^{+} = 143$ days and the outcome indicator Sick $= 0$.

Subject ID 0013 had one event, on 15 September 2003, five days after recruitment. Data row 2, represents this uncensored observation, with Visit $= 1$, Time $= 5$ and Sick $= 1$. Furthermore, since he had experienced the first event, he was at risk of the second event. Thus row 3 shows this censored observation, with Visit $= 2$ and Sick $= 0$. Time $= 138$ is the number of days from the first event (15 September 2003) to the censoring date.

Subject ID 6763 had two events; hence two uncensored and one censored observations in the data set. The values on the Visit variable run from 1 to 3. Subject ID 6744 had three events and therefore three uncensored observations in the data set. This participant was at risk of the fourth event. However, none of the subjects had more than three events and it is not necessary to create a censored observation in this case.

Once the data set is ready, it can be analysed using a Cox model with stratification on Visit and using the robust SE. Since the randomisation was stratified by centre, both the treatment variable and two dummy variables representing the three centres are included

Table 10.8 *PWP* model of recurrent time to clinic visit and standard Cox model of time to first clinic visit, (ACT03) Trial, The Gambia. (Data courtesy of Dr Paul Milligan, London School of Hygiene and Tropical Medicine)

Variables	Recurrent events			First event only		
	log(*HR*)	Robust SE	*p*-value	log(*HR*)	*SE*	*p*-value
Treatment *A*	0	—		0	—	
Treatment *B*	0.1099	0.1143	0.3360	0.0422	0.1207	0.7263
Centre 1	0	—		0	—	
Centre 2	−1.0751	0.0581	<0.0001	−1.1238	0.0588	<0.0001
Centre 3	−0.0159	0.1113	0.8867	0.0005	0.1295	0.9997

in the model as design variables in the manner discussed in Section 6.2. The results are shown in Table 10.8, together with the results of analysing time to first event. The findings from the two analyses are fairly similar in terms of the log(*HR*) estimates. However, the analysis based on all (recurrent) events gives smaller *SE*s even after adjustment for within subject correlation than the analysis based on first event only. This demonstrates that the full utilisation of multiple failure time data tends to give more power and precision than analysis of first event only. In this example the difference is not large because the majority of the events recorded were first events.

References

Aboulker JP and Swart AM (1993). Preliminary analysis of the Concorde Trial. *Lancet*, **341**, 889–890. [1]

Advanced Ovarian Cancer Trialists' Group (1991). Chemotherapy in advanced ovarian cancer: an overview of randomized clinical trials. *British Medical Journal*, **303**, 884–893. [10]

Allison PD (1995). *Survival Analysis Using the SAS System: A Practical Guide*. SAS Institute Inc, Cary, NC. [1]

Altman DG (1991). *Practical Statistics for Medical Research*. Chapman & Hall, London. [1]

Altman DG and de Stavola BL (1994). Practical problems in fitting a proportional hazards model to data with updated measurements of the covariates. *Statistics in Medicine*, **13**, 301–341. [7]

Altman DG, Lausen B, Sauerbrei W and Schumacher M (1994). Dangers of using "optimal" cutpoints in the evaluation of prognostic factors. *Journal of the National Cancer Institute*, **86**, 829-835 and 1798–1799. [6]

Altman DG, Machin D, Bryant TN and Gardner MJ (eds) (2000). *Statistics with Confidence*. British Medical Association, London. [1]

Altman DG and Royston P (2000). What do we mean by validating a prognostic model? *Statistics in Medicine*, **11**, 453–473. [8]

Ang ES-W, Lee S-T, Gan CS-G, See PG-J, Chan Y-H, Ng L-H and Machin D (2001). Evaluating the role of alternative therapy in burn wound management: randomized trial comparing most exposed burn ointment with conventional methods in the management of patients with second-degree burns. *Medscape General Medicine*, **6**, 3 [1].

Bland M (2000). *An Introduction to Medical Statistics* (3rd edn). Oxford University Press, Oxford. [1]

Bleehen NM and Stenning SP on behalf of the Medical Research Council Brain Tumour Working Party (1991). A Medical Research Council trial of two radiotherapy doses in the treatment of grades 3 and 4 astrocytoma. *British Journal of Cancer*, **64**, 769–774. [5, 8]

Bonacini M, Louie S, Bzowej N and Wohl AM (2004). Survival in patients with HIV infection and viral hepatitis B or C: a cohort study. *AIDS*, **18**, 2039–2045. [1]

Bradburn MJ, Clark TG, Love SB and Altman DG (2003a). Survival Analysis Part II: Multivariate data analysis—an introduction to concepts and methods. *British Journal of Cancer*, **89**, 431–436. [1]

Bradburn MJ, Clark TG, Love SB and Altman DG (2003b). Survival Analysis Part III: Multivariate data analysis—choosing a model and assessing its adequacy of fit. *British Journal of Cancer*, **89**, 605–611. [1]

Campbell MJ, Machin D and Walters SJ (2006). *Medical Statistics: A Commonsense Approach* (4th edn). Wiley, Chichester. [1]

Capra M, Hewitt M, Hayward J, Weston CL, Machin D and Radford M. Long term outcome and cure in children with Hodgkin's lymphoma: The UKCCSG HD82 trial. (Submitted) [10]

Cheingsong-Popov R, Panagiotidi C, Bowcock S, Aronstam A, Wadsworth J and Weber J (1991). Relation between humoral responses to HIV gag and end proteins at seroconversion and clinical outcome of HIV infection. *British Medical Journal*, **302**, 23–26. [3]

CheungYB (2000). Marital status and mortality in British women: a longitudinal study. *International Journal of Epidemiology*, **29**, 93–99. [5, 6]

Cheung YB, Gao F and Khoo K-S (2003). Age at diagnosis and the choice of survival analysis methods in cancer epidemiology. *Journal of Clinical Epidemiology*, **56**, 38–43. [7]

Cheung YB, Yip PSF and Karlberg JPE (2001a). Parametric modelling of neonatal mortality in relation to size at birth. *Statistics in Medicine* **20**, 2455–2466. [2, 7]

Cheung YB, Yip PSF and Karlberg JPE (2001b). Fetal growth, early postnatal growth and motor development in Pakistani infants. *International Journal of Epidemiology*, **30**, 66–74. [4]

Chiasson J-L, Josse RG, Gomis R, Hanefeld M, Karasik, Laakso M, for the STOP-NIDDM Trial Research Group (2002). Acarbose for prevention of type 2 diabetes mellitus: the STOP-NIDDM randomised trial. *Lancet*, **359**, 2072–2077. [1]

Chow PK-H, Tai B-C, Tan C-K, Machin D, Win K-M, Johnson PJ and Soo K-C (2002). High-dose tamoxifen in the treatment of inoperable hepatocellular carcinoma: A multicenter randomised controlled trial. *Hepatology*, **36**, 1221–1226 [2, 9].

Clark TG, Bradburn MJ, Love SB and Altman DG (2003a). Survival analysis part I: basic concepts and first analyses. *British Journal of Cancer*, **89**, 232–238. [1]

Clark TG, Bradburn MJ, Love SB and Altman DG (2003b). Survival analysis part IV: further concepts and methods in survival analysis. *British Journal of Cancer*, **89**, 781–786. [1]

Cleves MA, Gould WW and Gutierrez RG (2002). *An Introduction to Survival Analysis Using STATA*. Stata Press, College Station, TX. [1]

Collett D (2003). *Modelling Survival Data in Medical Research* (2nd edn). Chapman & Hall, London. [1, 4]

Coviello V and Boggess M (2004). Cumulative incidence estimation in the presence of competing risks. *The Stata Journal*, **4**, 103–12. [10]

Cox DR (1972). Regression models and life tables (with discussion). *Journal of the Royal Statistical Society*, **B34**, 187–220. [1, 5]

Cox DR and Oakes D (1984). *Analysis of Survival Data*. Chapman & Hall, London. [1]

Donner A and Klar NS (2000). *Design and Analysis of Cluster Randomisation Trials in Health Research*. Arnold, London. [10]

Elashoff JD (2000). *nQuery Advisor Version 4.0 User's Guide*. Los Angeles, CA. [1, 9]

Farewell VT (1979). An application of Cox's proportional hazards model to multiple infection data. *Applied Statistics*, **28**, 136–143. [7]

Farley TMM, Ali MM and Slaymaker E (2001). Competing approaches to analysis of failure times with competing risks. *Statistics in Medicine*, **20**, 3601–3610. [10]

Farley TMM, Rosenberg MJ, Rowe PJ, Chen J-H and Meirik O (1992). Intrauterine devices and pelvic inflammatory disease: an international perspective. *Lancet*, **339**, 785–788. [2]

Fisher B, Anderson S, Fisher ER, Redmond C, Wickerham DL, Wolmark N, Mamounas EP, Deutsch M and Margolese R (1991). Significance of ipsilateral breast tumour recurrence after lumpectomy. *Lancet*, **338**, 327–331. [5, 7]

Fisher B, Bryant J, Dignam JJ, Wickerham DL, Mamounas EP, Fisher ER, Margolese RG, Nesbitt L, Paik S, Pisansky TM, Wolmark N; National Surgical Adjuvant Breast and Bowel Project (2002). Tamoxifen, radiation therapy, or both for prevention of ipsilateral breast tumour recurrence after lumpectomy in women with invasive breast cancers of one centimeter or less. *Journal of Clinical Oncology*, **20**, 4141–4149. [10]

France LΛ, Lewis JA and Kay R (1991). The analysis of failure time data in crossover studies. *Statistics in Medicine*, **10**, 1099–1113. [10]

Gray R, James R, Mossman J and Stenning SP (1991). AXIS: a suitable case for treatment. *British Journal of Cancer*, **63**, 841–845. [5]

Hankey GJ, Slattery JM and Warlow CP (1991). Prognosis and prognostic factors of retinal infarction: a prospective cohort study. *British Medical Journal*, **302**, 499–504. [2]

Hayes RJ, Alexander ND, Bennett S and Cousens SN (2000). Design and analysis issues in cluster-randomized trials of interventions against infectious diseases. *Statistical Methods in Medical Research*, **9**, 95–116. [7]

Kalbfleisch JD and Prentice RL (2002). *The Statistical Analysis of Failure Time Data* (2nd edn). Wiley, New York. [1]

Kaplan EL and Meier P (1958). Nonparametric estimation from incomplete observations. *Journal of the American Statistical Association*, **53**, 457–481. [1, 2]

Kelly PJ and Lim LLY (2000). Survival analysis for recurrent event data: an application to childhood infectious diseases. *Statistics in Medicine*, **19**, 13–33. [10]

Khawaja HT, Campbell MJ and Weaver PC (1988). Effect of transdermal glyceryl trinitrate on the survival of peripheral intravenous infusions: a double-blind prospective clinical study. *British Journal of Surgery*, **75**, 1212–1215. [2]

Korenman S, Goldman N, Fu H (1997). Misclassification bias in estimates of bereavement effects. *American Journal of Epidemiology*, **145**, 995–1002. [6, 7]

Leonard RCF, Hayward RL, Prescott RJ and Wang JX (1991). The identification of discrete prognostic groups in low-grade non-Hodgkin's lymphoma. *Annals of Oncology*, **2**, 655–662. [8]

Mackie RM, Bufalino R, Morabito A, Sutherland C and Cascinelli N for the World Health Organization Melanoma Programme (1991). Lack of effect of pregnancy on outcome of melanoma. *Lancet*, **337**, 653–655. [7]

Machin D and Campbell MJ (2005). *Design of Studies for Medical Research*. Wiley, Chichester. [1]

Machin D, Campbell MJ, Fayers PM and Pinol APY (1997). *Statistical Tables for the Design of Clinical Trials* (2nd edn). Blackwell Scientific Publications, Oxford. [1, 9]

Maldonado G, Greenland S (1993). Simulation study of confounder-selection strategies. *American Journal of Epidemiology*, **138**, 923–936. [6]

Marubini E and Valsecchi MG (1995). *Analysing Survival Data from Clinical Trials and Observational Studies*. Wiley, Chichester. [1]

Mayo NE, Korner-Bitensky NA and Becker R (1991). Recovery time at independent function post-stroke. *American Journal of Physical Medicine and Rehabilitation*, **70**, 5–12. [1, 5]

McDiarmid T, Burns PN, Lewith GT and Machin D (1985). Ultrasound and the treatment of pressure sores: preliminary study. *Physiotherapy*, **71**, 66–70. [3]

McIllmurray MB and Turkie W (1987). Controlled trial of γ linolenic acid in Dukes' C colorectal cancer. *British Medical Journal*, **294**, 1260; **295**, 475. [2, 4]

Medical Research Council Brain Tumour Working Party (1990). Prognostic factors for malignant glioma: development of a prognostic index. *Journal of Neuro-Oncology*, **9**, 47–55. [8]

Medical Research Council Lung Cancer Working Party (1989a). Survival, adverse reactions and quality of life during combination chemotherapy compared with selective palliative treatment for small-cell lung cancer. *Respiratory Medicine*, **83**, 51–58. [5]

Medical Research Council Lung Cancer Working Party (1989b). Controlled trial of twelve versus six courses of chemotherapy in the treatment of small-cell lung cancer. *British Journal of Cancer*, **59**, 584–590. [5]

Medical Research Council Lung Cancer Working Party (1991). Inoperable non-small-cell lung cancer (NSCLC): a Medical Research Council randomised trial of palliative radiotherapy with two fractions or ten fractions. *British Journal of Cancer*, **63**, 265–270. [5]

Medical Research Council Lung Cancer Working Party (1992). A Medical Research Council (MRC) randomised trial of palliative radiotherapy with two fractions or a single fraction in patients with inoperable non-small-cell lung cancer (NSCLC) and poor performance status. *British Journal of Cancer*, **65**, 934–941. [5]

Medical Research Council Lung Cancer Working Party (1993). A randomised trial of 3 or 6 courses of etoposide, cyclophosphamide, methotrexate and vincristine, or 6 courses of etoposide and ifosfamide in small-cell lung cancer (SCLC). I: Survival and prognostic factors. *British Journal of Cancer*, **68**, 1150–1156. [5, 7]

Medical Research Council Lung Cancer Working Party (1996). The role of post-operative radiotherapy in non-small-cell lung cancer: a multicentre randomised trial in patients with pathologically staged T_{1-2}, N_{1-2}, M_0 disease. *British Journal of Cancer*, **74**, 632–639. [3]

Medical Research Council Working Party on Advanced Carcinoma of the Cervix (1993). A trial of Ro 03-8799 (pimonidazole) in carcinoma of the uterine cervix: an interim report from the Medical Research Council Working Party on advanced carcinoma of the cervix. *Radiotherapy and Oncology*, **26**, 93–103. [3, 4]

Medical Research Council Working Party on Misonidazole in Gliomas (1983). A study of the effect of misonidazole in conjunction with radiotherapy for the treatment of grades 3 and 4 astrocytomas. *British Journal of Radiology*, **56**, 673–682. [5, 6, 8]

Meng CD, Zhu JC, Chen ZW, Wong LT, Zhang GY, Hu YZ, Ding JH, Wang XH, Qian SZ, Wang C, Machin D, Pinol A and Waikes GMH (1988). Recovery of sperm production following the cessation of gossypol treatment: a two centre study in China. *International Journal of Andrology*, **11**, 1–11. [1, 5]

Moffatt CJ, Franks PJ, Oldroyd M, Bosanquet N, Brown P, Greenhalgh RM and McCollum CN (1992). Community clinics for leg ulcers and impact on healing. *British Medical Journal*, **305**, 1389–1392. [2]

Mufti GJ, Stevens JR, Oscier DG, Hamblin TJ and Machin D (1985). Myelodysplastic syndromes: a scoring system with prognostic significance. *British Journal of Haematology*, **59**, 425–433. [3]

Nash TP, Williams JD, Machin D (1990). TENS: does the type of stimulus really matter? *Pain Clinic*, **3**, 161–168. [3]

Nolan T, Debelle G, Oberklaid F and Coffey C (1991). Randomised trials of laxatives in treatment of childhood encopresis. *Lancet*, **338**, 523–527. [10]

Packer M, Carver JR, Rodeheffer RJ, Ivanhoe RJ, DiBianco R, Zeldis SM, Hendrix GH, Bommer WJ, Elkayam U, Kukin ML, Mallis GL, Sollano A, Shannon J, Tandon PK and DeMets DL for the PROMISE Study Research Group (1991). Effect of oral milrinone on mortality in severe chronic heart failure. *New England Journal of Medicine*, **325**, 1468–1475. [1, 3]

Peto J (1984). The calculation and interpretation of survival curves. In: Buyse ME, Staquet MJ and Sylvester RJ (eds), *Cancer Clinical Trials. Methods and Practice*. Oxford University Press, Oxford, pp. 361–380. [2]

Peto R, Pike MC, Armitage P, Breslow NE, Cox DR, Howard SV, Mantel N, MacPherson K, Peto J and Smith PG (1976). Design and analysis of randomised clinical trials requiring prolonged observation of each patient. I: introduction and design. *British Journal of Cancer*, **34**, 585–612. [1]

Peto R, Pike MC, Armitage P, Breslow NE, Cox DR, Howard SV, Mantel N, MacPherson K, Peto J and Smith PG (1977). Design and analysis of randomised clinical trials requiring prolonged observation of each patient. II: Analysis and examples. *British Journal of Cancer*, **35**, 1–39. [1]

Peduzzi P, Concato J, Kemper E, Holford TR and Feinstein AR (1996). A simulation study of the number of events per variable in logistic regression analysis. *Journal of Clinical Epidemiology*, **49**, 1372–1379. [9]

Piffarré A, Rosell R, Monzó M, De Anta JM, Moreno I, Sánchez JJ, Ariza A, Mate JL, Martínez E and Sánchez M (1997). Prognostic value of replication errors on chromosomes 2p and 3p in non-small-cell lung cancer. *British Journal of Cancer*, **75**, 184–189. [9]

Pocock SJ, Clayton TC and Altman DG (2002). Survival plots of time-to-event outcomes in clinical trials: good practice and pitfalls. *Lancet*, **359**, 1686–1689. [1]

Poon D, Yap S-P, Wong Z-W, Cheung Y-B, Leong S-S, Wee J, Tan T, Fong K-W, Chua E-T and Tan E-H (2004). Concurrent chemoradiotherapy in locoregionally recurrent nasopharyngeal carcinoma. *International Journal of Radiation Oncology, Biology and Physics*, **59**, 1312–1318. [4]

Remuzzi G, Lesti M, Gotti E, Ganeva M, Dimitrov BD, Ene-Iordache B, Gherardi G, Group (2004). Mycophenolate mofetil versus azathioprine for prevention of acute rejection in renal transplantation (MYSS): a randomised trial. *Lancet*, **364**, 503–512. [6]

Samanta A, Roy S and Woods KL (1991). Gold therapy in rheumatoid arthritis. *Lancet*, **338**, 642. [2]

Samuelson SO and Kongerud J (1994). Interval censoring in longitudinal data of respiratory symptoms in aluminium workers: a comparison of methods. *Statistics in Medicine*, **13**, 1771–1780. [5, 6]

Sauerbrei W, Royston P, Bojar H, Schmoor C and Schumacher M (1999). Modelling the effects of standard prognostic factors in node-negative breast cancer. *British Journal of Cancer*, **79**, 1752–1760. [8]

Schoenfeld D (1982). Partial residuals for the proportional hazards regression model. *Biometrika*, **69**, 239–241. [5]

Shuster JJ (1991). Median follow-up in clinical trials. *Journal of Clinical Oncology*, **9**, 191–192. [2]

Sposto R (2000). Cure model analysis in cancer: an application to data from the Children's Cancer Group. *Statistics in Medicine*, **21**, 293–312. [10]

StataCorp (2005). *Stata Statistical Software: Release 9.0*. StataCorp LP, College Station, Tx. [4, 10]

Stephens RJ, Girling DJ and Machin D (1994). Can patients at risk from death during treatment for small-cell lung cancer be identified? *Lung Cancer*, **11**, 259–274. [2]

Sun GW, Shook TL and Kay GL (1996). Inappropriate use of bivariable analysis to screen risk factors for use in multivariable analysis. *Journal of Clinical Epidemiology*, **49**, 907–916. [6]

Tai B-C, Peregoudov A and Machin D (2001). A competing risk approach to the analysis of trials of alternative intrauterine devices (IUDs) for fertility regulation. *Statistics in Medicine*, **20**, 3589–3600. [10]

Tai B-C, White I, Gebski V and Machin D (2001). Competing risks analysis of patients with osteosarcoma: a comparison of four different approaches. *Statistics in Medicine*, **20**, 661–684. [10]

Tan C-K, Law N-M, Ng N-S and Machin D (2003). Simple clinical prognostic model for hepatocellular carcinoma in developing countries and its validation. *Journal of Clinical Oncology*, **21**, 2294–2298. [8, 9]

The RISC Group (1990). Risk of myocardial infarction and death during treatment with low dose aspirin and intravenous heparin in men with unstable coronary artery disease. *Lancet*, **336**, 827–830. [3, 5]

Therneau TM and Grambsch PM (2000). *Modeling Survival Data: Extending the Cox Model*. Springer-Verlag, New York. [5]

Turnbull BW, Brown BW Jr and Hu M (1974). Survivorship analysis of heart transplant data. *Journal of the American Statistical Association*, **69**, 74–86. [1, 2, 7]

Umen AJ and Le CT (1986). Prognostic factors, models and related statistical problems in the survival of end-stage renal disease patients on haemodialysis. *Statistics in Medicine*, **5**, 637–652. [6]

Wallentin L, Wilcox RG, Weaver WD, Emanuelsson H, Goodvin A, Nyström P and Bylock A (2003). Oral ximelagatran for secondary prophylaxis after myocardial infarction: the ESTEEM randomised controlled trial. *Lancet*, **362**, 789–797. [1]

Valerius NH, Koch C and Hoiby N (1991). Prevention of chronic Pseudomonas aeruginosa colonisation in cystic fibrosis by early treatment. *Lancet*, **338**, 725–726. [9]

Venables WN and Ripley BD (1999). *Modern Applied Statistics with S-Plus* (3rd edn). Springer-Verlag, New York. [1]

Van Griensven GJP, Boucher EC, Roos M and Coutinho RA (1991). Expansion of AIDS case definition. *Lancet*, **338**, 1012–1013. [2]

Weston CL, Douglas C, Craft A, Lewis IJ, and Machin D (2004). Establishing long term survival and cure in young patients with Ewing's sarcoma. *British Journal of Cancer*, **91**, 225–232. [10]

World Health Organization Task Force on Long-acting Systemic Agents for Fertility Regulation. Special Programme of Research, Development and Research training in Human Reproduction (1988). A multicentred phase III comparative study of two hormonal contraceptive preparations given once-a-month by intramuscular injections. 1: contraceptive efficacy and side effects. *Contraception*, **37**, 1–20. [3]

World Health Organization Task Force on Long-acting Systemic Agents for Fertility Regulation (1990). Microdose intravaginal levenorgestrel contraception: a multicentre clinical trial. III. The relationship between pregnancy rate and body weight. *Contraception*, **41**, 143–150. [3]

Yudkin PL, Ellison GW, Chezzi A, Goodkin DE, Hughes RAC, McPherson K, Mertin J and Milanese C (1991). Overview of aziathioprine treatment in multiple sclerosis. *Lancet*, **338**, 1051–1055. [10]

Statistical Tables

Table T1 The Normal distribution. The value tabulated is the probability, α, that a Normally distributed random variable with mean zero and standard deviation 1 will be greater than $z_{1-\alpha/2}$ or less than $-z_{1-\alpha/2}$

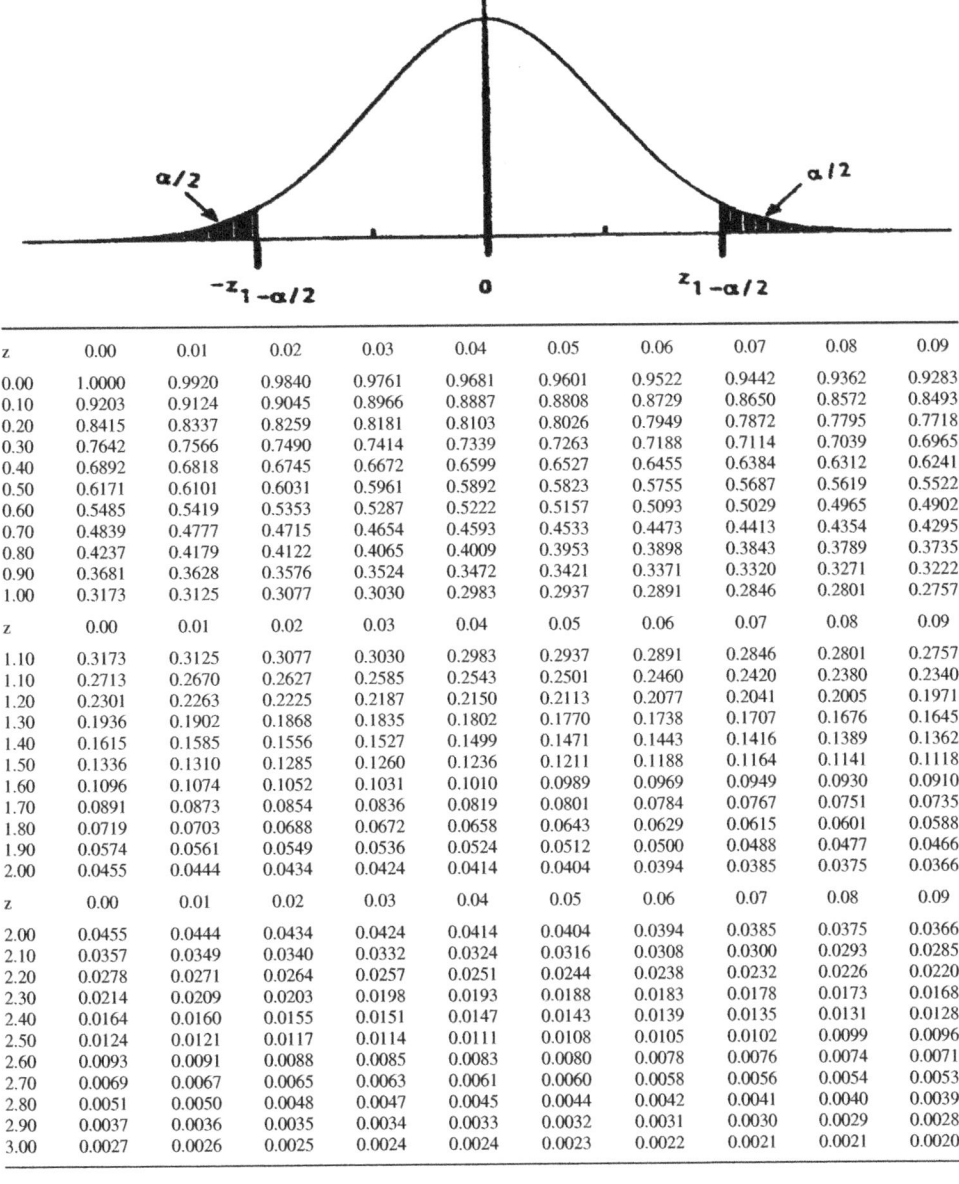

z	0.00	0.01	0.02	0.03	0.04	0.05	0.06	0.07	0.08	0.09
0.00	1.0000	0.9920	0.9840	0.9761	0.9681	0.9601	0.9522	0.9442	0.9362	0.9283
0.10	0.9203	0.9124	0.9045	0.8966	0.8887	0.8808	0.8729	0.8650	0.8572	0.8493
0.20	0.8415	0.8337	0.8259	0.8181	0.8103	0.8026	0.7949	0.7872	0.7795	0.7718
0.30	0.7642	0.7566	0.7490	0.7414	0.7339	0.7263	0.7188	0.7114	0.7039	0.6965
0.40	0.6892	0.6818	0.6745	0.6672	0.6599	0.6527	0.6455	0.6384	0.6312	0.6241
0.50	0.6171	0.6101	0.6031	0.5961	0.5892	0.5823	0.5755	0.5687	0.5619	0.5522
0.60	0.5485	0.5419	0.5353	0.5287	0.5222	0.5157	0.5093	0.5029	0.4965	0.4902
0.70	0.4839	0.4777	0.4715	0.4654	0.4593	0.4533	0.4473	0.4413	0.4354	0.4295
0.80	0.4237	0.4179	0.4122	0.4065	0.4009	0.3953	0.3898	0.3843	0.3789	0.3735
0.90	0.3681	0.3628	0.3576	0.3524	0.3472	0.3421	0.3371	0.3320	0.3271	0.3222
1.00	0.3173	0.3125	0.3077	0.3030	0.2983	0.2937	0.2891	0.2846	0.2801	0.2757

z	0.00	0.01	0.02	0.03	0.04	0.05	0.06	0.07	0.08	0.09
1.10	0.3173	0.3125	0.3077	0.3030	0.2983	0.2937	0.2891	0.2846	0.2801	0.2757
1.10	0.2713	0.2670	0.2627	0.2585	0.2543	0.2501	0.2460	0.2420	0.2380	0.2340
1.20	0.2301	0.2263	0.2225	0.2187	0.2150	0.2113	0.2077	0.2041	0.2005	0.1971
1.30	0.1936	0.1902	0.1868	0.1835	0.1802	0.1770	0.1738	0.1707	0.1676	0.1645
1.40	0.1615	0.1585	0.1556	0.1527	0.1499	0.1471	0.1443	0.1416	0.1389	0.1362
1.50	0.1336	0.1310	0.1285	0.1260	0.1236	0.1211	0.1188	0.1164	0.1141	0.1118
1.60	0.1096	0.1074	0.1052	0.1031	0.1010	0.0989	0.0969	0.0949	0.0930	0.0910
1.70	0.0891	0.0873	0.0854	0.0836	0.0819	0.0801	0.0784	0.0767	0.0751	0.0735
1.80	0.0719	0.0703	0.0688	0.0672	0.0658	0.0643	0.0629	0.0615	0.0601	0.0588
1.90	0.0574	0.0561	0.0549	0.0536	0.0524	0.0512	0.0500	0.0488	0.0477	0.0466
2.00	0.0455	0.0444	0.0434	0.0424	0.0414	0.0404	0.0394	0.0385	0.0375	0.0366

z	0.00	0.01	0.02	0.03	0.04	0.05	0.06	0.07	0.08	0.09
2.00	0.0455	0.0444	0.0434	0.0424	0.0414	0.0404	0.0394	0.0385	0.0375	0.0366
2.10	0.0357	0.0349	0.0340	0.0332	0.0324	0.0316	0.0308	0.0300	0.0293	0.0285
2.20	0.0278	0.0271	0.0264	0.0257	0.0251	0.0244	0.0238	0.0232	0.0226	0.0220
2.30	0.0214	0.0209	0.0203	0.0198	0.0193	0.0188	0.0183	0.0178	0.0173	0.0168
2.40	0.0164	0.0160	0.0155	0.0151	0.0147	0.0143	0.0139	0.0135	0.0131	0.0128
2.50	0.0124	0.0121	0.0117	0.0114	0.0111	0.0108	0.0105	0.0102	0.0099	0.0096
2.60	0.0093	0.0091	0.0088	0.0085	0.0083	0.0080	0.0078	0.0076	0.0074	0.0071
2.70	0.0069	0.0067	0.0065	0.0063	0.0061	0.0060	0.0058	0.0056	0.0054	0.0053
2.80	0.0051	0.0050	0.0048	0.0047	0.0045	0.0044	0.0042	0.0041	0.0040	0.0039
2.90	0.0037	0.0036	0.0035	0.0034	0.0033	0.0032	0.0031	0.0030	0.0029	0.0028
3.00	0.0027	0.0026	0.0025	0.0024	0.0024	0.0023	0.0022	0.0021	0.0021	0.0020

Survival Analysis Second Edition   David Machin, Yin Bun Cheung, Mahesh K.B. Parmar
© 2006 John Wiley & Sons, Ltd   ISBN: 0-470-87040-0

Table T2   Percentage points of the Normal distribution

1-sided α	z	2-sided α
0.0005	3.2905	0.0010
0.0025	2.8070	0.0050
0.0050	2.5758	0.0100
0.0100	2.3263	0.0200
0.0125	2.2414	0.0250
0.0250	1.9600	0.0500
0.0500	1.6449	0.1000
0.1000	1.2816	0.2000
0.1500	1.0364	0.3000
0.2000	0.8416	0.4000
0.2500	0.6745	0.5000
0.3000	0.5244	0.6000
0.3500	0.3853	0.7000
0.4000	0.2533	0.8000

Table T3 The χ^2 distribution. The value tabulated is $\chi^2(\alpha)$, such as that if X is distributed as a χ^2 with df degrees of freedom, then α is the probability that $X \geq \chi^2$

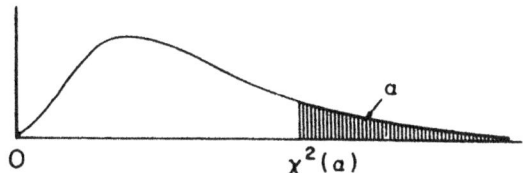

	0.2	0.1	0.05	0.04	0.03	0.02	0.01	0.001	0.0005
$df = 1$	1.64	2.71	3.84	4.22	4.71	5.41	6.63	10.83	12.12
2	3.22	4.61	5.99	6.44	7.01	7.82	9.21	13.82	15.20
3	4.64	6.25	7.81	8.31	8.95	9.84	11.34	16.27	17.73
4	5.99	7.78	9.49	10.03	10.71	11.67	13.28	18.47	20.00
5	7.29	9.24	11.07	11.64	12.37	13.39	15.09	20.52	22.11
6	8.56	10.64	12.59	13.20	13.97	15.03	16.81	22.46	24.10
7	9.80	12.02	14.07	14.70	15.51	16.62	18.48	24.32	26.02
8	11.03	13.36	15.51	16.17	17.01	18.17	20.09	26.13	27.87
9	12.24	14.68	16.92	17.61	18.48	19.68	21.67	27.88	29.67
10	13.44	15.99	18.31	19.02	19.92	21.16	23.21	29.59	31.42
11	14.63	17.28	19.68	20.41	21.34	22.62	24.73	31.26	33.14
12	15.81	18.55	21.03	21.79	22.74	24.05	26.22	32.91	34.82
13	16.98	19.81	22.36	23.14	24.12	25.47	27.69	34.53	36.48
14	18.15	21.06	23.68	24.49	25.49	26.87	29.14	36.12	38.11
15	19.31	22.31	25.00	25.82	26.85	28.26	30.58	37.70	39.72
16	20.47	23.54	26.30	27.14	28.19	29.63	32.00	39.25	41.31
17	21.61	24.77	27.59	28.45	29.52	31.00	33.41	40.79	42.88
18	22.76	25.99	28.87	29.75	30.84	32.35	34.81	42.31	44.43
19	23.90	27.20	30.14	31.04	32.16	33.69	36.19	43.82	45.97
20	25.04	28.41	31.41	32.32	33.46	35.02	37.57	45.32	47.50
21	26.17	29.61	32.67	33.60	34.75	36.34	38.91	47.00	49.01
22	27.30	30.81	33.92	34.87	36.04	37.65	40.32	48.41	50.51
23	28.43	32.01	35.18	36.13	37.33	38.97	41.61	49.81	52.00
24	29.55	33.19	36.41	37.39	38.62	40.26	43.02	51.22	53.48
25	30.67	34.38	37.65	38.65	39.88	41.55	44.30	52.63	54.95
26	31.79	35.56	38.88	39.88	41.14	42.84	45.65	54.03	56.41
27	32.91	36.74	40.12	41.14	42.40	44.13	47.00	55.44	57.86
28	34.03	37.92	41.35	42.37	43.66	45.42	48.29	56.84	59.30
29	35.14	39.09	42.56	43.60	44.92	46.71	49.58	58.25	60.73
30	36.25	40.25	43.78	44.83	46.15	47.97	50.87	59.66	62.16

Table T4   The total number of patients required to detect an improvement $\delta = (\pi_T - \pi_C)$ in survival over the survival rate of the standard therapy π_C, when $\alpha = 0.05$ and power $1 - \beta = 0.8$ (upper figure) and $1 - \beta = 0.9$ (lower figure)

π_C	δ									
	0.05	0.10	0.15	0.20	0.25	0.30	0.35	0.40	0.45	0.50
0.05	498	174	100	70	54	44	38	32	30	26
	664	232	134	92	72	58	50	44	38	36
0.10	964	296	156	102	74	58	48	40	36	32
	1290	396	208	136	98	76	64	54	46	42
0.15	1416	406	204	128	90	68	56	46	40	34
	1894	544	272	170	120	92	74	62	52	46
0.20	1828	506	246	150	104	78	62	50	42	36
	2446	676	328	200	138	104	82	66	56	48
0.25	2188	590	280	168	114	84	66	64	44	38
	2928	788	376	224	152	112	88	70	60	50
0.30	2488	658	308	182	122	90	68	56	46	40
	3330	880	412	244	164	118	92	74	60	52
0.35	2724	710	328	192	128	90	70	56	46	40
	3648	950	438	256	170	122	94	74	60	52
0.40	2896	744	340	196	130	92	70	56	46	38
	3876	996	454	262	172	124	94	74	60	50
0.45	3000	762	344	198	128	92	68	54	44	38
	4014	1020	460	264	172	122	92	72	58	48
0.50	3034	764	342	194	126	88	66	52	42	
	4062	1020	456	258	166	116	88	68	56	
0.55	3002	746	330	186	120	84	62	48		
	4018	998	442	248	158	110	82	64		
0.60	2900	714	312	174	110	76	56			
	3882	954	418	232	146	102	74			
0.65	2730	664	286	158	100	68				
	3654	886	382	210	132	90				
0.70	2494	596	254	138	86					
	3338	796	338	182	112					
0.75	2190	512	214	114						
	2930	684	284	150						
0.80	1822	414	168							
	2436	552	222							
0.85	1388	300								
	1854	398								
0.90	892									
	1190									

Index

Survival Analysis Second Edition   David Machin, Yin Bun Cheung, Mahesh K.B. Parmar
© 2006 John Wiley & Sons, Ltd   ISBN: 0-470-87040-0

Index prepared by Neil Manley

Printed and bound in the UK by
CPI Antony Rowe, Eastbourne

Printed and bound by CPI Group (UK) Ltd, Croydon, CR0 4YY

16/04/2025

14658506-0001